ORTHOPEDIC RESEARCH AND THERAPY

SCOLIOSIS

DIAGNOSIS, CLASSIFICATION AND MANAGEMENT OPTIONS

ORTHOPEDIC RESEARCH AND THERAPY

Additional books and e-books in this series can be found on Nova's website under the Series tab.

Orthopedic Research and Therapy

Scoliosis

Diagnosis, Classification and Management Options

**Federico Canavese
Antonio Andreacchio
and
Hongwen Xu**
Editors

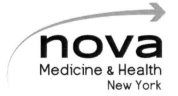

Copyright © 2018 by Nova Science Publishers, Inc.

All rights reserved. No part of this book may be reproduced, stored in a retrieval system or transmitted in any form or by any means: electronic, electrostatic, magnetic, tape, mechanical photocopying, recording or otherwise without the written permission of the Publisher.

We have partnered with Copyright Clearance Center to make it easy for you to obtain permissions to reuse content from this publication. Simply navigate to this publication's page on Nova's website and locate the "Get Permission" button below the title description. This button is linked directly to the title's permission page on copyright.com. Alternatively, you can visit copyright.com and search by title, ISBN, or ISSN.

For further questions about using the service on copyright.com, please contact:
Copyright Clearance Center
Phone: +1-(978) 750-8400   Fax: +1-(978) 750-4470   E-mail: info@copyright.com.

NOTICE TO THE READER

The Publisher has taken reasonable care in the preparation of this book, but makes no expressed or implied warranty of any kind and assumes no responsibility for any errors or omissions. No liability is assumed for incidental or consequential damages in connection with or arising out of information contained in this book. The Publisher shall not be liable for any special, consequential, or exemplary damages resulting, in whole or in part, from the readers' use of, or reliance upon, this material. Any parts of this book based on government reports are so indicated and copyright is claimed for those parts to the extent applicable to compilations of such works.

Independent verification should be sought for any data, advice or recommendations contained in this book. In addition, no responsibility is assumed by the publisher for any injury and/or damage to persons or property arising from any methods, products, instructions, ideas or otherwise contained in this publication.

This publication is designed to provide accurate and authoritative information with regard to the subject matter covered herein. It is sold with the clear understanding that the Publisher is not engaged in rendering legal or any other professional services. If legal or any other expert assistance is required, the services of a competent person should be sought. FROM A DECLARATION OF PARTICIPANTS JOINTLY ADOPTED BY A COMMITTEE OF THE AMERICAN BAR ASSOCIATION AND A COMMITTEE OF PUBLISHERS.

Additional color graphics may be available in the e-book version of this book.

Library of Congress Cataloging-in-Publication Data

ISBN: 978-1-53614-464-2

Published by Nova Science Publishers, Inc. † New York

CONTENTS

Preface		ix
Chapter 1	Growth of the Spine and Thorax *Alain Dimeglio, Federico Canavese and Francois Bonnel*	1
Chapter 2	Assessment of Maturation *Vito Pavone and Gianluca Testa*	13
Chapter 3	Classification of Early Onset Spinal Deformity *Mattia Cravino, Lorenza Marengo, Federico Canavese and Antonio Andreacchio*	27
Chapter 4	Classification of Adolescent Idiopathic Scoliosis *Lorenza Marengo, Mattia Cravino, Federico Canavese and Antonio Andreacchio*	35
Chapter 5	Serial Elongation Derotation Flexion Casting for Patients with Progressive Scoliosis *Federico Canavese and Alain Dimeglio*	45
Chapter 6	Halo Traction: When and How? *Zhaomin Zheng*	61
Chapter 7	EOS and Surgery: Techniques, Indications and Limitations *Ashok N. Johari*	69
Chapter 8	Growth Friendly Implants with Rib Anchors in Early Onset Scoliosis *Alaaeldin A. Ahmad, Loai J. Aker and Yahia B. Hanbali*	87
Chapter 9	Growth and Adolescent Idiopathic Scoliosis *Ismat Ghanem and Maroun Rizkallah*	101
Chapter 10	Physiotherapy and Scoliosis: What to Do and What to Reasonably Expect from It *Jacques Deslandes*	113

Chapter 11	The Scoliosis Specific Physical Orthopedic Test™: Creating Conservative Streams of Care for Youth with Adolescent Idopathic Scoliosis (AIS) Using Exercise, Lifestyle and Maintenance *Suzanne Clements Martin*	135
Chapter 12	Adolescent Idiopathic Scoliosis: Conservative Treatments *Andre J. Kaelin and Federico Canavese*	155
Chapter 13	Fusionless Techniques for Juvenile and Adolescent Idiopathic Scoliosis *Kedar Padhye and Ron El-Hawary*	175
Chapter 14	Instrumented Posterior Fusion in AIS: Indications, Preoperative Planning and Outcome *Xiaodong Qin and Zezhang Zhu*	199
Chapter 15	Anterior Instrumented Fusion in Adolescent Idiopathic Scoliosis: Indication, Preoperative Planning, and Outcome *Michael Ruf and Jörg Drumm*	217
Chapter 16	Posterior Minimally Invasive Surgery for the Treatment of Adolescent Idiopathic Scoliosis *Charlotte de Bodman, Anne Tabard-Fougère, Alexandre Ansorgue, Nicolas Amirghasemi and Romain Dayer*	231
Chapter 17	Pre- and Postoperative Sagittal Alignment in Patients with Adolescent Idiopathic Scoliosis *Mehmet Çetinkaya, Ali Eren and Alpaslan Senkoylu*	243
Chapter 18	Postoperative Shoulder Imbalance (PSI) and Adding-On Phenomenon *Ismail Daldal, Erdem Aktas and Alpaslan Senkoylu*	261
Chapter 19	How to Control Shoulder Balance and Prevent Imbalance in Patients with AIS Undergoing Surgery *Jun Jiang and Zezhang Zhu*	277
Chapter 20	Postoperative Deep Infections Following Scoliosis Surgery *Qiang Jie, Xiaowei Wang, Qingda Lu and Fei Su*	293
Chapter 21	Neuromonitoring Signal Decrement: What to Do *Qianyu Zhuang and Shujie Wang*	307
Chapter 22	Evaluation and Conservative Management of Spinal Deformities in Patients with Cerebral Palsy *Michèle Kläusler and Erich Rutz*	319
Chapter 23	Neuromuscular Scoliosis: Surgical Considerations and Management of Complications *Ismat Ghanem, Maroun Rizkallah and Federico Canavese*	331

Chapter 24	Radiographic Assessment and Follow-Up of Patients with Scoliosis *Mohsen Karami*	353
Chapter 25	Rasterstereography for the Follow-Up of AIS Patients *Anne Tabard-Fougère, Charlotte de Bodman, Alice Bonnefoy-Mazure and Romain Dayer*	365
Chapter 26	Anesthesia Considerations and Pain Management in Children Undergoing Scoliosis Surgery *Marie Granier and Xing Rong Song*	377
Chapter 27	Experimental Animal Models in Scoliosis: Incidence and Diagnosis of Idiopathic and Congenital Scoliosis in Rhesus Monkey (*Macaca mulatta*) through Evoked Potentials and Imaging Studies *Alejandra Ibáñez-Contreras, David Ducoing-Gonzalez, Janine Cardoso and Braulio Hernández-Godínez*	383

Editors Contact Information — 413

List of Contributors — 415

Index — 417

PREFACE

The importance of the initial diagnosis and subsequent management of scoliosis is crucial as it affects the patient's future. Initial diagnosis is highly important in orientating the patient and correlating available therapeutic means to the expected results.

Since the 1900s, the surgical approach to scoliosis has changed as thoughts and possibilities have evolved. Nowadays, progressive spinal deformities can be managed with specific orthopedic devices or vertebral arthrodesis surgery, depending on the age of the patient. Additionally, the type and extent of scoliotic deformity as well as on the presence of comorbidities have aided in the transforming of these methods. Arthrodesis is not considered the best treatment for younger patients; however, it becomes almost inevitable to cure important deformities of the spine in older children. Surgical fusion in patients with severe scoliosis can improve the deformity, but the spine is rendered more rigid and spinal growth is subsequently affected.

The information contained in this clinical book are derived from the valuable experience of over 40 authors and co-authors from all over the world, and we hope this format will help the reader at the critical junctures to which decisions must be made. All the participants provided their own analysis, and their therapeutic choices and contributions have served this project well. This book would not exist without their efforts, diligence and commitment.

This clinical book is an opportunity for every physician and surgeon dealing with children and adolescents with scoliosis to obtain updates concerning actual trends and knowledge in this field of study.

Federico Canavese
Antonio Andreacchio
HongWen Xu
Editors

Chapter 1

GROWTH OF THE SPINE AND THORAX

Alain Dimeglio[1], Federico Canavese[2], and *Francois Bonnel[1]*
[1]Université de Montpellier, Faculté de Médecine, Montpellier, France
[2]CHU Estaing, Service de Chirurgie Infantile, Clermont Ferrand, France

ABSTRACT

Only perfect knowledge of normal growth parameters allows a better understanding of both normal and abnormal spine growth and of the pathologic changes induced on a growing spine by an early onset spinal deformity. The growing spine is a mosaic of growth plates characterized by changes in rhythm. The most important growth occurs during the intra-uterine period. During post-natal growth, complex phenomena follow each other in very rapid succession. All growth plates are perfectly synchronized to maintain harmonious limb and spine relationships as growth does not occur simultaneously in the same magnitude or rate in the various body segments. The slightest error or modification can lead to a malformation or deformity (i.e., congenital scoliosis or early onset scoliosis) with negative effects on standing and sitting height, thoracic cage shape, volume and circumference, and lung development.

Keywords: spine growth, thoracic growth, scoliosis, surgery, brace

INTRODUCTION

The growing spine is a mosaic of growth plates and it is characterized by changes in rhythm. During growth, complex phenomena follow each other with significant speed. This succession of events, this setting up of elements is programmed according to a hierarchy. Growth is harmony and synchronization. The slightest error, the slightest slip or modification, can lead to a malformation or to a deformity. Abnormal growth alters this virtuous circle.

Only perfect knowledge of normal growth parameters allows a better understanding of the pathologic changes induced on a growing organism by an early onset spinal deformity

---

[*] Corresponding Author Email: Federico Canavese MD PhD Prof. Email: canavese_federico@yahoo.fr.

(Table 1). As the spinal deformity progresses, by a "domino effect", not only spinal growth is affected but size and shape of the thoracic cage are modified as well. This distortion of the thorax will interfere with lungs development. Over time, the spine disorder changes its nature: from a mainly orthopedic issue, it becomes a severe pediatric, systematic disease with Thoracic Insufficiency Syndrome [1, 2] Cor Pulmonale [3].

Table 1. Growth is a change in proportion. The Sitting Height/Lower Limb ratio varies with age: it is 4.5 during early pregnancy, 3 during late pregnancy, 1.9 at birth, 1.3 during childhood and 1 at skeletal maturity

Developmental Stage	Sitting Height		Lower Limb
	Head	Trunk	
Fetus (early pregnancy)	50%	32%	18%
Fetus (late pregnancy)	35%	40%	25%
Newborn	25%	40%	35%
Infant	23%	37%	40%
Child	20%	35%	45%
Young	18%	34%	48%
Adult	13%	40%	47%

Normal Growth of the Spine

In normal children, the longitudinal growth of the thoracic spine is about 1.3 cm/year between birth and 5 years, about 0.7 cm/year between the ages of five and ten and 1.1 cm/year during puberty. T1-T12 is the posterior pillar of the thoracic cage and it is a strategic segment (Table 2). A precocious arthrodesis of this segment can have repercussions on thoracic growth and lungs development. In young children with progressive deformity there is decrease of longitudinal growth and a loss of normal proportionality of trunk growth. Untreated progressive early onset spinal deformity has been associated with short trunk, short stature and often-respiratory insufficiency. In untreated patients, the loss of vital capacity in those with early onset scoliosis has been shown to be 15% greater than in those with adolescent idiopathic scoliosis [4-12]. Moreover, fusion is a cause of respiratory insufficiency and adds to the spinal deformity the loss of pulmonary function [13, 14]. Emans et al. showed that pelvic inlet width, measured by computerized tomograms or plain radiographs, is an age-independent predictor of the expected thoracic dimensions in unaffected children and adolescents [15, 16].

Microscopic Growth of the Spine

Symmetric and harmonious growth characterizes normal spines although spinal growth itself is the product of more than 130 growth plates working at different paces. In severe scoliosis (Figure 1), growth becomes asymmetrical as a result of growth plate disorganization. Complex spinal deformities alter the growth spine cartilage and vertebral bodies become progressively distorted and can perpetuate the disorder. Therefore, over time, many scoliotic deformities can become growth plate disorders [4-8, 12, 15].

Table 2. Evaluation of T1–T12 and L1–L5 spinal segments from birth to skeletal maturity. Values are expressed in cm and are average values

Developmental Stage	Spinal Segment			
	Boys		Girls	
	T1-T12	L1-L5	T1-T12	L1-L5
Newborn	11	7,5	11	7,5
Child	18	10,5	18	10,5
Young	22	12,5	22	12,5
Adult	28	16	26	15,5

The neurocentral synchondrosis is a physis in the spine located at the junction of the pedicle and the vertebral body and is important in the growth of both the vertebral body and the posterior arch. It has been shown in a growing pig model that unilateral transpedicular screw fixation which traverses the neurocentral synchondrosis can produce asymmetric growth of the synchondrosis and create scoliosis with the convexity on the side of the screw fixation. However, in humans, neurocentral synchondrosis fuses around age nine, and by five years of age the spinal canal has already grown to about 95% of its definitive size. Therefore, a perivertebral arthrodesis performed after age five should have no influence on the size of the spinal canal [4-8, 12, 15].

Macroscopic Growth of the Spine

T1-S1 Spinal Segment

Assessment of the T1-S1 spinal segment is important as many spinal deformities originate in this segment. At birth, the T1-S1 segment measures about 20 cm and reaches 45 cm at skeletal maturity. It should be recalled that the height of the spine accounts for 60% of total sitting height, with the head and the pelvis accounting for the remaining 40%. The T1-S1 segment accounts for approximately 50% of the sitting height, two-third for the thoracic spine and one-third for the lumbar spine. It grows around 10 cm during the first five years of life (2 cm/year), about 5 cm between age 5 and 10 (1 cm/year), and about 10 cm between age 10 and skeletal maturity (1.8 cm/year) [4-8, 12, 15].

T1-T12 Spinal Segment

T1-T12 is the posterior pillar of the thoracic cage and thus a strategic segment. It measures about 12 cm at birth, 18 cm at 5 years of age, and about 27 cm on an average at skeletal maturity. The thoracic spine makes up 30% of the sitting height and a single thoracic vertebra and its disc represents about 2.5% of the sitting height. In normal children, the longitudinal growth of the thoracic spine is about 1.3 cm/year between birth and 5 years, about 0.7 cm/year between the age of 5 and 10, and 1.1 cm/year during puberty. A precocious arthrodesis of this segment has effects on thoracic growth and lung development [4-8, 12, 15].

In young children with progressive deformity, there is a decrease of longitudinal growth and a loss of the normal proportionality of trunk growth. If untreated, progressive early-onset spinal deformity has been associated with short trunk, short stature and often respiratory insufficiency. In untreated patients, the loss of vital capacity in those with early onset scoliosis has been shown to be 15% greater than in those with adolescent idiopathic scoliosis [4-8, 12, 15].

L1-L5 Spinal Segment

L1-L5 length is approximately 7 cm at birth and 16 cm on an average at skeletal maturity. The lumbar spine makes up about 18% of the sitting height and a single lumbar vertebra and its disc represents 3.5% of the sitting height. At the age of 10 years, the lumbar spine reaches about 90% of its final height, but only 60% of its definitive volume. A perivertebral arthrodesis of the lumbar spine performed after the age of 10 years results in minimal loss of sitting height [4-8, 12, 15].

Other Growth Indicators

The best way to monitor and to evaluate growth is to repeat measurements: standing height, sitting height, thoracic perimeter, arm span, and weight should be assessed at each visit. It must be remembered that growth is not a linear process. It is characterized by periods of acceleration and deceleration that should be taken into account when treatment is planned.

Arm Span

The measurement of arm span is an indirect measurement to evaluate standing height and can be used to assess predicted height in non-ambulatory children with myelomeningocele or cerebral palsy. Arm span and standing height have an almost perfect linear correlation. Standing height corresponds approximately to 97% of arm span with a small gender difference; boys have an arm spam that is a greater proportion of total standing height than girls. This relationship persists throughout puberty and into adulthood. In 77% of healthy children, arm span will be 0 to 5 cm greater than standing height; in 22% it will be 5 to 10 cm greater; and in the remaining 1% it will be greater by 10 cm or more. As a rule of thumb, arm span divided by 2 is very close to the sitting height, and divided by 4 to the T1-S1 spinal segment [4-8, 12, 15].

The arm span is particularly helpful to estimate standing height in wheelchair-bounded individuals. It represents about 102% of the standing height and half of the arm span is very close to the sitting height.

Weight

Weight is another useful parameter for evaluating growth. Starting from birth to skeletal maturity, weight increases by 20-fold. At 5 years of age, weight is approximately 20 kg, 30 kg by 10 years of age, and reaches 60 kg or more by 16 years of age. It should also be kept in mind that during pubertal spurt, weight usually doubles [4-8, 12, 15].

Standing Height

Standing height does not perfectly reflect spine growth. It can be considered as a "global measurement" as it includes the lower limbs.

The gain in standing height is approximately 25 cm during the initial 1st year of life and around 12.5 cm during the 2nd year. Between the ages 2-3 and 3-4 years, the gain in standing height is approximately 9 and 7 cm/year, respectively. At 5 years of age, standing height increases by 5 to 5.5 cm each year in both boys and girls; at the beginning of puberty, remaining growth is about 18 cm for girls (11%) and 20 cm for boys (13%). Standing height is a global marker composed of two components: sitting height and subischial height. These two regions often grow at different rates and at different times. For this reason, standing height does not always exactly correlate with the trunk height loss of children with severe spinal deformities [4-8, 12, 15].

Sitting Height

Sitting height reflects the growth of the spine: it is a reliable and effective measurement.

Sitting height averages about 34 cm at birth, and 88 cm and 92 cm at the end of growth, for girls and boys respectively, and it correlates with the severity of a spinal deformity [4-8, 12, 15].

Skeletal Age Assessment

Skeletal age is important to evaluate remaining growth and the risk of progression of a scoliotic deformity. In 50% of normal children and adolescents bone age do not differ from chronological age. However, age is a difficult notion to define. Skeletal age is a valuable *indicator*, and it may reduce causes of error if measured repeatedly, *but* it is a purely conventional measure.

During puberty, skeletal age is an important tool when treating (conservatively or surgically) patients with spinal deformities. Skeletal age alone is not enough and must be assessed together with other clinical and radiological findings such as standing and sitting height, Risser sign, Tanner stages and annual growth rate. Puberty starts at 11 years of skeletal age and ends at 13 years of skeletal age in girls; in boys puberty starts two years later (13 years of skeletal age) and subsequently finishes at age 15 of skeletal age. Most current clinical and radiographic markers do not help paediatric orthopaedic surgeons to clearly distinguish maturity levels prior to Risser I [4-8].

Growth of the Thoracic Cage

The thoracic cage can be considered as the "fourth dimension" of the spine. When dealing with severe early onset scoliosis, the priority is to protect the development of the lungs and heart within the thoracic cage. At birth, thoracic cage volume represents about 6% of its definitive size. It becomes about 30% by age 5 and about 50% by age 10 years. Moreover, between age 10 and skeletal maturity, thoracic cage volume doubles and its volumetric growth ends up [4-8, 12, 15].

Table 3. Chest shape modification during growth. The overall thoracic cage shape evolves from ovoid at birth to elliptical at skeletal maturity. Values are expressed in mm and are average values

Developmental Stage	Chest Dimensions			Chest Shape
	Chest Depth	*Chest Width*	*Ratio Depth/Width*	
Birth	79	72	1.1	Ovoid-Round

5 years	132	150	0.9	Ovoid
10 years	160	220	0.7	Elliptical
Skeletal Maturity	210	280	0.7	Elliptical

The thoracic circumference corresponds to 95% of sitting height and increase more both during the first five years of life and during puberty. The thorax perimeter gives an idea of the growth of the spine and of thoracic cage on the transverse plane (horizontal plane development).

On average the newborn thoracic perimeter is 32.3 cm in boys and 31.5 cm in girls and it will attain a mean value of 89.2 cm and 85.4 cm respectively [4-8, 12, 15].

Thoracic cage shape varies with age (Table 3). At birth, the difference between thoracic depth and width is minimal and the ratio thoracic depth/thoracic width is close to 1. At skeletal maturity, on the other hand, the thoracic depth/thoracic width ratio is lower than 1 as width has grown more than depth. For this reason, the overall thoracic cage shape evolves from ovoid at birth to elliptical at skeletal maturity (Table 3). At the end of growth the thorax has an average thoracic depth of 21 cm in boys and 17.7 cm in girls and an average thoracic width of 28 cm and 24.7 cm respectively. At skeletal maturity, thoracic depth and thoracic depth represent about 20% and 30% of sitting height, respectively [4-8, 12, 15, 17].

Between birth and age 8 years, is the golden period for both thoracic spine and thoracic cage growth and it coincides with lungs development. The source of the potential respiratory failure is therefore double: intrinsic alveolar hypoplasia and extrinsic disturbances of the chest wall functions as thoracic cage deformities prevent hyperplasia of lungs tissues. It is important to preserve both thoracic growth and lungs volume during this critical period of life. Post-mortem studies showed that patients with early-onset deformities have fewer alveoli than expected, and that emphysematous changes in existing alveoli are present. These studies suggest that mechanical compression is not a factor in reducing the number of alveoli, and that this is probably due to a premature cessation of alveolar proliferation [18, 19]. Indeed, from zero to four years, the number of alveoli grows by a factor of 10, and the development of the bronchial tree ends around 8-9 years of age. Gollogly et al. showed on a CT scan study that lung parenchyma volume is a function of age. At birth lung parenchyma volume is 400 cc, at age 5 years is about 900 cc, at age 10 years is about 1500 cc and at skeletal maturity is about 4500 cc for boys and 3500 for girls [20]. An early-onset scoliosis therefore adversely affects thoracic growth in the critical period of maximum 'respiratory growth', which induces irreversible changes in the thoraco-pulmonary structure [4-8, 12, 15, 18-25].

Campbell et al. have described the Thoracic Insufficiency Syndrome which is the inability of the thorax to ensure normal breathing [1-3, 21, 22]; Dubousset et al. have shown that that severe spinal deformities lead to penetration of the apical portion of the deformity inside the thoracic cage ("endo-thoracic hump") and have described the "spinal penetration index" [22].

It is now known that deformations of the spine adversely affect the development of the thorax, by changing its shape and reducing its normal motility. In this respect, Canavese et al. have described the '*rib-vertebral-sternal complex*', which fits the thoracic cavity three-dimensionally, tends to constitute an elastic structural model, similar to a cube in shape, but in the presence of scoliosis it becomes flat and rigid and turns elliptical, thus preventing the lungs from expanding [17]. These deformations, which can be lethal in the most severe cases, result from mutual interactions and influences among the various skeletal and organic components of the thoracic cage. Alterations in some of these elements affect and change the development and growth of the others [5, 12, 17, 23-25]. Metha et al. have demonstrated that a unilateral deformity of the spine or the thorax induces scoliosis and thoracic cage deformity with asymmetrical lung volume [24]. Canavese et al. evaluated the consequences of a disturbed growth of vertebral bodies on the development of the other elements, i.e., ribs, sternum, and lungs, which are part of '*rib-vertebral-sternal complex*' [21]. These influences are much more evident when the arthrodesis is carried out in the 'critical portion' (T1-T6 segment) of the thoracic spine [12, 13, 15, 17, 20-24]. Early spine fusion especially if performed in the thoracic region, is cause of respiratory insufficiency and adds to the spinal deformity the loss of pulmonary function (Figure 1 and Figure 2). Karol et al. have shown as well that a thoracic spine height of 18-22 cm or more is necessary to avoid severe respiratory insufficiency. They have shown that children undergoing a precocious spinal fusion have a reduction of thoracic depth and a shorter T1-T12 segment compared to normal subjects. The forced vital capacity may decrease 50% of predicted volume if more than 60% of the thoracic spine is fused (i.e., 8 thoracic vertebrae) before the age of 8 years [13].

Therefore, arthrodesis carried out in the thoracic spine at an early age does not address the impact of the deformity on lung parenchyma development or preservation of pulmonary function. Even its effect on completely preventing deformity progression has been questioned. In children with spinal deformities with strong progression potential, expansible materials can be used to support the expansion of the thoracic cage and lung growth [1, 2, 17, 26-33].

Effects of Surgery

Modern techniques and instrumentations only control one plane of the deformity as distraction forces are applied to the spine or to the thoracic cage. Nowadays, there is no instrumentation able to control the tri-dimensional nature of early onset spinal deformities. To preserve thoracic motility and permit a normal development of the respiratory tree, the treatment should not focus on the spine only but should consider the '*rib-vertebral-sternal complex*' as a whole [5, 12, 17, 23-25].

Campbell et al. showed that the opening wedge thoracostomy can increase the thoracic volume ('parasol effect') [1, 2]. It is important to perform such procedure before the end of the development of the bronchial tree at age 8 years of age [18, 19]. However, those procedures have the inconvenience to increase the stiffness of the thoracic cage and to increase the amount of energy needed to breathe.

The crankshaft phenomenon is the progression of the spinal deformity when the anterior portion of the spine continues to grow, whereas the posterior portion is blocked by arthrodesis [25, 33]. Golberg et al. showed that early surgery, in patients that developed scoliosis before the age of 4, does not modify the deformation produced by scoliosis and does not preserve the respiratory function, even when the anterior growth of the spine is arrested [26, 34]. Therefore, it is very important for the surgeon to consider the state of skeletal maturity and the amount of growth remaining in the segment of the spine that is to be fused.

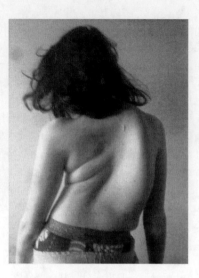

Figure 1. Severe scoliosis with significant deformity of the thoracic cage.

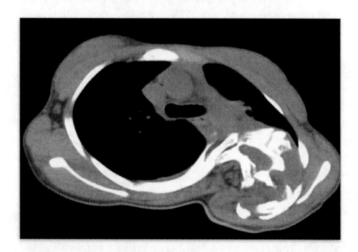

Figure 2. Effects of spinal deformity on chest size and shape. Severe scoliosis with chest cage deformity. Computed Tomography scan (transverse section): penetration of the vertebrae inside the thorax with crushing of the lung on the concave side.

New techniques have been recently developed, such as the Shilla procedure. The most curved portion in the center of the spine is held straight and fused. Ends of the rods are not fused, but held in place with growing screws, allowing the spine to lengthen without additional trips to the operating room. The screws capture the rods, but slide as the patient grows. This procedure seems to reduce the number of surgeries compared to traditional techniques [32]. However, the Shilla procedure is very new and experimental; whether it has a long-term future in the treatment of severe scoliosis is still undetermined. Surgery should be as much limited as possible and extensive arthrodesis of the spine should be avoided.

Does a Deformed Spine Grow Normally?

Both spinal and thoracic growth adhere to strict rules and can be controlled only by following their requirements. Only critical analysis of all growth parameters over time, allow unmasking and understanding the magnitude of the deficits induced by an early onset spinal deformity.

Four different scenarios can be identified:

1. The clinical picture gets worse. Abnormal growth leads to a deficit that sustains the deformity ("snow ball effect"). Hypotrophy due to weight loss, weakens – among others - the respiratory muscle making breathing more difficult (Figure 1).
2. The clinical picture is stable.
3. The clinical picture gets slightly better with improvement of different clinical parameters such as weight, vital capacity, sitting height.
4. The clinical picture gets back to normal. In this "ideal" scenario, all clinical parameters catch-up the deficit induced by the deformity. Unfortunately, this is not likely to happen as most of the children with severe spinal deformities will end up at skeletal maturity with a short trunk, a significant loss of vital capacity and disproportionate body habitus.

Therefore, surgical strategies should consider the whole life span of the patient and should provide answer to two basic questions: 1) For what functional benefit? 2) For what morbidity?

The thoracic cage is part of the deformity. There is a normal interaction between the organic components of the spine, the thoracic cage and the lungs. Both early onset spinal deformities and precocious spinal arthrodesis alter spinal growth and affect thorax development by changing its shape and reducing its normal mobility.

Challenging the growing spine means to preserve thoracic spine, thoracic cage and lungs growth without reducing spinal motion.

The principle that a short straight spine, produced by an early fusion is better that a long curved spine, is no longer generally accepted.

What Have We Learned from Growth?

1. Offensive strategy is essential when dealing with severe thoracic congenital scoliosis during the first 5 years of life. Respiratory function is a priority!
2. In patients with early onset scoliosis, treatment must be adjusted according to the growth parameters. Surgery, bracing or casting depend upon the etiology, the severity and the aggressiveness of the curve;
3. Growth is a three-dimensional process. As it, spinal deformity should be assessed in all planes;
4. If thoracic cage is sufficiently developed, the severity of the deformity as per Cobb's angle values, is not the key-element;
5. The suppleness of the curve is another essential parameter. If the curve is supple, whatever the angulation, it is possible to perform only one surgery at the beginning of puberty. The complete correction of the curve will compensate for the deficit of the trunk induced by spine surgery;

6. Physiotherapy has an important place in the treatment of patients with severe scoliosis. The goal is to stimulate the inspiratory and the expiratory muscles, in order to preserve thorax cage motion. More than 100 muscles (large and very small muscles together) set up the network surrounding the spine.
7. Decision for definitive fusion needs a critical analysis of all growth parameters. When dealing with a curve exceeding 50° at the beginning of pubertal growth spurt, there is no reason to wait for deformity progression and surgery is indicated; As for point 5, correction of the curve will compensate for the deficit of the trunk induced by spine surgery;
8. In patients with early onset scoliosis, the goal of treatment is to achieve:
   - Vital Capacity more than 50%
   - Weight more than 40 Kg
   - T1-S1 more than 30 cm
   - T1-T12 more than 22 cm

REFERENCES

[1] Campbell, RM; Smith, MD; Mayes, TC; et al. The characteristics of thoracic insufficiency associated with fused ribs and congenital scoliosis. *J Bone Joint Surg Am*, 2003, 85, 399-408.
[2] Campbell, MR; Hell-Vocke, AK. Growth of the thoracic spine in Congenital Scoliosis after expansion thoracoplasty. *J Bone Joint Surg Am*, 2003, 85, 409-20.
[3] Swank, SM; Winter, RB; Moe, JH. Scoliosis and cor pulmonale. *Spine*, 1982, 7, 343-54.
[4] Dimeglio, A; Canavese, F. The growing spine. How spinal deformities influence normal thorax and spine growth. *Eur Spine J*, 2012, 21, 64-70.
[5] Dimeglio, A; Bonnel, F. (1990). *Le rachis en croissance*. [*The growing spine.*] Springer Verlag, Paris, France.
[6] Canavese, F; Dimeglio, A. Normal and abnormal spine and thoracic cage development. *World J Orthop*, 2013, 4(4), 167-174.
[7] Dimeglio, A. Growth in Pediatric Orthopedics. *J Pediatr Orthop*, 2001, 21, 545-55.
[8] Charles, YP; Dimeglio, A; Marcoul, A; et al. Influence of idiopathic scoliosis on Three-dimensional thoracic growth spine. *Spine*, 2008, 33 (11), 1209-18.
[9] Shapiro, BK; Green, P; Krick, J. Growth of severely impaired children: neurological versus nutritional factors. *Dev Med Child Neurol*, 1986, 28, 729-33.
[10] Stallings, VA; Charney, EB; Davies, JC; et al. Nutrition-related growth failure of children with quadriplegic cerebral palsy. *Dev Med Child Neurol*, 1993, 35, 126-38.
[11] Skaggs, DL; Sankar, WN; Albrektson, J; et al. Weight gain following vertical expandable prosthetic titanium ribs surgery in children with thoracic insufficiency syndrome. *Spine*, 2008, 34, 2530-3.

[12] Canavese, F; Dimeglio, A; Volpatti, D; et al. Dorsal arthrodesis of thoracic spine and effects on thorax growth in prepubertal *New Zealand White rabbits*. *Spine*, 2007, 32, E443-E450.

[13] Karol, L; Johston, C; Mladenov, K; et al. Pulmonary function following early thoracic fusion in non neuromuscular scoliosis. *J Bone Joint Surg Am*, 2008, 90, 1272-81

[14] Pehrsson, K; Larsson, S; Oden, A; et al. Long-term follow-up of patients with untreated scoliosis. A study of mortality causes of death, and symptoms. *Spine*, 1992, 17, 1091-6.

[15] Canavese, F; Dimeglio, A; D'Amato, C; et al. (2010). Dorsal arthrodesis in prepubertal New Zealand White rabbits followed to skeletal maturity: effect on thoracic dimensions, spine growth and neural elements. *Indian J Orthop*, 2010, 44, 14-22.

[16] Emans, JB; Ciarlo, M; Callahan, M; et al. Prediction of thoracic dimensions and spine length based on individual pelvic dimensions in children and adolescents. *Spine*, 2005, 30, 2824-9.

[17] Canavese, F; Dimeglio, A; Granier, M; et al. Arthrodesis of the first six dorsal vertebrae in prepubertal *New Zealand White* rabbits and thoracic growth to skeletal maturity: the role of the "Rib-Vertebral-Sternal complex". *Minerva Ortop Traumatol,* 2007, 58, 369-78.

[18] Berend, N; Rynell, AC; Ward, HE. A Structure of a human pulmonary acinus. *Thorax*, 1991, 46, 117-21.

[19] de Groodt, EG; van Pelt, W; Borsboom, GI. Growth of the lung and thorax dimensions during the pubertal growth spurt. *Eur Respir J*, 1988, 1, 102-8.

[20] Gollogly, S; Smith, JT; White, SK; et al. The volume of lung parenchyma as a function of age: a review of 1050 normal CT scans of the chest with three-dimensional volumetric reconstruction of the pulmonary system. *Spine*, 2004, 29, 2061-7.

[21] Rizzi, PE; Winter, RB; Lonstein, JE; et al. (1997). Adult spinal deformity and respiratory failure. Surgical results in 35 patients. *Spine*, 1997, 22, 2517-30.

[22] Dubousset, J; Wicart, P; Pomero, V; Scolisoes thoraciques: les gibbosités exo et endo-thoraciques et l'index de penetration rachidienne. [Thoracic scolioes: the exo and endo-thoracic gibbosities and the spinal penetration index.] *Rev Chir Orthop Reparatrice Appar Mot*, 2002, 88, 9-18.

[23] Canavese, F; Dimeglio, A; Granier, M; et al. Influence de l'arthrodèse vertébrale sélective T1-T6 sur la croissance thoracique: étude expérimentale chez des lapins New Zealand White prépubertaires. [Influence of T1-T6 selective vertebral arthrodesis on thoracic growth: an experimental study in prepubertal New Zealand White rabbits.] *Rev Chir Orthop Reparatrice Appar Mot*, 2008, 94, 490-7.

[24] Mehta, HP; Snyder, BD; Callender, NN; et al. The reciprocal relationship between thoracic and spinal deformity and its effect on pulmonary function in a rabbit model: a pilot study. *Spine*, 2006, 31, 2654-64.

[25] Dubousset, J. (1973). Recidive d'une scoliose lombaire et d'un basin oblique après fusion precoce: le phénomène du Villebrequin. [Recurrence of lumbar scoliosis and oblique pelvis after premature fusion: the phenomenon of the Cranberry.] *Proceeding Group Etude de la Scoliose*; Paris, France.

[26] Goldberg, CJ; Gillic, I; Connaughton, O; et al. Respiratory function and cosmesis at maturity in infantile-onset scoliosis. *Spine*, 2003, 28, 2397-406.

[27] Coleman, SS. The effect of posterior spinal fusion on vertebral growth in dogs. *J Bone Joint Surg Am*, 1968, 50, 879.

[28] Ponseti, IV; Friedman, B. Changes in the scoliotic spine after fusion. *J Bone Joint Surg (Am)*, 1950, 32, 751-66.

[29] Kioschos, HC; Asher, MA; Lark, RG; et al. Overpowering the crankshaft mechanism. The effect of posterior spinal fusion with and without stiff transpedicular fixation on anterior column growth in immature canines. *Spine*, 1996, 21, 1168-73.

[30] Hell, AK; Campbell, RM; Hefti, F. The vertical expandable prosthetic titanium rib implant for the treatment of thoracic insufficiency syndrome associated with congenital scoliosis and neuromuscular scoliosis in young children. *J Pediatr Orthop B*, 2005, 14, 286-92.

[31] Emans, JB; Caubet, JF; Ordonez, CL; et al. The treatment of the spine and chest wall deformities with fused ribs by expansion thracostomy and insertion of vertical expandable prosthetic titanium rib: growth of thoracic spine and improvement of lung volume. *Spine*, 2005, 30S (17), 58-68.

[32] Akbarnia, B; Yazici, M; Thompson, G. (2011). *Growing Spine; Management of Spine Deformities in Young Children*. Springer, Berlin.

[33] Zhang, H; Sucato, D. Unilateral pedicle screw epiphysiodesis of the neurocentral synchondrosis. Production of idiopathic-like scoliosis in an immature animal model. *J Bone Joint Surg Am*, 2008, 90, 2460-9.

[34] Hefti, FL; McMaster, MJ. The effect of the adolescent growth spurt on early posterior spinal fusion in infantile and juvenile idiopathic scoliosis. *J Bone Joint Surg Br*, 1983, 65, 247-54.

Chapter 2

ASSESSMENT OF MATURATION

Vito Pavone and Gianluca Testa
Department of General Surgery and Medical Surgical Specialties,
Section of Orthopedics and Traumatology, University of Catania, Catania, Italy

ABSTRACT

Idiopathic scoliosis is a spine disorder for which effective treatment requires an accurate estimation of skeletal maturation. A thorough understanding of developmental growth parameters, including weight, height, bone age, and pubertal stages is paramount for predicting curve progression and facilitate the selection of the most promising treatment approach. Radiographs of the hand, wrist, and elbow enable digital skeletal, distal radius, and ulna classification, in addition to elbow ossification center, calcaneal apophysis classification and Risser sign determination. Going forward, additional indicators must be identified that can distinguish ethnic and sex-based variations towards maximizing the therapeutic outcome for patients with scoliosis.

Keywords: weight, height, chronological age, bone age, Tanner classification, hand and wrist radiograph, Risser sign

INTRODUCTION

Pediatric growth can be divided into three phases: 1) birth to five years old; 2) five to ten years old; 3) ten years old to skeletal maturity. Over the course of these three phases, spine length increases up to three-fold. These milestones can vary based on ethnicity, sex, and puberty onset. Variation up to four years in chronological age has been described [1]. Growth and skeletal maturation are essential, correlated elements that play a key role in orthopedic disorders during the developmental age. Specifically, early-onset scoliosis is strictly associated with the first two phases of growth while idiopathic adolescent-onset scoliosis affects the third phase [2]. Several growth parameters are used to evaluate skeletal maturity that can be divided into clinical or radiological methodologies. Clinical approaches involve the stages of puberty,

CLINICAL PARAMETERS

Stages of Puberty and Tanner Classification

Puberty is the most important growth phase. It is characterized by a gradual onset and persists over a period of two years beginning at a bone age of 11 and 13 years in girls and boys respectively. Puberty consists of an acceleration phase with two years of rapid growth and a deceleration phase with three years of steady reduction in growth rate [1, 3]. These two phases inform the appropriate use of bracing for the management of scoliosis. Brace treatment must be initiated at peak height velocity (PHV) to prevent curve worsening. When deceleration phase occurs, curve progression is significantly reduced and the overuse of bracing and associated complications can be prevented [4]. The risk of scoliosis is higher during the acceleration phase of puberty. The main curve progression occurs in conjunction with rapid adolescent skeletal growth, which is between 11 and 13 years of bone age in girls and 13 and 15 years of bone age in boys [4].

Table 1. Tanner stages

	Stage I	*Stage II*	*Stage III*	*Stage IV*	*Stage V*
Female Pubic Hair Growth	Vellos hair develops over the pubes	Sparse, long, pigmented, downy hair appears along the labia	Darker, coarser, and curlier sexual hair appears over the junction of the pubes	Adult hair distribution with lower quantity (no spread to the thighs medial surface	Adult hair and presence of inverse triangle of the classically feminine type.
Male Pubic Hair Growth	Vellos hair appears over the pubes	Sparse development of long pigmented downy hair, which is only slightly curled or straight. at the base of penis	darker, coarser, and curlier pubic hair over the junction of the pubes	Adult hair distribution with lower quantity (no spread thighs medial surface)	Adult hair distribution and presence of inverse triangle.
Females Breast Development	Only the papilla is elevated above the level of the chest wall	Elevation of the breasts and papillae may occur as small mounds along with some increased diameter of the areolae.	The breasts and areolae continue to enlarge, although they show no separation of contour	The areolae and papillae elevate above the level of the breasts and form secondary mounds with further development of the overall breast tissue	Mature female breasts, The papillae may extend slightly above the contour of the breasts
Male Genitalia Development	The testes, scrotal sac, and penis size and proportion similar to those seen in early childhood	Enlargement of the scrotum and testes and change in the texture of the scrotal skin.	Further growth of the penis, testes and scrotum	The penis significantly enlarged in length and circumference, with further development of the glans penis.	Adult genitalia with regard to size and shape

Specifically, during puberty's acceleration phase, a 5° curve is associated with a 10% risk of progression, a 10° curve with a 20% risk, a 20° curve with a 30% risk, and a 30° curve raises the risk of progression to nearly 100%. During this period, an increase in spinal curvature of 1° each month (12°/year) is considered progressive and requires treatment; a curve that increases by 0.5°/month is considered as mild [4].

At the onset of puberty, growth velocity determines stature size, upper and lower body length, and the development of sexual features. These characteristic changes were classified by Tanner [5] in 1976 and are represented in Table 1. The Tanner staging for secondary sexual characteristics (breast and pubic hair development in girls, scrotum and pubic hair in boys) can be used to identify the rapid height gain phase [6]. Nevertheless, it cannot pinpoint PHV, which occurs at Tanner stages 2 or 3 for girls and Tanner stages 3 to 5 for boys [7]. Instead, menarche is the most commonly used parameter for growth prediction because it usually occurs after PHV is reached. In the treatment of scoliosis, menarche onset indicates that the ideal time for bracing has passed, though a delayed menarche may misinform projections of peak growth termination [8].

Weight

Body weight is one of the best indicators of health during infancy and childhood. Weight is always changing and should be measured frequently to evaluate maturation. The weight of a five-year-old child should be at least 20 kg, increasing to 30 kg by ten years of age, and 60 kg by the age of 16. At skeletal maturity, weight can be up to 20-fold higher than at birth.

Weight gain can have differential effects on scoliosis. This disorder is associated with a lower weight, Body Mass Index (BMI), and bone mass compared to age-matched, healthy controls [9]. In patients with idiopathic scoliosis, there is a high prevalence of lower weight, typically present in adolescents suffering from eating disorders (e.g., anorexia), which is predictive of worse treatment outcomes [10]. Lower weight and BMI result in lower levels of leptin in skeletal and adipose tissue [11], osteopenia and low bone density, and increased scoliosis curve magnitude [12].

Higher weight in patients with adolescent idiopathic scoliosis, as demonstrated in a study by Li et al. [13], also contributes to increased curve magnitude at presentation to an orthopedic surgeon, and can negatively affect surgical duration time and post-operative complications. During the pubertal spurt, body weight increases about 5 kg/year; a gain-rate over 10% above this average renders brace treatment less effective [14]. Moreover, elevated BMI (more than 25 Kg/m^2) plays a key-role in etiology, kyphosis progression, delayed diagnosis, and operative morbidity [15].

Height

Height is another important indicator of child maturation. From birth to skeletal maturity, the stature increases up to 1.3 m.

Standing height encompasses both sitting height and subischial height; both must be considered because their growth is unrelated and changes at different ages.

Arm span is used to evaluate standing height since the two are known to correlate. In over 70% of healthy children, arm span is 5 cm less than standing height. [16]. This parameter is useful in cases of spine deformity, allowing for the assessment of pulmonary function and the diagnosis of disorders characterized by limb-trunk disproportion (Figure 1). The distance between the T1 and S1 spinal segments is close to a quarter of arm span [16]. A single measurement of standing height is not sufficiently informative in patients with spinal deformities, as it does not reflect decreases in trunk height.

Sitting height, defined as the distance from the highest point on the head to the base-sitting surface, is used to accurately quantify trunk length (Figure 2). Sitting height enables estimation of puberty onset, which occurs at approximately 75 cm in girls and 78 cm in boys. At 84 cm, this measurement becomes indicative of a girl's menarche. Despite not always being recorded, sitting height is an important parameter affecting the treatment of scoliosis. Changes to sitting height are often associated with angular spinal changes, and thus can illuminate a progressive curve. During the acceleration phase of puberty, a spinal curve that increases by 1°/month necessitates prompt treatment; alternatively, curves with less than a 0.5°/month gain require less aggressive treatment [17].

Subischial leg length refers to the difference between stature and sitting height. This parameter is important to consider because it reflects the growth dynamics of the lower extremities (Figure 3).

At the end of the active growth phase, the average subischial leg length is over 81 cm in boys and 74.5 cm in girls and represents a great percentage of height growth [16].

During puberty, standing height increases by approximately 1 cm/month. At the puberty onset, males have a remaining standing height growth of above 14%, approximately 22.5 cm, whose 13 cm of sitting height and 9.5 cm of subischial leg length. In contrast, females have 12% of their standing height left to grow, approximately 20.5 cm on average, roughly divided between 12 cm of sitting height and 8.5 cm of subischial leg length [5].

Despite the importance of height in determining growth, as previously discussed, it is not predicative of future growth [1].

In regards to the distal-to-proximal growth gradient, the distal portion of the body experiences its pubertal growth spurt earlier [5]. Therefore, *foot length* is used as an early indicator of peak growth velocity. Differences in shoe size can serve as an alternative but its use for curve progression prediction is limited due to variations in brands, recall bias, and its mismatch with sitting height [18].

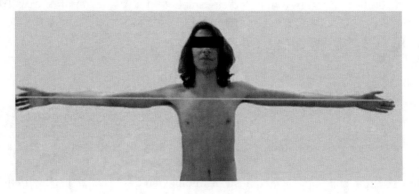

Figure 1. Arm span.

Assessment of Maturation

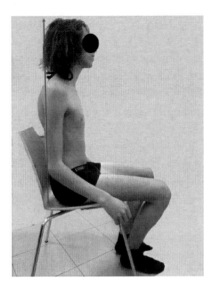

Figure 2. Sitting height.

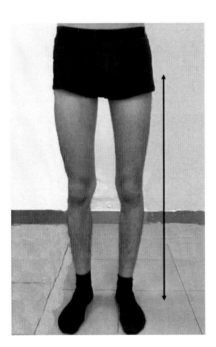

Figure 3. Subischial leg length.

RADIOLOGICAL INDICATORS

Bone age is predictive of remaining growth potential and is determined using different techniques and radiographs. Bone age approximations enable the prevention of scoliosis curve progression and the identification of optimal bracing time, with the aid of the following radiological indicators.

Risser Sign

Ossification of the iliac apophysis is most commonly used radiographic indicator of skeletal maturity. This important indirect measure is referred to as the Risser sign, named after Joseph Risser who first described the phenomenon in 1958 [19].

Two versions of the Risser staging system have been used. The U.S. version includes five stages based on the maturation of the iliac crest into the four quarters visible on an anteroposterior radiograph (Figure 4); the French version only contains four stages, which are designated by dividing the apophysis into thirds (Table 2) [20]. Risser sign is an easily available parameter calculated from the same spine radiograph used for initial diagnosis. The Risser sign is employed to measure skeletal maturity because the chronological age of the patient is considered as inaccurate.

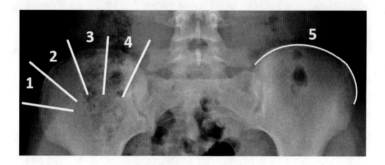

Figure 4. Risser stages (US version): 1) Ossification of the anterior lateral quarter; 2) Ossification of the anterolateral half; 3) Ossification of the anterior three quarters; 4) complete ossification; 5) fusion to the ilium.

Table 2. Risser stages - French version

Risser 1	Ossification of the lateral third
Risser 2	Ossification of the middle third
Risser 3	Ossification of the medial third
Risser 4	Ossification/fusion of the apophysis

Limitations include the prevalence of posteroanterior spine radiographs that reduces the view of the sign and the risk of false interpretation in patients with posteromedial to anteromedial development of iliac apophysis, which typically ossifies at the anterosuperior iliac spine and extends behind the posterior superior iliac spine [21]. However, the Risser sign has another drawback: inability to predict PHV, a feature critical for determining the optimal timing of brace treatment [22]. To address this issue and enable peak growth prediction, Risser 0 is divided into two stages, based on the triradiate cartilage closure [23]. At Risser sign I there is a 10% risk of progression for a 20° curve and a 60% risk for a 30° curve; at Risser sign II there is a 2% risk for a 20° curve and 30% risk for a 30° curve; at Risser III there is a 12% risk for a 30° curve; at Risser sign IV the risk of progression is markedly decreased; at Risser sign V skeletal maturation has ended [23].

Furthermore, a study on the Risser staging system revealed that in three-quarters of the cases, apophyseal capping was not associated with growth cessation [22]. Indeed, two-thirds of the pubertal growth spurt has since been shown to occur prior to Risser stage I. The iliac apophysis does not always fuse until adulthood; therefore, evidence of Risser stage IV does not necessarily reflect the remaining growth potential accurately [24].

Furthermore, many cases of early growth cessation have been described at Risser stage III [25]. Therefore, the Risser sign does not accurately predict further growth. Clinically, this means that the Risser staging system cannot be used as a predictor for brace weaning in the treatment of idiopathic scoliosis. Bone age, growth rate, and the onset of secondary sexual characteristics are considered to be more reliable parameters. However, the Risser sign remains the most commonly used tool for the assessment of skeletal maturity due to its simplicity, the ease of pelvic visualization in radiographs, and its ability to correctly signal the end of the risk period for curve progression.

Hand and Wrist Radiograph

Morphological changes in the epiphysis and metaphysis of the digital bones of the non-dominant hand, typically visualized in an antero-posterior hand and wrist radiograph, is the most used measure of bone age. Changes to the digital bone, distal radius, and ulna more accurately than other radiographic signs determine and predict growth in children under 9-12 years of age [26].

The development of skeletal maturity involves bony complex fusions between the epiphyseal and metaphyseal regions. The order of this fusion is specific, beginning with the distal phalanges, followed by the metacarpals, proximal phalange, and finally the middle phalange. There is no significant correlation between fusion order and growth rate, and the progression is not linear. Therefore, bone age does not correspond to chronological age but reflects maturity in healthy children compared to children with developmental disabilities [27].

Two main techniques have been developed to measure skeletal maturity using hand and wrist radiographs, proposed by Tanner and Whitehouse (TW) [28] and Greulich and Pyle (GP) [29].

The TW1 method, based on data collected from 3,000 British children, was developed in 1962, modified into the TW2 in 1975, and into the TW3 in 2002 [28]. The revisions involved changes to the scoring of each stage and the inclusion of sex-specific standards respectively. A total of twenty bone complexes, including the radius, are included in this scoring system. The final score, when matched to a table, approximates bone age.

The TW3 describes the prototypical characteristics of the bones in the hand and their development over time. Two analysis schemes have been described for the TW3 method: the RUS method uses 13 bones (the phalanges, radius, and ulna) and the TW2 method uses 20 bones (the 13 bones in RUS method plus the seven bones of the carpal region).

Maturity stage for each bone in TW3 is calculated from linguistic statements using a similar process for all bones. Six features must be defined to aptly classify each stage (Table 3):

1. Presence of epiphysis: if this is absent, the output is stage A. If it is present but small and barely visible, the output is stage B. If it is present and easily visible, the output stages range from C to I.
2. Separation: relative position of epiphysis and metaphysis: separated (stages B, C, D, E, F, and G), capped (stage H), or partially fused (stage I).

3. Shape of epiphysis I: oval (stage C) or sharp (stages D-I).
4. Diameter: ratio between metaphysis and epiphysis.
5. Shape of epiphysis II: "sharp" epiphysis can have a regular outline (stages D and E), be adapted to the metaphysis shape (stage F), or have an articulated form (stages G, H, and I).
6. Representation of inner surfaces: either absent (stages B, C, and D) or present as a white line (stage E), two white lines (stage F), or c-shaped (stages G, H, and I).

Table 3. TW3 maturity stages

Stage	Presence	Separation	Shape I	Diameters	Shape II	Surface
A	No					
B	Small	(Yes)	(oval)	>2		(no)
C	Yes	Yes	oval	>2		no
D	Yes	Yes	sharp	≤2	regular	no
E	Yes	Yes	sharp	≤2	regular	1 line
F	Yes	Yes	sharp	≤2	adapted	2 lines
G	Yes	Yes	sharp	≤2	articulation	c-shape
H	Yes	capping	sharp	≤2	articulation	c-shape
I	Yes	fusion	sharp	≤2	articulation	c-shape

The GP technique, introduced by Todd in 1959 in the U.S., is a more simple but subjective method [30]. It involves the determination of the morphological changes to the 28 hand bones followed by comparison to an atlas reference image of a hand. The GP technique has some limitations in the assessment of maturity, especially during puberty. This method is based on the assumption that the hand and wrist bone complexes mature at the same rate.

Hand and wrist AP radiographs from girls between 11 and 13 years old and boys between 13 and 15 years old are difficult to evaluate and images from 11.5 and 12.5 years of bone age (girls) and 14.5 years of bone age (boys) are not included in the atlas [31].

Both techniques described here are limited in their accuracy and clinical application, as reflected by high intraobserver disagreement, which can be up to 0.5 years for the TW3 method and 0.82 years for the GP method [32].

Therefore, in 2008, Sanders et al. [33] tried to simplify bone age assessment by introducing a new approach derived from the TW3 method. It consists of eight stages, encompassing the period when girls and boys are 8 and 12 years old respectively until maturity (Figure 4). In particular, stages 3 and 4, characterized by phalangeal capping, represent the early and late stages of adolescent rapid growth, corresponding to the acceleration phase and PHV. Stage 8 corresponds to skeletal maturity, similar to Risser grade V.

This method is closely aligned with the progression of scoliosis curvature, more so than the Risser, TW3, and GP techniques. A limitation includes the need for physeal assessment of all digits, which can be time-consuming, complex, and not well suited for a busy clinic setting [33].

Wrist Radiograph

Wrist radiographs allow for the morphological evaluation of the two physeal plates of the distal radius and ulna (DRU) and classification of growth phases [34] using 11 radius grades and 9 ulna grades (Table 4). These grades are evenly distributed throughout pubertal age. For example, peak growth spurt is indicated by the medial capping of the distal radius (R7) and the appearance of an ulna styloid with a defined head that is denser than a styloid (U5). Maturation and the subsequent longitudinal growth cessation is represented by the complete fusion of the distal radial growth plate (R11) and ulna epiphysis (U9). This wrist-based classification provides 80% sensitivity and 80% specificity and is more accurate than the Risser staging system and menarche age, both of which only weakly correlate to PHV and poorly predict growth cessation [25].

Table 4. DRU classification [35]

Radial stage		Ulnar stage		TW3 stage
R1	Epiphysis appears as single or multiple spots	U1	The epiphysis appears at single/multiple spots.	B
R2	Distinct and oval shaped epiphysis	U2	A rounded shape epiphysis.	C
R3	Maximal diameter is more than half the width of metaphyseal	U3	The epiphysis is at least half the width of metaphysis.	D
R4	Double line at the distal border of epiphysis, represent palmar and dorsal surface	U4	The styloid is visible on the medial end of the epiphysis.	E
R5	Proximal border of epiphysis visible as an irregular thickened white line, more pronounced on the medial side; proximal boarder assuming concave shape; width of epiphysia not as wide as metaphysis	U5	The head of the ulna is distinctly defined and denser than styloid; the border adjacent to the radial epiphysis is flattened.	F
R6	Either medial part of epiphysis overhangs the metaphysis, lateral border wider than metaphysis, or both; medial border develops articulation with the ulna.	U6	The epiphysis is as wide as the metaphysis; the proximal border of the epiphysis overlaps with the metaphysis at the center third.	G
R7	Epiphysis capping on the medial side while the lateral side is rounded	U7	Narrowing of the medial physeal plate; the medial border of the epiphysis and the metaphysis form a smooth curve line (articulation with radius); fusion may be seen on the medial half.	H
R8	Squaring/cap seen on lateral proximal corner; physeal plate still well visible. Its medial and lateral ends are wider than the center	U8	Unfused growth plate visible proximal to styloid process; in a rotated film, the medial and lateral border appear fused but the physeal space can be seen under the styloid.	
		U9	Complete fusion	
R9	The epiphysis strongly capping the metaphysis with sclerosis of the physeal space; the growth plate is visible but blurred; the epiphysis almost touches the metaphysis at the medial and lateral end.			I
R10	The growth plate is completely obliterated, forming a sclerotic line, at times appearing as a broken line; the notch is visible at the medial or lateral end of the growth plate.			
R11	Complete fusion with the lateral/medial edge of the physeal line rounded; growth plate scar may still be visible			

DRU classification is straightforward enough for clinical use and has been proven robust with excellent intra- and interobserver reliability. To understand these developmental stages and their influence in treatment options is useful for scoliosis patient management. A thorough and accurate understanding of growth peak and cessation informs brace initiation timing, curve progression prediction, and is particularly relevant for patients with early-onset scoliosis [34].

Elbow Radiograph

The elbow is a joint with six secondary ossification centers that appear and fuse at different ages, thereby reflecting the bone age of a child. The ossification centers always appear in a specific sequence, following the well-known acronym "CRITOE" (capitellum, radial head, internal epicondyle, trochlea, olecranon, external epicondyle). The ages at which these ossification centers first appear are highly variable (Table 5) but the "1-3-5-7-9-11 years" sequence can serve as a general guide [35].

The elbow undergoes typical morphological changes at the distal epiphysis ossification centers. The method for inferring bone age from radiographs of the elbow was developed by Sauvegrain et al. [36] in 1962 and simplified by Dimeglio et al. [31] in 2005. Elbow radiographs are accurate for studying skeletal age around and during the pubertal spurt, thereby providing information from bone age 10-13 years in girls and 12-15 years boys. Specifically, every six months, expected morphological changes in olecranon apophysis could be observed [31]. Each stage corresponds to a characteristic morphology that is related to a specific age. Stage 1 represents the start of puberty and stage 5 occurs at the end of PHV and the resulting end of the pubertal spurt (Figure 5).

This method is reliable, easy to learn, and provides pediatric orthopedics with a robust assessment tool for the first two years of puberty Moreover, it determines the risk for spinal deformity progression when combined with curve magnitude and annual curve progression velocity [31].

Table 5. Elbow ossification center and age of their appearance

Ossification Center	Girls (yr)	Boys (yr)
Capitellum	1	1
Radial head	4	5
Internal epicondyle	5	7
Trochlea	8	8
Olecranon	8	10
External epicondyle	11	12

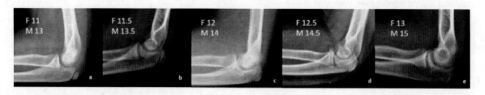

Figure 5. Olecranon apophysis maturation classification: a) double ossification center; b) half-moon shape; c) rectangular shape; d) beginning of fusion: e) Complete fusion.

Calcaneal Radiograph

Lateral radiographs of the hind foot allow for visualizing of calcaneal apophysis ossification, a useful for the assessment of skeletal maturity and PHV physiologically. Six stages of apophyseal ossification can be distinguished (Figure 6). Four of the six stages of calcaneal apophyseal ossification occur before PHV has been reached: stage 3 occurs about 0.9 years before PHV and stage 4 approximately 0.5 years after PHV [37].

The calcaneal system is similar to the Risser staging system, whose simplicity has solidified its continued use in skeletal maturity assessment [24, 25]. The benefits of the calcaneal system are that the ossification stages occur both before and after reaching PHV, unlike the Risser signs that occur exclusively after PHV and have substantial overlap between stages. In addition to the effective delineation of concrete stages of skeletal maturity in relation to PHV, calcaneal radiographs avoid gonadal exposure to radiation [37].

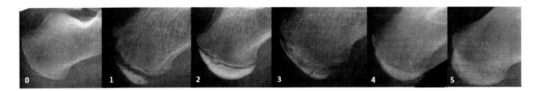

Figure 6. Calcaneal apophysis maturation classification: *stage 0*: no ossification of the apophysis is evident; *stage 1*: the apophysis extends more quickly over the plantar than dorsal surface, covering about <50% of the metaphysis; *stage 2*: the apophysis covers ≥50% of the metaphysis but has not extended to the plantar edge; *stage 3*: complete extension over the plantar surface is seen when the apophysis extends within 2 mm of the plantar edge of the calcaneal concavity; *stage 4*: fusion of the apophysis is occurring, but there are still visible intervals between the apophysis and metaphysis. Fusion begins in the central region of the interval between the apophysis and metaphysis; *stage 5*: complete fusion of the apophysis.

CONCLUSION

Accurate growth assessment is the key to effectively predicting the risk of scoliosis progression. These sex- and ethnicity-dependent factors are invaluable when selecting optimal treatment approaches for scoliosis patients.

Since chronological age is insufficiently informative, bone age must be determined by correlation to clinical and radiological parameters. Knowledge of the phases of puberty is needed to identify the accelerating growth phase, the crucial period in curve progression. Elbow radiography enables visualization of olecranon morphology and represents the most straightforward and reliable method for assessing bone age during the acceleration phase of puberty. Correlation-based prediction methods were first based on the Risser staging system, sitting and standing height measurements, and the Tanner stages. Specifically, an increase in sitting height, in the absence of spinal curvature worsening, is predictive of a positive patient outcome; conversely, an increase in sitting height accompanied by worsening of the curvature is indicative of an ineffective treatment strategy.

The accurate prediction of growth dynamics is paramount for effective strategy selection. Orthopedic surgeons should determine treatment efficacy and switch to surgery (if necessary) as early as possible, prior to puberty cessation.

Despite their accuracy and utility, these parameters could never substitute for the insight of a pediatric orthopedic clinician in selecting the treatment strategy most likely to optimize patient outcome.

REFERENCES

[1] Cheung, J. P. Y., Luk, K. D. (2017). Managing the Pediatric Spine: Growth Assessment. *Asian Spine J* 11 (5): 804-816.

[2] Dimeglio, A., Canavese, F. (2013). Progression or not progression? How to deal with adolescent idiopathic scoliosis during puberty. *J Child Orthop* 7 (1): 43-49.

[3] Duval-Beaupe're, G., Lamireau, T. (1985). Scoliosis at less 30°. Properties of the evolutivity (risk of progression). *Spine (Phila Pa 1976)* 10 (5): 421–424.

[4] Cheung, K. M., Cheng, E. Y., Chan, S. C., Yeung, K. W., Luk, K. D. (2007). Outcome assessment of bracing in adolescent idiopathic scoliosis by the use of the SRS-22 questionnaire. *Int Orthop* 31 (4): 507-511.

[5] Tanner, J. M., Whitehouse, R. H. (1976). Clinical longitudinal standards for height, weight, height velocity and weight velocity and the stages of puberty. *Arch Dis Child* 51 (3): 170–179.

[6] Grumbach, M. M. (2000). The role of estrogen in the male and female: evidence from mutations in synthesis and action. *Horm Res* 53(Suppl 3): 23-24.

[7] Sanders, J. O., Browne, R. H., Cooney, T. E., Finegold, D. N., McConnell, S. J., Margraf, S. A. (2006). Correlates of the peak height velocity in girls with idiopathic scoliosis. *Spine (Phila Pa 1976)* 31 (20): 2289-2295.

[8] Chang, S. H., Tzeng, S. J., Cheng, J. Y., Chie, W. C. (2000). Height and weight change across menarche of schoolgirls with early menarche. *Arch Pediatr Adolesc Med* 154 (9): 880-884.

[9] Lee, W. T., Cheung, C. S., Tse, Y. K., Guo, X., Qin, L., Ho, S. C., Lau, J., Cheng, J.C. (2005). Generalized low bone mass of girls with adolescent idiopathic scoliosis is related to inadequate calcium intake and weight bearing physical activity in peripubertal period. *Osteoporos Int* 16 (9): 1024-1035.

[10] Smith, F. M., Latchford, G., Hall, R. M., Millner, P. A., Dickson, R. A. (2002). Indications of disordered eating behaviour in adolescent patients with idiopathic scoliosis. *J Bone Joint Surg Br* 84 (3): 392-394.

[11] Qiu, Y., Sun, X., Qiu, X., Li, W., Zhu, Z., Zhu, F., Wang, B., Yu, Y., Qian, B. (2007). Decreased circulating leptin level and its association with body and bone mass in girls with adolescent idiopathic scoliosis. *Spine (Phila Pa 1976)* 32 (24): 2703-2710.

[12] Lee, W. T., Cheung, C. S., Tse, Y. K., Guo X, Qin, L., Lam, T. P., Ng, B. K., Cheng, J. C. (2005). Association of osteopenia with curve severity in adolescent idiopathic scoliosis: a study of 919 girls. *Osteoporos Int* 16 (12): 1924-1932.

[13] Li, Y., Binkowski, L., Grzywna, A., Robbins, C. B., Caird, M. S., Farley, F. A., Glotzbecker, M. (2017). Is Obesity in Adolescent Idiopathic Scoliosis Associated With Larger Curves and Worse Surgical Outcomes? *Spine (Phila Pa 1976)* 42 (3):E156-E162.

[14] Dimeglio, A., Canavese, F. (2012). The growing spine: how spinal deformities influence normal spine and thoracic cage growth. *Eur Spine J* 21 (1): 64–70.

[15] Lonner, B. S., Toombs, C. S., Husain, Q. M., Sponseller, P., Shufflebarger, H., Shah, S. A., Samdani, A. F., Betz, R.R., Cahill, P.J., Yaszay, B., Newton, P.O. (2015). Body Mass Index in Adolescent Spinal Deformity: Comparison of Scheuermann's Kyphosis, Adolescent Idiopathic Scoliosis, and Normal Controls. *Spine Deform* 3 (4): 318-326.

[16] Dimeglio, A., Bonnel, F., Canavese, F. (2011). Normal growth of the spine and thorax. In: Akbarnia, B. A. et al. (eds) *The growing spine*, 1st edn. Springer, Berlin, pp 13–42.

[17] Dimeglio, A. (2005). Growth in pediatric orthopaedics. In: Morrissy T, Weinstein SL (eds) *Lovell & Winter's pediatric orthopaedics*, 6th edn. Lippincott, William & Wilkins, Philadelphia, pp 35–61.

[18] Busscher, I., Kingma, I., Wapstra, F. H., Bulstra, S. K., Verkerke, G. J., Veldhuizen, A. G. (2011). The value of shoe size for prediction of the timing of the pubertal growth spurt. *Scoliosis* 6 (1): 1.

[19] Risser J. C. (2010). The classic: The iliac apophysis: an invaluable sign in the management of scoliosis. 1958. *Clin Orthop Relat Res* 468 (3): 643-653.

[20] Bitan, F. D., Veliskakis, K. P., Campbell, B. C. (2005). Differences in the Risser grading systems in the United States and France. *Clin Orthop Relat Res* (436): 190-195.

[21] Shuren, N., Kasser, J. R., Emans, J. B., Rand, F. (1992). Reevaluation of the use of the Risser sign in idiopathic scoliosis. *Spine (Phila Pa 1976)* 17 (3): 359-361.

[22] Hoppenfeld, S., Lonner, B., Murthy, V., Gu, Y. (2004). The rib epiphysis and other growth centers as indicators of the end of spinal growth. *Spine (Phila Pa 1976)* 29 (1): 47-50.

[23] Nault, M. L., Parent, S., Phan, P., Roy-Beaudry, M., Labelle, H., Rivard, M. (2010). A modified Risser grading system predicts the curve acceleration phase of female adolescent idiopathic scoliosis. *J Bone Joint Surg Am* 92 (5): 1073-1081.

[24] Wang, W. W., Xia, C. W., Zhu, F., Zhu, Z. Z., Wang, B., Wang, S. F., Yeung, B. H., Lee, S. K., Cheng, J. C., Qiu, Y. (2009). Correlation of Risser sign, radiographs of hand and wrist with the histological grade of iliac crest apophysis in girls with adolescent idiopathic scoliosis. *Spine (Phila Pa 1976)* 34 (17): 1849-1854.

[25] Cheung, J. P., Cheung, P. W., Samartzis, D., Cheung, K. M., Luk, K. D. (2016). The use of the distal radius and ulna classification for the prediction of growth: peak growth spurt and growth cessation. *Bone Joint J* 98B (12): 1689-1696.

[26] Pietka, E., Gertych, A., Pospiech, S., Cao, F., Huang, H. K., Gilsanz, V. (2001). Computer-assisted bone age assessment: image preprocessing and epiphyseal/metaphyseal ROI extraction. *IEEE Trans Med Imaging* 20 (8): 715-729.

[27] Parfitt, A. M. (2002). Misconceptions (1): epiphyseal fusion causes cessation of growth. *Bone* 30 (2): 337-339.

[28] Aja-Fernandez, S., De Luis-Garcia, R., Martin-Fernandez, M. A., Alberola-Lopez, C. (2004). A computational TW3 classifier for skeletal maturity assessment. A Computing with Words approach. *J Biomed Inform* 37 (2): 99-107.

[29] Greliuch, W. W., Pyle, S. I. (1959). *Radiographis atlas of skeletal development of the hand and wrist.* 2nd edition. Stanford: Stanford University Press.

[30] Todd, T. W. (1937). *Atlas of skeletal maturation (hand).* St. Louis: C. V. Mosby Co.

[31] Diméglio, A., Charles, Y. P., Daures, J. P., de Rosa, V., Kaboré, B. (2005). Accuracy of the Sauvegrain method in determining skeletal age during puberty. *J Bone Joint Surg Am* 87 (8): 1689–1696.

[32] Thodberg, H. H., Kreiborg, S., Juul, A., Pedersen, K. D. (2009). The BoneXpert method for automated determination of skeletal maturity. *IEEE Trans Med Imaging* 28 (1): 52-66.

[33] Sanders, J. O., Khoury, J. G., Kishan, S., Browne, R. H., Mooney, J. F. 3rd, Arnold, K. D., McConnell, S. J., Bauman, J. A., Finegold, D. N. (2008). Predicting scoliosis progression from skeletal maturity: a simplified classification during adolescence. *J Bone Joint Surg Am* 90 (3): 540-553.

[34] Luk, K. D., Saw, L. B., Grozman, S., Cheung, K. M., Samartzis, D. (2014). Assessment of skeletal maturity in scoliosis patients to determine clinical management: a new classification scheme using distal radius and ulna radiographs. *Spine J* 14 (2): 315-325.

[35] De Boeck, H. (1996). Radiology of the elbow in children. *Acta Orthop Belg* 62(Suppl 1): 34-40.

[36] Sauvegrain, J., Nahm, H., Bronstein, N. (1962) Etude de la maturation osseuse du coude. [Study of bone maturation of the elbow.] *Ann Radiol* 5: 542–550.

[37] Nicholson, A. D., Liu, R. W., Sanders, J. O., Cooperman, D. R. (2015). Relationship of Calcaneal and Iliac Apophysis Ossification to Peak Height Velocity Timing in Children. *J Bone Joint Surg Am* 97 (2): 147-154.

Chapter 3

CLASSIFICATION OF EARLY ONSET SPINAL DEFORMITY

Mattia Cravino[1], Lorenza Marengo[1], Federico Canavese[2] and Antonio Andreacchio[1]

[1]Department of Pediatric Orthopedics,
Regina Margherita Children's Hospital, Torino, Italy
[2]Department of Pediatric Surgery, University Hospital Estaing,
University of Clermont Auvergne, Faculty of Medicine,
Clermont Ferrand, France

ABSTRACT

Early-onset spinal deformities are a wide group of scoliosis that occur before age 10. If not treated, they may evolve to a thoracic insufficiency syndrome. These types of scoliosis can be classified in four separate groups due to: congenital deformity, neuromuscular, syndromic and idiopathic scoliosis. It is crucial to have an early diagnosis, independently of the type of cause, in order to start the proper treatments and avoid thoracic insufficiency syndrome onset.

Keywords: classification, scoliosis, congenital, neuromuscular, syndromic, idiopathic

INTRODUCTION

Although early onset scoliosis (EOS) is clearly not a new condition, it was described for the first time only 30 years ago.

The first definition of EOS was by Dickson who, for the first time, identified in his book in 1994 a group of scoliosis that not only included the idiopathic form in children younger than 5 years of age, but also those children with neuromuscular, congenital or syndromic scoliosis.

He moreover divided this group of scoliosis into two groups: *Infantile scoliosis*, in which the diagnosis is made between birth and 3 years of age, and *Juvenile scoliosis*, in which the diagnosis is made between 4 and 10 years of age.

This classification criticized the previous one by the Scoliosis Research Society (SRS) focused on the spinal deformity and age of diagnosis rather than on the physiological effects that this disease made on the patients. SRS indeed, suggests differentiating scoliosis according to its age of onset and radiological issues in: infantile (0-3 years; IIS), juvenile (3-10 years; JIS), adolescent (10-18 years; AID) and adult (>18 years).

Recently, the Chest Wall and Spine Deformity Study Group (CWSDSG) has developed a new and more inclusive classification of EOS, which compensates for the lack of consensus in the scientific community for the definition of this group of diseases [1].

As we know, classification systems are utilized for guiding management, optimizing communication between colleagues and facilitating research leading to a common language. The complexity in etiologies, associations and manifestations of EOS does not completely lead itself to previous classification systems used for scoliosis. For these reasons, CWSDSG developed a classification system for early onset scoliosis based on the input of a group of experienced clinicians in this area with a minimum of ten years of clinical experience.

They created a classification system consisting in 5 variables: age (as continuous prefix), three core variables: etiology (congenital, neuromuscular, syndromic, idiopathic), major curve angle (<20°, 20-50°, 51-90°, >90°), kyphosis (<20°, 20-50°, >50°) and an optional modifier: annual progression rate of the curve (APR: <10°/yr, 10-20°/yr, >20°/yr).

This classification provide a fundamental nomenclature for EOS and, furthermore, it is a dynamic evaluation tool because it categorize all patients with early onset scoliosis throughout their clinical course prior to surgical intervention as other classification systems do.

The common element that pool together all this kind of scoliosis is, therefore, not only the age of onset but also the risk of developing a pulmonar disease better know with the name of thoracic insufficiency syndrome.

As we know, spinal development is closely linked to pulmonar growth. Both pulmonar intraparenchymal and extraparenchymal develops during growth with the chest wall. This compliance decrease with time and it is particularly restricted by external compression due to spinal or thoracic cage deformity. Lung "growth," described as hyperplasia and airway expansion, is essentially completed by the age of 8 years, with the maximal growth occurring before 5 years.

This explained that respiratory failure due to untreated scoliosis before ten years of age double the mortality rate as in the general population [3, 4], in contrast patients with adolescent scoliosis have the same rate as in the health people.

The increased morbidity and mortality recognized in patients with early-onset scoliosis justify to classify such patients as a separate group in which the emphasis, as we said before, is in not necessary in treating the spine itself but on maintaining growth of the thorax to lead the increment of lung volume, in particular in the first, more critical, decade of life [2].

Early-onset spinal deformity can be therefore defined as scoliosis with onset at the age of less than ten years, due to a wide spectrum of etiologies, associations and manifestations that all leads to a common pathway: thoracic insufficiency syndrome.

Classification of Early Onset Spinal Deformity

As described in CWSDSG classification system, early-onset spinal deformity can be classified in the following categories: congenital deformity, neuromuscular, syndromic and idiopathic.

Congenital Deformity

Spine congenital deformities include a spectrum of condition that range from pure scoliosis through kyphoscoliosis to kyphosis. These pathologies are the results of failure in the longitudinal development of one or more vertebrae. This failure can lead to an unbalanced growth of the spine that can turn in a benign curve that need no surgical treatment but only clinical observation or brace, until very aggressive and progressive deformities with consequent functional, cosmetic, respiratory and neurological complications [5].

Our aim, as pediatric orthopedic doctors, is to understand in advance which curves will progress in order to use the best treatment as soon as possible.

The prevalence in the general population of congenital deformities of the spine is 1 in 1,000 live births, with a reported familial incident of 1 to 5%. Girls are more affected than boys.

Pure scoliosis are nearly 80% of congenital deformities, while kyphoscoliosis represents the 14% and kyphosis only the 6% [6].

The causes of congenital vertebral anomalies are an association of *genetic factors*, like disorders of the Notch 1 gene, abnormal HOX gene expression, translocations of chromosome 13 and 17, and *environmental factors* like exposure to toxins including carbon monoxide, the use of antiepileptic medication and maternal diabetes.

Scoliosis caused by congenital deformity can be classified in:

- *Failure of vertebral segmentation* that produces an un-segmented bar and can be bilateral or unilateral. This defect can involve one or more vertebrae, either in the vertebral bodies, in the posterior elements, or in both. Un-segmented bar have the worst prognosis for progression and deformity. If the bar affected the lateral part of two or more vertebrae causes a scoliosis, if it affected the posterior elements causes a fixed lordosis, if anterior part of the body causes a kyphosis.
- *Failure of vertebra formation* that can be complete or incomplete. Hemivertebra caused by failure of complete unilateral formation can be non-segmented, semi-segmented or segmented from the adjacent vertebrae. A non-segmented hemivertebra is completed fused with the vertebra above and below with no disc or vertebral growth plates. If the growth is symmetrical this condition does not lead progressive spinal deformity. A semi-segmental hemivertebra has only one end plate and disc and is fused on the controlateral side (above or below). Due to some asymmetry of growth there is likelihood of progressive spinal deformity. A fully segmented hemivertebra is completely separated from the adjacent vertebrae, with an intact vertebra growth plates and discs (Figure 1, 2). This condition can lead to a sever scoliosis most of all if there are more than one hemivertebra on one side. Instead two hemivertebra on different level and on opposite side can balance the growth and the degree of curvature is less progressive.

- *Mixed anomalies* that can affect different areas of the spine with a combination of the two types describe above. The resultant scoliosis can be very severe.

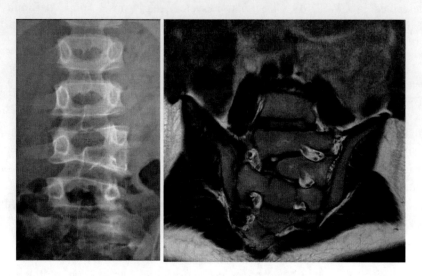

Figure 1. Failure of formation: XR and MRI of a fully segmented hemivertebra completely separated from the adjacent vertebrae.

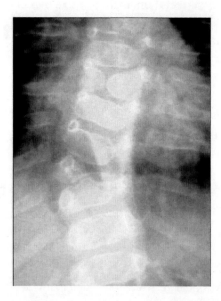

Figure 2. Failure of formation: XR of a fully segmented hemivertebra with a butterfly vertebra three levels above.

The natural history of all these kind of spine anomalies depends on the type, numbers and location of deformities. Maximal progression must be expected during the first 3 years of life and during pre-pubertal and pubertal years, where the skeletal growth is faster [7, 8].

Neuromuscular Scoliosis

The term neuromuscular scoliosis appears as a separate and well-defined group of diseases in 1990 in the 10th Revision of the International Classification of Diseases, approved by the 43rd World Health Assembly.

This definition is clearly applied to a wide range of conditions and disorders that can be assemble in 5 groups: cerebral palsy, Friederich's ataxia, poliomyelitis, other type of neuromuscular disorders and pediatric spinal cord injury (SCI).

Neuromuscular scoliosis is caused by disorders of the brain, spinal cord, and muscular system. Nerves and muscles are unable to maintain appropriate balance and alignment of the spine.

This kind of scoliosis is often associated with skin breakdown, pulmonary compromise, functional decline and kyphosis, they classically involve the entire thoracolumbar spine, often extending to the pelvis and causing pelvic obliquity.

Actually the scientific literature agrees on the fact that it's very difficult to predict the emergency and progression of scoliosis in children with severe neuromuscular pathologies. As in the other form of early onset scoliosis the onset age in strictly correlated to the possibility of curve progression. Saito et al. found that when scoliosis started before the age of 10 years, it progressed rapidly during the adolescent growth period, continuing to increase after this growth period ended. They also published that a curve of more than 40 degrees of Cobb's angle before 15 years of age are associated to a significantly worse progression over time [9].

Regarding scoliosis due to a SCI, the age when the injury occurs, is the only significant predictor of worst curve and of progression to spinal fusion [10].

Syndromic Scoliosis

Syndromic scoliosis is a compound of spinal deformity and genetic disorders. This deformity can be evident at birth or take place during growth. They can be classified according to:

- Genetic condition: Rett syndrome, Prader-Willi syndrome, neurofibromatosis, VACTERL (vertebral, anal, cardiac, trachea-esophageal fistula, renal dysplasia, limb defect), achondroplasia, arthrogryposis, spondyloepiphyseal dysplasia, diastrophic dysplasia, Down's syndrome.
- Dystonia: genetic, cerebral palsy associated, metabolic
- Malformations: Chiari malformation, syringomyelia, spinal dysraphism.
- Inborn errors of metabolism: mucopolysaccaridoses, lucolipidoses.
- Collagen disorders: Marfan syndrome, Ehlers-Danlos syndrome (Figures 3, 4).

Idiopathic Scoliosis

Scoliosis is defined idiopathically with an early onset when it occurs in a child before they reach ten years old, but a real cause is not found. This category is probably the more underhand because of the complexity of predicting the real prognosis and curve evolution.

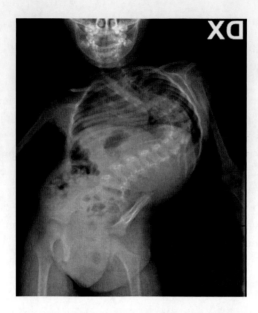

Figure 3. XR of a syndromic early onset scoliosis in Ehlers-Danlos syndrome.

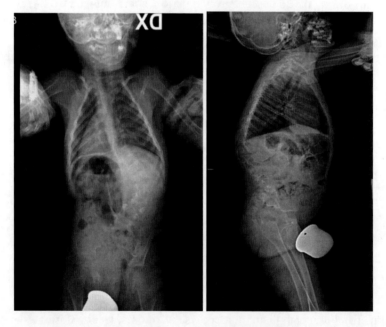

Figure 4. XR of a syndromic early onset scoliosis in collagen disorders.

Idiopathic scoliosis can be divided by the age of onset in: Infantile (that manifest between birth and 3 years of age), juvenile (that occurs between the ages of 4 and 10 years of age) and adolescent scoliosis (in children older than 10 years of age).

While adolescent idiopathic scoliosis is well described in the orthopedic literature for regarding natural history and treatment, little has been written about the infantile and juvenile forms.

As the adolescent forms, the early onset one may manifest as a spontaneous resolving curves, a slowly progressive curves that responds to nonoperative treatments or a progressive curves that requires surgical treatments.

The literature reports that 12% to 21% of idiopathic scoliosis are EOS. Male are affected more commonly than female (range 2:1 to 4:1), even if in younger child, between 3 and 6 years of age, the female-male ratio is 1:1.

In contrast to late-onset idiopathic scoliosis, three quarters of thoracic curves are convex to the left. Figueiredo and James found that 13% of their patients has positive family histories for scoliosis. They also found that 12% of their patients with idiopathic EOS had mental deficiencies and 2% had epilepsy [11].

More young is the patient at the age of onset more frequent is the rate of spontaneous correction of the curve during growth. Some authors also describe that thoracic and thoracolumbar curves tend to resolve, but double structural with a thoracic component have a potential defined progression.

Obviously initial curve size and the amount of associated rotation are also prognostic factors. Females with right-side thoracic curves have a worse prognosis [12].

A unique characteristic of idiopathic EOS, in comparison with the adolescent forms, is the tendency to progression during the relative plateau of growth that occurs between the age of 5 and 10 years.

As predictable, due to the significant amount of spinal growth remaining in these patients, approximately 70% of these curves progress and require a surgical treatment.

REFERENCES

[1] Brendan A. Williams, MD, Hiroko Matsumoto, MA, Daren J. McCalla, BS, Behrooz A. Akbarnia, MD, Laurel C. Blakemore, MD, Randal R. Betz, MD, John M. Flynn, MD, Charles E. Johnston, MD, Richard E. McCarthy, MD, David P. Roye Jr., MD, David L. Skaggs, MD, John T. Smith, MD, Brian D. Snyder, MD, PhD, Paul D. Sponseller, MD, MBA, Peter F. Sturm, MD, George H. Thompson, MD, Muharrem Yazici, MD, and Michael G. Vitale, MD, MPH. 2014. "Development and Initial Validation of the Classification of Early Onset Scoliosis (C-EOS)." *JBJS* 96:1359-67.

[2] Herrenstein RJ. 1930. "Die Skoliose bei Saueglingen und ihre behandlung." [Scoliosis in infants and their treatment.] *Z. Orthop Chir* 52:1-40.

[3] Grassi V, Tantucci C. 1993. "Respiratory prognosis in chest wall diseases." *Monaldi Arch Chest Dis* 48:183.

[4] Branthwaite MA. 1986. "Cardiorespiratory consequences of unfused idiopathic scoliosis." *Br J Dis Chest* 80:360-369.

[5] Kawakami N, Tsuji T, Imagama S, Lenke LG, Puno RM, Kuklo TR. 2009. "Classification of congenital scoliosis and kyphosis: a new approach to the three-dimensional classification for progressive vertebral anomalies requiring operative treatment." *Spinal Deformity Study Group. Spine* Aug 1;34(17):1756-65.

[6] Morin B, Poitras B, Duhaime M, Rivard CH, Marton D. 1985 "Congenital kyphosis by segmentation defect: etiologic and pathogenic studies." *J Pediatr Orthop* May-Jun 5(3):309-14.

[7] Mohanty S, Kumar N. 2000. "Patterns of presentation of congenital scoliosis." *J Orthop Surg* Dec 8(2):33-37.

[8] Shahcheraghi GH, Hobbi MH. 1999. "Patterns and progression in congenital scoliosis." *J Pediatr Orthop*. Nov-Dec 19(6):766-75.

[9] Saito N, Ebara S, Ohotsuka K, Kumeta H, Takaoka K. 1998. "Natural history of scoliosis in spastic cerebral palsy." *Lancet* 351:1687-1692.

[10] Injury MJ. Mulcahey, PhD, John P. Gaughan, PhD, Randal R. Betz, MD, Amer F. Samdani, MD, Nadia Barakat PhD, and Louis N. Hunter PT, 2013. "Neuromuscular Scoliosis in Children with Spinal Cord." *Top Spinal Cord Inj Rehabil. Spring* 19(2): 96–103.

[11] Figueiredo UM, James JIP. 1981. "Juvanile idiopathic scoliosis." *JBJS [Br]* 63: 61-66.

[12] Thompson SK, Bentley G. 1980. "Prognosis in infantile idiopatich scoliosis." *J Bone Joint Surg* [Br] 47:524-525.

[13] Dickson RA. 1994 *"Early onset scoliosis."* Vol I. New York: Raven.

In: Scoliosis: Diagnosis, Classification and Management Options   ISBN: 978-1-53614-464-2
Editors: F. Canavese, A. Andreacchio and H. Xu   © 2018 Nova Science Publishers, Inc.

Chapter 4

CLASSIFICATION OF ADOLESCENT IDIOPATHIC SCOLIOSIS

Lorenza Marengo[1],*, MD, Mattia Cravino[1], MD, Federico Canavese[2], MD, PhD and Antonio Andreacchio[1], MD

[1]Pediatric Orthopeadic and Traumatology Department,
Regina Margherita Hospital, Turin, Italy
[2]Department of Pediatric Surgery, University Hospital Estaing,
Clermont Ferrand, France

ABSTRACT

Adolescent idiopathic scoliosis is the most common type of scoliosis. Several classification systems have been developed in order to identify the different subtypes; to support communication; to provide treatment guidelines; and to prognosticate the outcome. In 1905, Schulthess described the first classification system for scoliotic curves, based on curve location. In 1983, King et al. described the first classification system for scoliosis based on treatment guidelines. They identified five thoracic curve patterns and recommended different fusion levels for different curve patterns when Harrington instrumentation was used. However, when more modern instrumentation systems are used, King classification fails to give accurate guidelines in determining the proper levels for fusion, being also not comprehensive enough to categorize all scoliosis patterns. In 2001, Lenke proposed a new classification system for scoliotic curve based on curve location, magnitude, and flexibility, as well as on a lumbar and a sagittal modifier. Lenke classification represents a useful tool for determining the extent of spinal fusion and shows a higher intra- and interobserver reliability. However, it does not take into account the rotational dimension of the deformity. Recently, three dimensional classification systems for AIS have been proposed, but their real clinical application is far from being defined.

Keywords: scoliosis, classification, idiopathic, sagittal plane, adolescent

---

* Corresponding Author Email: Lorenza Marengo, lorenzamarengo@libero.it.

Introduction

Scoliosis deformity can arise from a variety of causes. According to the etiology, the deformity can be classified as neuromuscular (if associated with neuromuscular disorders, such as cerebral palsy, muscular dystrophy, spina bifida, and others), syndrome-related (if associated with generalized diseases and syndromes, such as neurofibromatosis, Marfan syndrome, and bone dysplasia), congenital (if caused by failure in vertebral formation or segmentation), and idiopathic. Idiopathic scoliosis is the most common type of spinal deformity, accounting for about 75% of all cases of scoliosis [1]. Its diagnosis of exclusion can be made only when a thorough physical examination and radiographic analysis have ruled out other causes.

Scoliosis can also be classified based on age at onset into: infantile (0–3 years), juvenile (3–10 years), adolescent (>10 years and before skeletal maturity), and adult (after skeletal maturity). Adolescent idiopathic scoliosis is the most common type of scoliosis.

Several factors contribute in determining the natural history of the disorder, including radiologic deformity features.

A good classification system should identify and rank different deformity patterns and subtypes in order to:

- provide a universal language and help communication
- guide strategies for treatment
- prognosticate the disease

Several classification systems have been developed for adolescent idiopathic scoliosis. All of them include an x-ray assessment. A high quality image is important to allow for a reliable evaluation since the correct determination of the measuring points (upper and lower neutral vertebra, apex vertebra, terminal vertebra) is crucial.

Schulthess Classification

The first classification system for scoliosis was described by Schulthess in 1905 [2]. It was based on the curve location and identified 5 different types of scoliosis [2]:

1) *Cervicothoracic* type: when the curve apex is between C7-T1.
2) *Thoracic* type when the curve apex is between T2 and T11.
3) *Thoracolumbar* type when the curve apex is between T12 and L1.
4) *Lumbar* type when the curve apex is below L1.
5) *Combined double primary* type with two primary curves in the thoracic and lumbar spine.

PONSETI-FRIEDMANN CLASSIFICATION

Ponseti and Friedman proposed a classification system, taking into account coronal curve type and location, according to the apical level (see Schulthess classification) [3]. They claimed that curve type and location are important predictors of the natural history of the deformity and should be considered central to any classification system. These authors identified five different patterns. A further curve pattern was added by Moe.

1) *Single major lumbar curve:* the curve has the apex between L1-2 disc and L4.
2) *Single major thoracolumbar curve:* the curve apex is between T12 and L1.
3) *Combined thoracic and lumbar curve:* is a double major curve.
4) *Single major thoracic curve:* it is a thoracic curve the generally has a convex right pattern.
5) *Single major high thoracic curve:* it is a rare pattern. The curve apex is usually at T3.
6) *Double major thoracic curve:* it is a short upper thoracic curve associated with lower thoracic curve.

Thoracolumbar and lumbar curves have a higher risk of deformity progression compared to thoracic curves, and double curves have a higher risk of deformity progression than single curves.

However, this classification system, based on coronal curve type and location alone, cannot accurately identify and differentiate between curve patterns, and provide information to address deformity management.

KING CLASSIFICATION

In 1983, King and co-workers presented a classification system for AIS, based on Moe experience in the surgical treatment of AIS with the Harrington rod instrumentation [4]. It considered curve pattern and magnitude, and flexibility of the scoliosis deformity. The authors introduced the definition of "stable vertebra", as the vertebra that is most closely bisected by the central sacral vertical line (CSVL) (the line drawn perpendicular to the level of iliac crests and through the center of the sacrum).

Five different curves types were identified:

1) *Type I*: combined thoracic and lumbar curves, in which both curves crossed the CSVL, with the lumbar curve larger than the thoracic one;
2) *Type II*: combined thoracic and lumbar curves, in which both curves crossed the CSVL, with the thoracic curve equal or larger than the lumbar one;
3) *Type III*: thoracic curve with a compensatory, flexible lumbar curve not crossing the CSVL and with a plumbline directly centred over the sacrum (Figure 1);
4) *Type IV*: long thoracic curve with L5 centred over the sacrum and L4 tilted into the long thoracic curve;
5) *Type V:* double thoracic curve, with T1 tilted into the upper thoracic curve.

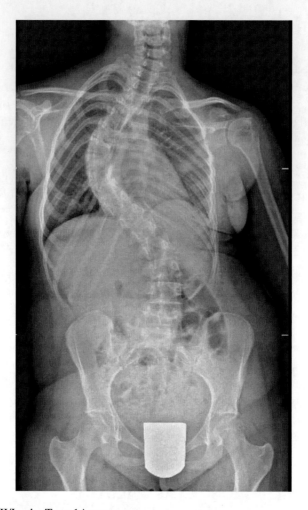

Figure 1. King type III/Lenke Type 1A curve.

According to the curve type, these authors recommended which levels should be instrumented with the Harrington rod to minimize the length of fusion and to preserve motion as much as possible. They suggested fusion from one level above the upper end vertebra to the stable vertebra, and selective thoracic fusion for King's type II curves.

However, when used with more modern instrumentation systems, King classification failed to give accurate guidelines in determining the proper levels for fusions [5, 6]. In particular, selective thoracic fusion for all King's type II curves was reported to have a high lumbar decompensation rate when used with the current segmental instrumentation systems. Also, it is not comprehensive enough to categorize all scoliosis patterns, by not including thoracolumbar, lumbar, and double and triple major curves (Figure 2).

Lastly, several papers reported poor to fair intra- and inter-observer reliability [7-9]. It appears that disagreement as for the existence of structural upper thoracic and lumbar curves is the main reason for poor reliability [9]. Moreover, intra- and interobserver agreement is independent of the observer's experience.

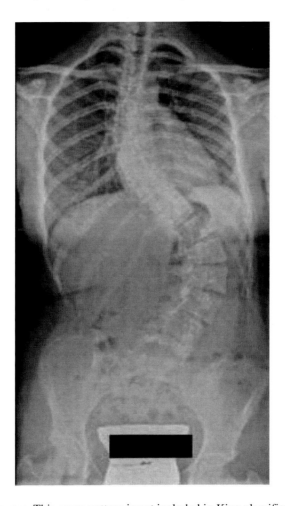

Figure 2. Lenke type 5 curve. This curve pattern is not included in King classification.

LENKE CLASSIFICATION

Lenke proposed a classification system with the intent to be comprehensive for all curve types, to guide deformity treatment, and to be easily understood and applied [10]. This triad classification system appears complete since it combines curve type with a lumbar modifier, along with a sagittal thoracic modifier, and is the first classification system that considers both the coronal and the sagittal plane deformity (Table 1).

In order to define the curve type, three curves should be identified on the coronal plane: the proximal thoracic (PT), the main thoracic (MT), and the thoracolumbar/lumbar (TL/L) curves. The PT curve has the apex between T2 and T5, the MT curve between T6 and T11-12 disc, the TL curve between T12 and L1, the lumbar curve between L1-2 disc and L4.

Table 1. Curve types, lumbar spine modifier and sagittal thoracic modifier combined in Lenke classification system

Lenke Classification System				
		PT	MT	TL/L
Curve Types	Type 1	ns	S	ns
	Type 2	s	S	ns
	Type 3	ns	S	s
	Type 4	s	S	S
	Type 5	ns	ns	S
	Type 6	ns	s	S
Lumbar modifier	A	CSVL intersects the apex vertebra, between the pedicles		
	B	CSVL touches the apical vertebral pedicle		
	C	CSVL falls medially to the apical vertebra		
Thoracic modifier	(-)	lateral T5-T12 Cobb angle < 10°		
	N	lateral T5-T12 Cobb angle 10-40°		
	(+)	lateral T5-T12 Cobb angle > 40°		

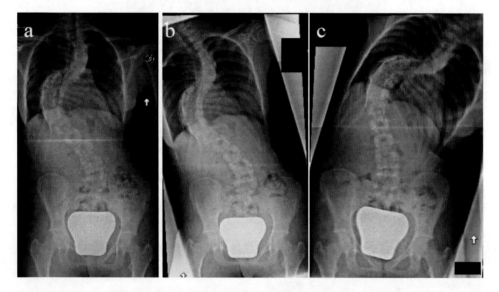

Figure 3. Lenke type 2 deformity (a). The bending radiographs demonstrate that the proximal thoracic curve is structural, while the lumbar curve is nonstructural.

The major curve is defined as the curve with the greatest magnitude, and the others two curves are defined as minor curves. The minor curves are defined structural if they have a residual side bending magnitude of at least 25° in the coronal plane, as well as sagittal hyperkyphosis of >20° in T2-T5 or T10-L2 regions. Otherwise, the minor curve is defined as non-structural (Figure 3). By combining all these factors, six different curve types are identified:

1) *Type 1*: the MT curve is the major and the only structural curve (Figure 1).
2) *Type 2*: double thoracic curve, with the MT curve as the major curve and PT curve as structural minor curve. The TL/L curves are non-structural (Figure 3).

3) *Type 3*: double major curve, with the MT curve as the major curve and TL/L curve as structural minor curve. The PT curve is non-structural. If the MT curve and the TL/L curve have the same Cobb measurement, than the MT curve is considered the major curve
4) *Type 4*: triple major curve, with MT or TL/L curve as the major one. The other two curves are structural minor curves.
5) *Type 5:* the TL/L curve is the major curve and the only structural curve (Figure 2).
6) Type 6: TL/L curve is the major curve and measures at least 5° more than the MT curve, which is structural.

To these curve types, a lumbar spine modifier and a thoracic modifier are added, to further differentiate curve patterns. The lumbar spine modifier is based on the relationship between the CSVL and the apical vertebra of the TL/L curve (Figure 4). The lumbar modifier A is designated if the CSVL passes between the pedicles of the apical vertebra of the TL/L curve. The curve must have a thoracic apex cephalad to T12. Therefore modifier A can be used only for a MT curve (Type 1-2-3-4). The lumbar modifier B is designated if the CSVL touches the pedicles of the lumbar apical vertebra. All these curves have an apex in the MT region, so, again, modifier B can be used only for a MT curve (Type 1-2-3-4). The lumbar modifier C is designated if the CSVL lies medially to the lumbar apical vertebra. These curves may have a major curve in MT, TL and L regions.

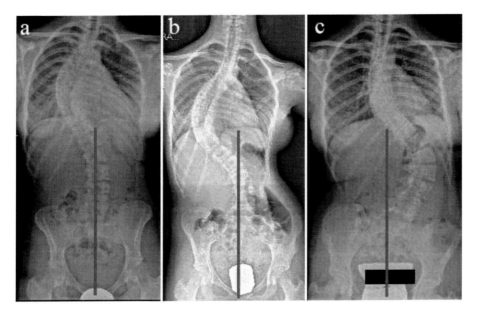

Figure 4. Three different types of lumbar modifier: the lumbar modifier A is designated if the central sacral vertical line (CSVL) passes between the pedicles of the apical vertebra of the TL/L curve (a), the lumbar modifier B if the CVLS touches the pedicles of the lumbar apical vertebra (b), the lumbar modifier C if the CSVL lies medially to the lumbar apical vertebra (c). (The red line represents the CSVL).

The sagittal thoracic modifier is based on the measurement of the T5-T12 lateral Cobb angle. If the thoracic kyphosis measured less than 10° a minus (-) or hypokyphotic modifier is added. If the thoracic kyphosis measured between 10 and 40° an N or normokyphotic modifier is added. If the thoracic kyphosis measured more than 40° a plus (+) or hyperkyphotic modifier is added.

According to the curve pattern, Lenke classification provides a standardized framework for determining fusion levels. The major curves is always included in the fusion, and minor curves should be included only if structural. In patients with lumbar modifier A or B, a selective thoracic fusion is recommended, unless a kyphosis of ≥20° in the thoracolumbar region is present.

Lenke classification provides a more comprehensive classification since it separates the King type II curves to Lenke's type 1 and type 3 curves, it includes thoracolumbar, lumbar, double and triple major curves, and takes into account the sagittal alignment. Also, it shows a higher inter and intra-observer reliability, compared to King classification (Table 2).

However, there is a significant variability in the selection of fusion levels [11], with a violation of the basic rules of Lenke Classification in 15% of the time, because of specific deformity features and patient clinical factors. In fact, Lenke recommends to combine his classification systems with patient clinical features and surgeon's experience to optimize fusion levels selection [12].

Table 2. Comparison between King's and Lenke classifications features

Features	King's Classification	Lenke's classification
Treatment based	+	+
It takes into consideration:		
- thoracic curves	+	+
- thoracolumbar curves	-	+
- lumbar curves	-	+
- double/triple major curves	-	+
- coronal plane deformity	+	+
- sagittal plane deformity	-	+
- rotational deformity	-	-
- curve flexibility	+	+
Intraobserver and interobserver reliability	fair/moderate	good

THREE-DIMENSIONAL CLASSIFICATION

Lenke classification considers only the coronal and sagittal deformity. However, scoliosis is a three dimensional deformity. Recently, increasing attention has been focused on the rotational dimension of the deformity. Innovative technologies also offer to the surgeon the opportunity to address the third dimension of the spine. Three dimensional classification systems for AIS have recently been presented [2]. However, real clinical application is far from being defined. Further efforts are needed to developed a three dimensional classification system that can guide surgeons in a three dimensional approach to AIS.

REFERENCES

[1] The Terminology Committee of the Scoliosis Research Society. A glossary of scoliosis terms. *Spine* 1976; 1: 57–58.

[2] Donzelli S, Poma S, Balzarini L, Borboni A, Respizzi S, Villafane JH, Zaina F, Negrini S. State of the art of current 3-D scoliosis classifications: a systematic review from a clinical perspective. *J Neuroeng Rehabil* 2015; 12: 91.

[3] Ponseti IV, Friedman B. Prognosis in idiopathic scoliosis. *J Bone Joint Surg Am* 1950; 32-A: 381-95.

[4] King HA, Moe JH, Bradford DS, Winter RB. The selection of fusion levels in thoracic idiopathic scoliosis. *J Bone Joint Surg Am* 1983; 65-A: 1302-13.

[5] Richards BS. Lumbar curve response in type II idiopathic scoliosis after posterior instrumentation of the thoracic curve. *Spine* 1992; 17: S282–86.

[6] Roye DP Jr, Farcy JP, Rickert JB, Godfried D. Results of spinal instrumentation of adolescent idiopathic scoliosis by King type. *Spine* 1992; 17:S270–73.

[7] Cummings RJ, Loveless EA, Campbell J, et al. Interobserver reliability and intraobserver reproducibility of the system of King et al. for the classification of adolescent idiopathic scoliosis. *J Bone Joint Surg Am* 1998; 80: 1107–11.

[8] Lenke LG, Betz RR, Bridwell KH, et al. Intraobserver and interobserver reliability of the classification of thoracic adolescent idiopathic scoliosis. *J Bone Joint Surg Am* 1998; 80:1097–106.

[9] Behensky H, Giesinger K, Ogon M, et al. Multisurgeon assessment of coronal pattern classification systems for adolescent idiopathic scoliosis: Reliability and error analysis. *Spine* 2002; 27: 762–67.

[10] Lenke LG, Betz RR, Harms J, et al. Adolescent idiopathic scoliosis a new classification to determine extent of spinal arthrodesis. *J Bone Joint Surg Am* 2001; 83-A: 1169-81.

[11] Newton PO, Faro FD, Lenke LG, et al. Factors involved in the decision to perform a selective versus nonselective fusion for Lenke 1B and 1C (King-Moe II) curves in adolescent idiopathic scoliosis. *Spine* 2003; 28: S217–23.

[12] Lenke LG. Lenke classification system of adolescent idiopathic scoliosis: treatment recommendations. *Instr Course Lect.* 2005; 54: 537-42.

In: Scoliosis: Diagnosis, Classification and Management Options ISBN: 978-1-53614-464-2
Editors: F. Canavese, A. Andreacchio and H. Xu © 2018 Nova Science Publishers, Inc.

Chapter 5

SERIAL ELONGATION DEROTATION FLEXION CASTING FOR PATIENTS WITH PROGRESSIVE SCOLIOSIS

Federico Canavese[1],*, MD and Alain Dimeglio[2],†, MD
[1]CHU Estaing, Service de Chirurgie Infantile,
Clermont Ferrand, France
[2]Université de Montpellier, Faculté de Médecine, Montpellier, France

ABSTRACT

Infantile and juvenile scoliosis, among different types of spinal deformity, still remain a challenge for pediatric orthopedic surgeons. Growth is an essential parameter when dealing with patients with early onset spinal deformities (i.e., infantile scoliosis) or juvenile deformities.

The ideal treatment of infantile and juvenile scoliosis has not yet been identified. In 1964, Morel and Cotrel improved the Risser technique by adding a third dimension, known as the flexion, to elongation and derotation. The Elongation, Derotation and Flexion (EDF) casting technique is a custom-made thoracolumbar cast based on a three dimensional correction concept. This cast offers three-dimensional correction and can control the evolution of the deformity in some cases. The EDF technique has the ability to correct scoliosis three-dimensionally.

This chapter aimed to provide a comprehensive review of how infantile and juvenile scoliosis can affect a normal spine and thorax, and how these deformities can be treated with a serial EDF casting technique.

Keywords: infantile scoliosis, juvenile scoliosis, early onset scoliosis, Elongation Derotation Flexion, casting, conservative

---

* Corresponding Author Email: canavese_federico@yahoo.fr.
† None of the Authors Received Financial Support for This Study.

INTRODUCTION

Scoliosis is a three-dimensional deformity of the spine with lateral, antero-posterior and rotational components. In most cases, the disease is idiopathic and affects children during adolescence. On the other hand, infantile (IS) and juvenile scoliosis (JS) have onset prior to age 5 and 10 years, respectively and are much rarer compared to adolescent scoliosis (AS). IS and JS have distinct presentation when compared to AS. In addition to age at onset, differences exist in associated anomalies, and frequency and rate of deformity progression [1-3].

IS and JS are some of the most challenging conditions in pediatric orthopedics with the potential for severe adverse consequences. Severe and progressive IS and JS represent a serious condition that can ultimately become life threatening if not properly treated. In particular, pathologic changes induced on a growing organism by an early onset spinal deformity can be dramatic and, in most severe cases, can lead to death. A vertebral column not permitted to grow normally, will affect the growth potential of the whole upper body, resulting in a short trunk, a disproportionate body habitus and an underdeveloped thoracic cage [1-6]. In addition, complication rates for all surgical techniques for treatment of IS and JS remain high because of the chronic and repetitive nature of lengthening surgeries, the implant bulk, and the stresses placed on any instrumentation in a mobile spine.

The goal of any treatment is to break this vicious circle; it is necessary to correct quickly all distortions secondary to distorted spinal growth: short height and disproportionate body habitus, underdeveloped thoracic cage and inability to ensure normal breathing, low weight and cardiac dysfunctions. Tachypnea, ventricular tachycardia, dyspnea, tracheomalacia, weight loss or chronic obstructive pulmonary diseases are often more worrisome elements than the distortion of the vertebral column itself [1-8].

THE IDEAL TREATMENT HAS NOT YET BEEN IDENTIFIED

Casting has been used since early XX century, primarily to address spinal curves in infantile, juvenile, adolescents and adult patients prior to surgery. However, with the advent of modern surgical techniques, casting has been used in selected cases only. In young and very young patients, the morbidity related to surgical procedures has favored the coming back of conservative treatment, i.e., serial EDF casting. In particular, even if "growth sparing" devices are implanted at reasonable distance from the spine, auto fusion of ribs and vertebral bodies may make definitive instrumented fusion more challenging [1, 2].

The ideal treatment of IS and JS has not yet been identified as both clinicians and surgeons still face multiple challenges including preservation of the thoracic spine, thoracic cage, lung growth and cardiac function without reducing spinal motion [1, 2, 5, 7, 8].

Spinal deformities associated with rib cage anomalies requiring fusion have highest risk of developing restrictive pulmonary disease. Early spine fusion is not the answer when dealing with progressive spinal deformities occurring in young and very young children. Arthrodesis carried out in the thoracic spine at an early age does not address the impact of the deformity on thoracic cage shape, lung parenchyma development or preservation of cardio-pulmonary function. Moreover, early spinal fusion, especially if performed in the thoracic region, is a cause of respiratory insufficiency and adds loss of pulmonary function to the pre-existing spinal deformity [1, 2, 5-7].

Elongation, Derotation and Flexion (EDF) casting technique is a custom-made thoracolumbar cast based on a three dimensional correction concept. This cast offers three-dimensional correction and can control the evolution of the deformity in some cases. Spinal growth can be guided by EDF casting as it can influence the initially curved spine to grow straighter [1, 2, 9, 10]. It can be used as a "positive" force to guide spinal growth [1, 2, 4, 6, 7, 9].

This article aimed to provide a comprehensive review of how IS and JS can affect normal spine and thorax and how these deformities can be treated with serial EDF casting technique. A current literature review is mandatory in order to understand the principles of the serial EDF casting technique and the effectiveness of conservative treatment in young and very young patients [1, 2, 6, 7, 9].

GROWTH HOLDS THE BASIC

Growth is an essential parameter that must be taken into account when dealing with young and very young patients with scoliosis.

The First Five Years of Age Are Crucial

Many changes occur during the first five years of life. The first five to ten years of life are critical for spine and thoracic cage growth [1-3, 5, 7, 9].

When dealing with severe scoliosis in young and very young patients, the priority is to protect the development of the lungs and the heart. Any severe deformity of the spine during this very crucial period must be considered first as a major risk for lung function and development.

In particular, as the spinal deformity progresses, by a "domino effect," not only spinal growth is affected but size and shape of the thoracic cage are modified as well. This distortion of the thorax will interfere with lungs development: constriction of the thoracic cage as a result of a spinal deformity significantly restricts lung growth and may contribute to serious pulmonary complications. In untreated patients, the loss of vital capacity in those with early onset scoliosis has been shown to be 15% greater than in those with adolescent idiopathic scoliosis. Moreover, Karol et al. have shown also that a thoracic spine height of 18 to 22 cm or more is necessary to avoid severe respiratory insufficiency [1, 2, 6, 8-13].

Over time, the spine disorder changes its nature: from a mainly orthopedic issue, it becomes a severe pediatric, systematic disease with Thoracic Insufficiency Syndrome, Cor Pulmonale and, in most severe cases, death [1-8, 11-13].

In particular, Pehrsson et al. analyzed the mortality and causes of death in 115 patients with untreated scoliosis compared to the expected according to official Swedish statistics. They found that the mortality was significantly increased in IS and JS but not in AS [1, 2, 7, 10-13].

From Age 5 Years to the Beginning of Puberty

Puberty starts at 11 years of age for girls and 13 years of age for boys. Prior to puberty, spinal growth slows down. The annual growth velocity on the standing height is 5.5 cm by year: 3.5 cm in the lower extremities and about 2 cm in the trunk. T1-S1 gain is about 1 cm/year and each vertebra grows approximately 1 mm/year.

When casting a juvenile scoliosis, the goal is not only to buy some time prior to definitive fusion but also to protect the thoracic cage. Many distraction devices can be used but the effects are limited. Moreover, the risk of crankshaft phenomenon is high. In addition, during this same period, vertebral bodies are poorly ossified and mainly cartilaginous. Moreover, distraction alone cannot control the horizontal plan of the spin.

Puberty Is a Turning Point

During puberty, the thoracic cage volume will double although there is not an increase of the overall number of alveoli. The beginning of puberty must be detected soon, to decide an effective strategy: the key point is anticipation. The standing height will increase about 18 to 20 cm: 12 to 14 cm at the level of the trunk (2/3) and 6 to 8 cm at the level of the lower limbs (1/3). Most of growth occurs during the first two years of puberty. The last 3 years are characterized by a reduction of annual growth rate.

GROWTH OF A DISTORTED SPINE

During growth, complex phenomena follow each other in very rapid succession. These events are well synchronized to maintain harmonious limb and spine relationships, as growth does not occur simultaneously in the same magnitude or rate in the various body segments. The slightest error or modification can lead to a malformation or deformity with negative effects on standing and sitting height, thoracic cage shape, volume and circumference, and lung development. In severe scoliosis, growth becomes asymmetrical as a result of growth plate disorganization. Complex spinal deformities alter growth spine cartilage and vertebral bodies become progressively distorted and can perpetuate the disorder by modifying thoracic cage shape and motility and altering lung growth.

In humans, untreated progressive early onset spinal deformities as well as those surgically treated before the age of 7 to 9 years have been reported to be associated with short stature, short trunk, and a deformed spinal column [1-3, 6].

In untreated patients, the inability of the thorax to ensure normal breathing and the accompanying serious respiratory insufficiency is characterized by the Thoracic Insufficiency Syndrome. This clinical picture can be linked to costo-vertebral malformations (e.g., fused ribs, hemivertebra, congenital bars), neuromuscular disease (e.g., expiratory congenital hypotonia), or syndromes such as Jeune and Jarcho-Levin.

Similarly, thoracic cage size modification following precocious spinal arthrodesis (50% to 75% fusion of the thoracic spine before the age of 7) appears to be a progressive process involving multiple skeletal parameters simultaneously. In young children with progressive deformity, there is a decrease of longitudinal growth and a loss of the normal proportionality of trunk growth. In young and very young children with progressive spinal deformity, there is a decrease of longitudinal growth and a loss of the normal proportionality of trunk growth. Moreover, in every operated patient with early onset scoliosis, the crankshaft phenomenon is a major concern. There is no ideal device able to control all the growth plates implicated in the spinal curvature.

CHEST KINEMATICS (BREATHING) IS IMPACTED BY PROGRESSIVE SCOLIOSIS

Previous works have shown that breathing is a function of movement involving ribs, clavicles, sternum, spine, diaphragm and abdominal wall and that these elements are strictly correlated. Alterations in one of these anatomical elements can induce deformity and loss of function in the others. The three dimensional anatomical distortion of the chest is thought to disturb the mechanics of breathing. In particular, scoliosis, kyphosis, and lordosis of the thoracic spine contribute to poor thoracic cage excursion and loss of thoracic cage compliance. Moreover, surgical fusion in patients with severe scoliosis can improve the deformity, but the spine is rendered more rigid, further decreasing the mechanical breathing efficiency. Karol et al. showed a marked decrease in pulmonary function at maturity in children with early onset scoliosis who underwent thoracic spinal fusion prior to age eight. Moreover, they showed that a thoracic spine height of 18 to 22 cm or more is necessary to avoid severe respiratory insufficiency [1, 2, 6, 8-13]. In addition, when thoracic growth is inhibited by congenital spinal deformity associated with rib fusions a significant decrease in the space available for lung growth can occur and chest the chest becomes stiff.

SERIAL ELONGATION, DEROTATION, AND FLEXION EDF CASTING: BRIEF HISTORY AND TECHNIQUE

The US orthopedic surgeon Joseph Risser introduced the frame that bears his name to treat scoliosis with casting. The technique is based on the principles of elongation and derotation in order to correct the spinal curvature [1, 2, 13].

In 1964, French surgeons Yves Cotrel and Georges Morel, improved the Risser technique by adding the third dimension, called flexion and popularized the EDF casting technique [2, 6, 10].

Between 1975 and 2000, United Kingdom physician Min Mehta, modified the EDF technique created by Cotrel and Morel and introduced the concept of serial casting. With the Metha's protocol, EDF casts are changed every 8 to 12 weeks under general anesthesia [1, 6, 7, 10-13].

Technique

MRI is indicated in all patients with IS and JS in order to detect an underlying spinal dysraphism. Untreated spinal dysraphism is a contraindication to any form of distraction treatment. A tethered low lying cord, syringomyelia, fatty filum terminale, Arnold Chiari malformation and/or split cord malformation may need neurosurgical intervention prior to the scoliosis treatment as distraction can lead to neurological deterioration.

EDF stands for elongation, derotation, and flexion. It is a method of orthopedic reduction of the scoliotic deformity on a specific reduction frame by traction, postero-lateral compression and rotation, the application of a thoraco-lumbo-sacral plaster cast and finally lateral manual compression [1, 2, 10].

The reduction apparatus is the Cotrel frame that is used to realize an axial correction of the spine, with the proximal point of traction being the chin and the occiput and the distal point the iliac crests, employing of harnesses and bands and measuring the amount of traction [2, 4, 6-9] (Figure 1 and Figure 2).

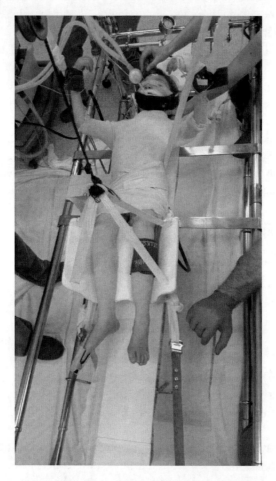

Figure 1. Positioning of the patient on a Cotrel frame. The proximal point of traction is the chin and the distal point is represented by the iliac crests, employing of harnesses and bands and measuring the amount of traction. The patient is initially supported by two metal bars, one under the shoulders and the other sustaining the pelvis. In the same time a band which surround the patient on the convex side of the scoliostic deformity is tensioned in order to reduce it, applying simultaneously a lateral and a posterior reduction forces.

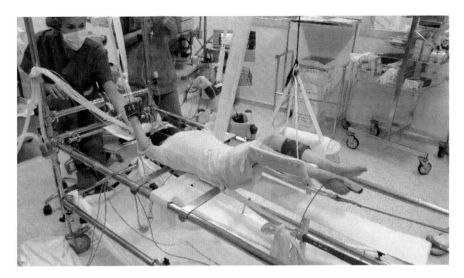

Figure 2. Position of the patient on Cotrel frame (bottom view).

The frame offers gentle traction of the spine and it provides support to hips and torso while allowing enough room for the surgeon to apply the cast and to correct all components of the scoliosis deformity. Serial EDF casting has been shown to be an excellent first line of defense by providing progressive, non-invasive, gentle and permanent correction of infantile and juvenile deformities; moreover, its effectiveness for controlling progressive IS and JS is well documented.

In particular, two horizontal metal bars support the patient, one under the shoulders and the other sustaining the pelvis. In the same time a band, which surrounds the patient on the convex side of the scoliosis curve, is tensioned in order to reduce it, applying simultaneously a lateral and a posterior reduction force. In the case of an "S" curve a second band can be applied in the opposite direction and side, on the level of this second convexity (Figure 3). Next, the two support bars are removed and the plaster is applied over the bands, well molded, especially in regard of the iliac crests. While the plaster is still malleable, one hand lateral pressure is applied on the convexity side and two hand counter-pressures is applied on the concavity side as close as possible to the end vertebrae and maintained until the plaster hardens (Figure 4). The cast is then reinforced by a few layers synthetic fiberglass and thoraco-abdominal window is cut as to obtain a decompression of the anterior abdomen (stomach and bowels) and a better expansion of the thoracic cage (Figure 4). The casts are changed at intervals of 8 to 12 weeks [2, 6].

At first sight, cast may appear as a constrictive force applied to the thoracic cage, limiting its expansion. Indeed, if well molded it does not compress the thoracic cage and respiratory movements are allowed. In particular, Dhawale et al. investigated the effects of casting on ventilation in IS. They reviewed data from 37 serial EDF casts. They found that casting induced transient restrictive pulmonary process: peak inspiratory pressure increased by 106% at cast application. After thoraco-abdominal winds were cut off, peak inspiratory pressure reduced to values close to baseline [1, 2, 14].

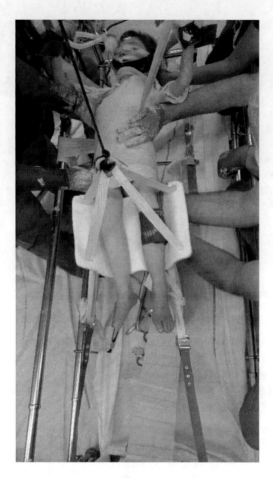

Figure 3. Spinal deformity correction. While the plaster still malleable, one hand pressure in applied on the convexity (apical vertebra) and two-hands counter-pressures is applied on the concavity as close as possible to the end vertebrae, and maintained until plaster hardens.

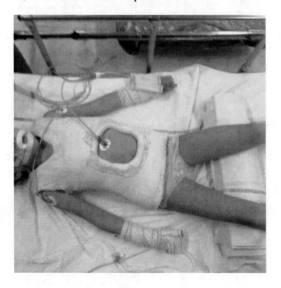

Figure 4. EDF plaster. Final result.

DELAYING TACTIC OR DEFINITIVE TREATMENT OPTION?

Challenging the growing spine means to preserve the thoracic spine, thoracic cage, and lung growth without reducing spinal motion.

The "scoliotic risk" depends upon the amount of remaining growth. The more remaining growth of the spine, the higher is the risk of progression of the deformity. At 5 years of age, the remaining growth of the trunk is about 30 cm; it is about 15 cm at T1–S1, 10 cm at T1-T12, and about 5 cm at L1-L5. These figures must be kept in mind when deciding in early onset scoliosis.

The serial EDF casting technique can be used either as *delaying tactic*, in order to prevent progression of the deformity for several years prior to definitive fusion, or as *definitive treatment* option. Serial EDF casting is an excellent, non-invasive, first line of defense that provides progressive, gentle and permanent correction of infantile and juvenile deformities. Serial EDF casting is a non-surgical option that can be considered in the management of the young and very young child with IS and JS. At what exact point, following EDF casting, should surgery be offered remains, however, a very subjective decision based on the age of the patient, magnitude of the deformity, co-morbidities present and the experience and expertise of the treating surgeon.

The main advantage of EDF casting is that the spine is left alone. Implantation of growth sparing devices, nearby and/or at the level of the spine can affect spinal growth as demonstrated by both experimental and clinical studies [2-4, 6]. Opposite to surgery, serial EDF casting is an alternative, which does not negatively affect spinal growth. Serial EDF casting does not further alter spinal growth and it can be used a "positive" corrective force as it plays an important role in delaying or even eliminating, in some cases, the need for growth sparing surgery. However, serial EDF casting is not effective for all types of IS and JS [1, 2, 11, 16].

The key to successful treatment is to anticipate curve progression, to recognize poor prognosis and apply prophylactic treatment, i.e., serial EDF casting technique. Factors influencing management are many and heterogeneous: age, curve magnitude, respiratory impairment, and pain, loss of function, patients' and/or parents' concerns on appearance due to spine and chest deformity, cardiac function, nutritional and neurological status. Metha reviewed 136 patients treated by a modified version of the EDF-technique introduced by Morel and Cotrel in 1964. Metha reported that patients casted aggressively before age twenty months for curves averaging 30 degrees had their scoliosis non-progressing and/or reducing 10 degrees or less at skeletal maturity; in particular casts were changed under general anesthesia every 8 to 16 weeks. On the other hand, children undergoing cast treatment after age 30 months for curves averaging 50 degrees did not gain significant correction, but their spinal curvature did not progress [1, 2, 11]. Fletcher et al. showed that serial casting is a viable alternative to surgical growth sparing techniques in moderate-to-severe early onset scoliosis and may help delay eventual surgical intervention [1, 2, 14-18]. More recently, van Hessem et al. found that serial casting is also effective for the management of patients with JS. They showed that serial casting can stop curve progression and it can eliminate the need for surgery [1, 2, 16].

THORACIC CAGE DEFORMITY FOLLOWING EDF CASTING TREATMENT

Chest wall and rib deformation commonly occurs if serial EDF casting is performed at ages where the chest is very plastic and easily deformed with drooping of the ribs on the convexity of the scoliosis, where corrective forces are applied.

When EDF cast treatment is completed, the rib cage deformity tend to disappear disappears spontaneously. However, if full-time bracing for a numbers of years follows EDF treatment, chest wall and rib deformation may become permanent and may not completely reverse.

REVIEW OF THE LITERATURE

The ideal treatment of IS and JS has not been identified. Management strategies must take into account the complete life span of the patient, and the effects of treatment on distorted spinal and chest growth must be considered as well. Advancement in growth-friendly surgical procedures are providing orthopedic surgeons multiple treatment options for children with IS and JS. Distraction-based (Vertebral Expandable Prosthetic Titanium Rib, Dual Growing rods) compression-based (vertebral body stapling), and growth-guided techniques (Shilla technique, Luque trolley) can be used to treat infantile and juvenile onset spinal deformities. However, because of the lack of evidence-based research, there is significant variation among surgeons' opinions when treatment options are being considered [1, 2, 19]. No single algorithm for treating EOS has been proposed. Numerous obstacles, including small, heterogeneous patient populations and regulatory challenges in prospectively studying off-label devices, make rigorous clinical research challenging in this area. In part for these reasons, the comparative effectiveness of various treatment strategies is not well elucidated. In most cases, growth-sparing surgery is not an isolated act as it can be peppered with numerous complications. The rate of surgical complications ranges from 8 to 50%; skin problems, wound and anesthetic complications, device migration, fractures, auto fusion, hardware failure, infections, and decompensation have all been reported. In particular, Mackenzie et al. reported that surgical site infection rate in patients with infantile deformities treated with growing constructs increase from 0% at insertion to up-to 29% during lengthening and/or revision procedures [1, 2, 20]. Moreover, repeated hospitalizations for lengthening and for unplanned surgical procedures increase the child's time away from school and can have repercussions on the child's psychological well-being [1, 2, 17, 21].

Despite those findings, there are various articles published during the last few years, which consider growth-sparing surgery as the *gold standard* for the management of severe scoliosis in patients younger than 10 years of age [1, 2, 22].

Serial EDF casting should be considered a valuable low risk treatment modality [1, 2, 6, 7, 15, 23], as well as an alternative to surgery, for patients with IS and JS. Unlike surgery, serial EDF casting is an alternative that does not negatively affect or further alter spinal growth, and it can be used as a "positive" corrective force to guide spinal growth. Serial EDF casting cannot control all types of curves and the technique is not able to completely arrest curve progression and to erase the potential need for surgery in this patient's population. However, it is effective in delaying or even eliminating, in some cases, the need for growth-sparing surgery. In particular, serial EDF casting has been proven to be effective in controlling curve progression in patients with IS and JS. Unfortunately, there is a lack of scientific publications reporting outcomes of serial EDF casting. Presently, less than fifteen works report clinical and radiological outcomes in patients with IS and JS treated by serial casting. On the other hand, more than one hundred publications report surgical outcomes in this patients' population.

Between early 50's and late 60's few works have been published in the English literature. Scott and Morgan reported that resolving curves are not uncommon [24] while Conner demonstrated that early onset deformities associated with developmental anomalies are likely to progress [25]. However, James et al. [26] and Lloyd-Roberts and Pilcher [27] could not identify absolute criteria for distinguishing between resolving and progressive curves [1, 2].

In 1972, Mehta showed that patients casted aggressively before age 20 months for curves averaging 30 degrees had the curve not progressing and/or reducing 10 degrees or less at skeletal maturity. On the other hand, children undergoing cast treatment after age 30 months for curve averaging 50 degrees had the curve stabilized [28]. Ceballos et al. confirmed Mehta's prognostic criteria. After reviewing 113 patients with IS, they concluded the relationship of the rib head and its corresponding vertebral body at the apex of the curve is the most reliable prognostic sign [1, 6, 7, 29].

In a later work, Mehta reviewed 136 children with IS. Although all children were treated the same way, results were not uniform. In 94 children treated before age 2 years the scoliosis resolved. On the other hand, in 42 patients treated after the age of 2 years and 6 months treatment could only reduce but not resolve the deformity. The rate of surgery in this subgroup was 35.7%. Mehta pointed out that avoidance of delay in treatment is of crucial importance [1, 2, 6, 7, 9].

Sanders et al. reviewed 55 patients with progressive infantile scoliosis treated by means of derotational casting. Forty-six out of 55 patients (83%) responded to treatment and, at the time of publication, did not require surgery. Sanders et al. confirmed Mehta's findings [6, 9, 26-30] and reported that initiation of cast correction at a younger age, moderate curve size, and an idiopathic diagnosis carry a better prognosis than an older age of initiation, curve over 60 degrees, and a non-idiopathic diagnosis. They concluded derotational cast correction seems to play a role in the treatment of progressive IS with cures in young patients and reductions in curve size with a delay in surgery in older and syndromic patients [1, 2, 30].

Similarly, Fletcher et al. have retrospectively reviewed a group of 29 patients with IS treated with derotational casting. They reported an average 39 months of delay of surgery and found that, at the time of publication, 21 out of 29 patients (72%) did not require surgery. Although a cure could not be obtained in this cohort of patients, Fletcher et al. concluded that serial casting is a viable alternative to surgical growth sparing techniques in moderate-to-severe early onset scoliosis and may help delay eventual surgical intervention [1, 2, 15].

Baulesh et al. reviewed 36 patients with early onset spinal deformity and reported an average 25 months of delay of surgery and found that, at the time of publication, 25 out of 36 patients (69%) did not require surgery [2, 6, 31]. They showed that serial casting is able to preserve normal longitudinal thoracic growth in patients with early onset scoliosis. Although about one third of patients required surgery, Baulesh et al. concluded that the increased thoracic height may have positive implications on ultimate pulmonary function [1, 2, 6, 7, 31].

More recently, Morin and Kulkarni reported that serial EDF casting for the treatment of progressive idiopathic IS is an effective tool for the Metha's benign-type of curves [1, 2, 11, 25] and spinal fusion can be avoided in about two third of cases [2, 6, 22].

Johnston et al. reviewed 27 patients with IS and JS treated with serial casting. The mean Cobb angle remained stable after a mean duration of treatment of 2.4 years. However, no distinction was made between infantile and juvenile patients, nor were the results of the idiopathic patients described separately from those of the patients with syndromic diagnoses. Despite study limitations, Johnston et al. concluded that cast treatment is a valuable delaying tactic for children with early onset scoliosis as it can adequately control spine deformity, it does not compromise spinal length and it avoids surgical complications associated with early growth sparing surgery [1, 2, 32].

On the other hand, casting and especially bracing has been less successful in JS compared to IS, with reported surgery rates ranging from 27% to 100% after conservative treatment. JS is a rare disease with diversity in clinical presentation. As a consequence, an extremely low number of studies reporting clinical and/or radiological outcomes of patients with JS treated by serial casting are available. Most studies published to date have evaluated the efficacy of rigid brace systems. In particular, studies evaluating the efficacy of rigid brace systems showed a slow loss of correction from the fitting point until the end of the treatment, when the curve is similar to the beginning of the treatment, and this is followed by an aggravation after the weaning point [2, 6, 33-36].

Tolo and Gillespie found 27% of their patients treated with the Milwaukee brace needed surgery [37]. Dabney and Browen found similar results with 33% of surgery recommendations [36]. Coillard et al. using a SpineCor orthosis reported 37% of surgical procedures in patients with JS [38]. Other authors have reported higher percentages of patients who needed surgery despite bracing, ranging from 40% to 100% [1, 2, 6, 7, 39-40].

However, more favorable results have been reported recently by van Hessem et al. and Canavese et al. in patients with JS scoliosis treated by serial casting [12, 34]. Van Hessem et al. reviewed 7 patients with JS treated by casting and/or bracing. They found that casting with patients awake is effective for the management of JS. They reported Cobb's angle was reduced by 32%, decreasing from 37 degrees to 25 degrees. In addition, none of the patients required surgery at a mean follow-up of 4.6 years [1, 7, 14].

More recently, Canavese et al. reviewed a cohort of 44 patients with JS. They reported that serial EDF casting under general anesthesia with neuromuscular-blocking drugs, i.e., curare, is more effective in controlling curve progression in patients with JS, compared to EDF casting under general anesthesia alone or no anesthesia. Canavese et al. hypothesized that complete muscle relaxation allows the surgeon to better derotate the spine while straightening it [2, 6, 39-42]; curve magnitude according to Cobb [40], rib vertebral angle difference according to Mehta [28] and apical vertebral degree according to Nash and Moe improved [43]. Rib vertebral angle difference and apical vertebral degree are expression of vertebral rotation and can be used to better characterize the spinal deformity and/or to evaluate effects of brace or surgical treatment [2, 44].

Demirkiran et al. have recently applied the principles of serial derotational casting to young and very young patients with congenital spine deformities. In particular, they reviewed 11 patients with progressive congenital scoliosis. During treatment period none of the patients developed complication nor required surgery for curve progression. Demirkiran et al. concluded that serial derotational casting is a safe and effective buying strategy to delay the surgical intervention in congenital deformities in the short term follow-up. [1, 6, 45].

There is an obvious lack of scientific publications reporting outcomes of serial EDF casting in patients with IS and JS. Presently, less than fifteen works report clinical and/or radiological outcomes in patients with IS and JS treated by serial casting. On the other hand, more than one hundred publications report surgical outcomes in this patients' population.

EDF casting is a safe technique that can modify the natural evolution of the infantile and juvenile-type scoliosis by reducing and slowing curve progression in both frontal and transverse plane [1, 2, 6].

Table 1. Studies reporting outcome of patients with IS and JS treated with serial casting. Only two studies are available to date reporting outcomes in patients with JS

Author	Infantile Scoliosis (IS) or Juvenile Scoliosis (JS)	Number of patients	Idiopathic/ Non-Idiopathic	Delay in surgery	% of surgery
Scott and Morgan, 1955	IS	28	-	N/A	N/A
James et al., 1959	IS	212	-	N/A	N/A
Lloyd-Roberts and Pilcher, 1965	IS	100	-	N/A	N/A
Conner, 1969	IS	61	-	N/A	N/A
Mehta, 1972	IS	64	64/0	N/A	N/A
Ceballos et al., 1980	IS	113	113/0	3.5 years	N/A
Mehta, 2005	IS	94*/42** (136)	100/36	*11 years **8 years	*0% **35.7%
Sanders et al., 2009	IS	55	41/14	2.1 years	17%
Fletcher et al., 2012	IS	29	12/17	3.3 years	28%
Baulesh et al., 2012	IS	36	19/17	2.1 years	31%
Johnston et al., 2013	IS/JS	27	11/16	20 months	55%
Van Hessem et al., 2014	JS	7	7/0	4.6 years	0%
Canavese et al., 2015	JS	44	36/8	2 years[1-3]	15%[1] 25%[2] 33%[3]
Demirkiran et al., 2015	Congenital Scoliosis°	11	N/A	2.1 years°	0%

*Children treated before age 2 years.
**Children treated after age 2 years and 6 months.
[1-3]Preliminary results, ongoing study; 2 years follow-up; [1]cast under general anesthesia and neuro-muscular blocking drugs; [2]cast under general anesthesia alone; [3]cast with patients awake.
°Preliminary results. Average age of patients at time of cast application was 3 years and 4 months.

REFERENCES

[1] Canavese F, Rousset M, Samba A, et al. Serial elongation, derotation and flexion (EDF) casting in patients with infantile and juvenile scoliosis. *Minerva Pediatrica* 2016; 68(1): 56-65.

[2] Canavese F, Samba A, Dimeglio A, et al. Serial elongation-derotation-flexion casting for children with early-onset scoliosis. *World J Orthop* 2015; 6(11): 935-43.

[3] Kopp SE. Infantile and juvenile idiopathic scoliosis. *Clin Orthop North Am* 1988; 19(2): 331-7.

[4] Canavese F, Dimeglio A, Stebel M, et al. Thoracic Cage Plasticity in prepubertal New Zealand White Rabbits Submitted to T1-T12 Dorsal Arthrodesis: Computed Tomography Evaluation, Echocardiographic Assessment and Cardio-pulmonary Measurements. *Eur Spine J* 2013; 22(5): 1101-12.

[5] Dimeglio A, Bonnel F. *Le rachis en croissance*. [*The growing spine*.] Paris, France: Springer Verlag 1990.

[6] Dimeglio A, Canavese F. The growing spine: how spinal deformities influence normal spine and thoracic cage growth. *Eur Spine J* 2012; 21(1): 64-70.

[7] Canavese F, Dimeglio A, Volpatti D, et al. Dorsal arthrodesis of thoracic spine and effects on thorax growth in prepubertal New Zealand white rabbits. *Spine* 2007; 32: E443-E450.

[8] Karol LA, Johnston CE, Mladenov K, et al. Pulmonary function following early thoracic fusion in non-neuromuscular scoliosis. *J Bone Joint Surg Am* 2008; 90: 1272-1281.

[9] Dimeglio A. Growth of the spine before age 5 years. *J Pediatr Orthop B* 1992; 1: 102-7.

[10] Cotrel Y, Morel G. The elongation-derotation-flexion technique in the correction of scoliosis. *Rev Chir Orthop Reparatrice Appar Mot* 1964; 50: 59-75.

[11] Metha MH. Growth as a corrective force in early treatment of progressive infantile scoliosis. *J Bone Joint Surg Br* 2005 87: 1237-1247.

[12] Pehrsson K, Larsson S, Oden A, et al. Long-term follow-up of patients with untreated scoliosis. A study of mortality causes of death, and symptoms. *Spine* 1992; 17: 1091-6.

[13] Risser JC. The application of body casts for the correction of scoliosis. *Instructional Course Lectures* 1955; 12: 255-9.

[14] Dhawale AA, Shah S, Reichard S, et al. Casting for infantile scoliosis: the pitfall of increased peak inspiratory pressure. *J Pediatr Orthop* 2013; 33: 63-7.

[15] Fletcher ND, McClung A, Rathjen KE, et al. Serial casting as a delaying tactic in the treatment of moderate-to-severe early onset scoliosis. *J Pediatr Orthop* 2012; 32(7): 664-71.

[16] Van Hessem L, Schimmel JJ, Graat HC, et al. Effective nonoperative treatment in juvenile idiopathic scoliosis. *J Pediatr Orthop B* 2014; 23: 454-60.

[17] Lattig F, Taurman L, Hell AK. Treatment of Early Onset Spinal Deformity (EOSD) with VEPTR: A Challenge for the Final Correction Spondylodesis: A Case Series. *J Spinal Disord Tech* 2012 [Epub ahead of print].

[18] Zivkovic V, Buchler P, Ovadia D, et al. Extraspinal ossifications after implantation of vertical expandable prosthetic titanium ribs (VEPTRs). *J Child Orthop* 2014; 8:237–244.

[19] Yang JS, McElroy MJ, Akbarnia BA et al. Growing rods for spinal deformity: characterizing consensus and variation in current use. *J Pediatr Orthop* 2010; 30: 264–270.

[20] Mackenzie WG, Matsumoto H, Williams BA, et al. Surgical site infection following spinal instrumentation for scoliosis. *J Bone Joint Surg Am* 2013; 95 (9): 800-6.

[21] Bess S, Akbarnia BA, Thompson GH et al. Complications of growing rod treatment for early-onset scoliosis: analysis of one hundred and forty patients. *J Bone Joint Surg Am* 2010; 92: 2533-43.

[22] Morin C, Kulkarni S. ED plaster-of-Paris jacket for infantile scoliosis. *Eur Spine J* 2014; 23 (Suppl. 4): S412-8.

[23] Badlani N, Korenblit A, Hammemberg K. Subclavian vein thrombosis after application of body cast. *J Pediatr Orthop* 2013; 33: e1-e3.

[24] Scott JL, Morgan TH. The natural history and prognosis of infantile idiopathic scoliosis. *J Bone Joint Surg Br* 1955; 37: 400-13.

[25] Conner AN. Developmental anomalies and prognosis in infantile idiopathic scoliosis. *J Bone Joint Surg Br* 1969; 51: 711.

[26] James JIP, Lloyd-Roberts GC, Pilcher MF. Infantile structural scoliosis. *J Bone Joint Surg Br* 1959; 41: 719.

[27] Lloyd-Roberts GC, Pilcher MF. Structural idiopathic scoliosis in infancy. *J Bone Joint Surg Br* 1955; 47: 520.

[28] Mehta MH. The rib-vertebral angle in the early diagnosis between resolving and progressive infantile scoliosis. *J Bone Joint Surg Br* 1972; 54: 230-43.

[29] Ceballos T, Ferrer-Torrelles M, Castillo F, et al. Prognosis in infantile idiopathic scoliosis. *J Bone Joint Surg Am* 1980; 62: 863-75.

[30] Sanders JO, D'Astous J, Fitgerald M, et al. Derotational casting for progressive infantile scoliosis. *J Pediatr Orthop* 2009; 29(6): 581-7.

[31] Baulesh DM, Huh J, Judkins T, et al. The role of serial casting in early-onset scoliosis (EOS). *J Pediatr Orthop* 2012; 32(7): 658-63.

[32] Johnston CE, McClung AM, Thompson GH, Poe-Kochert C, Sanders JO. Comparison of growing rod instrumentation versus serial cast treatment of early-onset scoliosis. *Spine Deform* 2013; 1:339-42.

[33] Grivas TB, Kaspiris A. European braces widely used for conservative scoliosis treatment. *Stud Health Technol Inform* 2010; 158: 157-66.

[34] Lonstein JE, Winter RB. The Milwaukee brace for the treatment of adolescent idiopathic scoliosis. A review of one thousand and twenty patients. *J Bone Joint Surg Am* 1994; 76: 1207-21.

[35] Gabos PG, Bojescul JA, Bowen JR, et al. Long-term follow-up of female patients with idiopathic scoliosis treated with the Wilmington orthosis. *J Bone Joint Surg Am* 2004; 86: 1891-9.

[36] Dabney KW, Browen JR. Juvenile idiopathic scoliosis. *Semin Spine Surg* 1991; 3: 524-30.

[37] Tolo VT, Gillespie R. The characteristics of juvenile idiopathic scoliosis and results of treatment. *J Bone Joint Surg Br* 1978; 60: 181-188.

[38] Coillard C, Leroux MA, Zabjek KF, et al. SpineCor non-rigid brace for the treatment of idiopathic scoliosis: post-treatment results. *Eur Spine J* 2003; 12: 141-8.

[39] Robinson CM, McMaster MJ. Juvenile idiopathic scoliosis. Curve patterns and prognosis in one hundred and nine patients. *J Bone Joint Surg Am* 1996; 78(8): 1140-8.

[40] Kahanovitz N, Levine DB, Lardone J. The part-time Milwaukee brace treatment of juvenile idiopathic scoliosis. Long-term follow-up. *Clin Orthop Rel Res* 1982; 167: 145-51.

[41] Canavese F, Botnari A, Dimeglio A, et al. Serial elongation, derotation and flexion (EDF) casting under general anesthesia and neuromuscular blocking drugs improve outcome in patients with juvenile scoliosis: preliminary results. *Eur Spine J* 2016; 25(2): 487-94.

[42] Cobb JR. Outline for the study of scoliosis. *Instructional Course Lectures* 5: 261-75.

[43] Nash CL Jr, Moe JH. A study of vertebral rotation. *J Bone Joint Surg Am* 1969; 51: 223-9.

[44] Canavese F, Holveck J, De Coulon G, et al. Analysis of concave and convex rib-vertebral angle, angle difference and angle ratio in patients with Lenke type I main thoracic adolescent idiopathic scoliosis treated by observation, bracing or posterior fusion and instrumentation. *J Spinal Dis Techniques* 2011; 24: 506-13.

[45] Demirkiran HG, Beccmez S, Celilov R, et al. Serial derotational casting in congenital scoliosis as a time buying strategy. *J Pedaitr Orthop* 2015; 35: 43-9.

Chapter 6

HALO TRACTION: WHEN AND HOW?

Zhaomin Zheng
Department of Spine Surgery, Sun Yat-Sen University, Guangzhou, China

ABSTRACT

Despite great technical improvement and modern instrumentation, surgical treatment of severe spinal deformity remains a challenge. Halo traction has been used as an adjunctive method in surgical treatment of severe and rigid spinal deformity. In this chapter, the indication, techniques, clinical effects and complication of Halo traction will be introduced.

Keywords: spinal deformity, halo traction, preoperative correction, complication

INTRODUCTION

Traction is one of the oldest methods for correction of spinal deformity. As early as 1876, Sayre described gravity-assisted traction before corrective casting for scoliosis correction. In the 1950s, Harrington invented the Harrington rod to obtain and maintain correction as an internal traction system. In 1959, Nickel and Perry developed the halo device to stabilize the head and cervical spine for cervical spinal fusion. In 1960, Cotrel introduced the concept of dynamic traction to treat adolescent idiopathic scoliosis and loosen up rigid curves before surgery. In 1967, Kane devised halo-femoral traction and in 1969 Stagnara for the first time introduced halo-gravity traction for the correction of scoliosis. Different types of traction have been used for most types of spinal deformity and gained positive clinical effects on peraoperative care and deformity correction [1]. In the modern concept, halo-gravity, halo-femoral and halo-pelvis traction are the most frequently used tranction systems.

APPLICATION TECHNIQUES

Halo-Gravity Traction

Halo-gravity traction can be used in all sorts of spinal deformity without contraindication. In children younger than 2 years of age, because of their thin calvarium, 10 to 12 pins should be used, and the torque should not exceed 2 inch-pounds or finger tightness [2]. Multiple pins (4-6 pins) should be used in older patient, and 6 to 8 inch-pounds of torque are applied. The pins are placed under general anesthesia if the child's overall condition allows. Two pins are placed anterolateral, in the lateral third of the eyebrow region, just above the brow. We placed 2 more posterolateral pins just behind the upper, outer region of the earlobe. The appropriate amount of torque was used to insert the pins. Traction is usually started immediately with a low amount of weight with either 3 to 5 pounds. Traction is gradually increased at a rate of 2 to 3 pounds per day as tolerated. The goal is to reach a maximum traction of 33% to 50% of body weight depending on how well it is tolerated. Traction is applied for a minimum of 12 hours per day, with the weight lessened by 50% to 75% when the patient is sleeping to avoid proximal migration in bed at nighttime. Traction is applied while in bed, a wheelchair, or standing apparatus. Neurologic checks are performed once every 8-hour shift. Daily cranial nerve and upper/lower extremity neurologic examinations are performed [3].

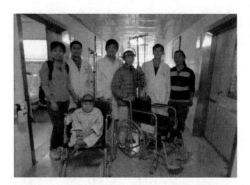

Figure 1. Patients during halo traction treatment.

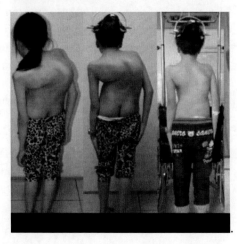

Figure 2. Halo traction: outcome.

Halo-Femoral Traction

Halo-femoral traction is mostly used as intraoperative traction for maintanace of the trunk balane and preoperative correction effect. Halo application was as described above. For femoral traction, a 0.32-mm K-wire was placed in the corresponding distal femur, from medial to lateral, avoiding the posteriorly located neurovascular bundle, for femoral traction on the elevated pelvis side. The patient was then positioned prone, with an average of 15 lbs placed on the halo, increasing femoral traction to an average of 25 lbs (range 15 – 40) until the pelvic obliquity was leveled.

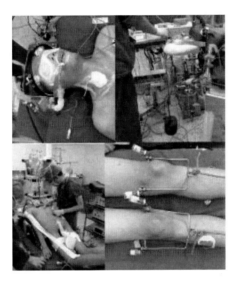

Figure 3. Halo-femoral traction.

Halo-Pelvis Traction

The device is consisted of a halo ring, a pelvic ring, pins to fix them in the cranial and iliac bone and correcting rods to align the two rings and distract the spine The halo-pelvic ring was placed under regional anesthesia. Pins in the cranial bone were placed with the same method as a halo ring. Two pins on the pelvic ring were inserted in the iliac crest and 2 in the posterior superior iliac spine. The correcting rods were used to connect the halo and pelvic rings, and were adjusted 3 to 5mm a day to distract the spine between the 2 rings. Daily cranial nerve and upper/lower extremity neurologic examinations are performed.

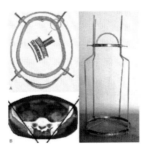

Figure 4. Halo-pelvis.

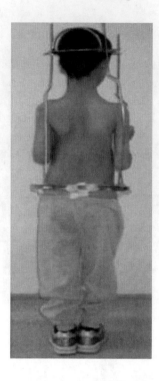

Figure 5. Patient with halo-pelvis.

Contraindications

Relative contraindications include short sharp rigid kyphosis, C-spine abnormalities or instability because of their obvious neurologic implications, cranial defects or thin skull, and age younger than 18 months because of pin penetration problems. Traction should be cautisouly applied when patients with spinal cord abnormaltiy and started with minimum weight.

Clinical Outcomes

Despite great technical improvement and modern instrumentation, surgical treatment of severe spinal deformity remains a challenge.

Halo-gravity traction had been used as an adjunctive method in surgical treatment of severe and rigid spinal deformity. In a meta-analysis about halo-gravity traction for deformity correction, it reported that with the help of halo-gravity traction, the correction rate after final spinal fusion was 51.1% in the coronal plane and 30.4% in the sagittal plane. Correction due to traction was 24.1% in the coronal plane and 19.3% in the sagittal plane, indicating that with halo-gravity traction partial correction can be achieved preoperatively. First of all, it can help improve preoperative pulmonary function and better tolerance for the aggressive procedure could be expected subsequently [4, 5]. Second, less correction is needed during surgery, and therefore, aggressive procedures such as vertebral column resection may be avoided [6]. Risk of massive blood loss and neurologic compromise might also decrease subsequently [7, 8]. The gradual traction preoperatively might also help evaluate the neurologic function and estimate the amount of correction that can safely reached. More important, there was also evidence that the preoperative curve correction may help improve neurologic function [4]. These factors, in turn, may contribute to reduction of risk of neurologic injury.

The issue of optimal duration of halo-gravity traction is currently with no gold standard. The duration of halo-gravity traction varied from 2 to 12 weeks in most studies and the maximum was 107 days. Watanabe et al. [9] noted 63.6% of preoperative correction within 1 week, 84.7% within 3 weeks. Park et al. [10] found that 66% of the preoperative correction occurred within 2 weeks, 88% within 3 weeks and 96% within 4 weeks. Nemani et al. [11] noted that the correction plateaued after approximately 2 months after rapid initial correction. Thus, in terms of curve correction, it is reasonable to think that the duration of traction should not exceed 2 months. As for pulmonary function, Koller et al. [4] showed that prolonged traction might not further improve the pulmonary function. However, no studies referred to the effect of traction on the general health (e.g., nutritional status). Thus, the existing evidence was not enough to provide information for the optimal duration of traction. Further studies should explore this important issue.

Halo-femoral traction is mostly used as intraoperative traction for maintanace of the trunk balane and preoperative correction effect. Qiu et al. reported that with intraoperative halo-femoral traction, both idiopathic and congenital scoliosis could achieve better correction rate and less complication rate after a anterior release procedure [12]. Keeler et al. more recently reported that when intraoperative halo-femoral traction is used, PSF-only surgery for Neuromuscular Scoliosis can provide excellent curve correction and spinal balance. In this study, the PSF-only group had shorter OR time, lower EBL, lower frequency of postoperative intubation, and fewer cases of pneumonias when compared with A/PSF with similar radiographic outcomes at 2-year follow-up [13].

The Halo-pelvic ring traction had been applied in the presurgical treatment of various spinal deformities since the 1970s, and some authors reported satisfactory results from those applications [14, 15]. However, there are few reports on halo-pelvic traction since the beginning of the 21st century. It is possibly because of the reluctance of patients to receive long periods of external fixation due to its inconvenience and unflattering appearance [16]. A recent study reported that halo-pelvic traction group achieved significantly better results than direct surgical treatment group by means of the time of surgery, intraoperative blood loss, correction of Cobb angle, change in patient height (9.4 ± 4.0cm vs 6.8 ± 3.8cm, $P = .024$) [17].

Complications

Traction-related complications were common. The most common was pin-related complications, such as pin loosening necessitating exchange or replacement of halo ring, superficial pin-site infection needing oral antibiotics, cleaning the pin site, or debridement. Other complications included cervical pain or discomfort, nystagmus, dizziness, and nausea, which could usually be relieved by decreasing the weight of traction. Traction-related complications were common and the prevalence was 22%. Although these complications were usually not severe, it should be noted that there were three neurologic complications related to traction were recorded. Janus et al. [18] observed that one patients with halo-gravity traction developed hyperreflexia of the legs, which disappeared after reducing the traction weight. Sink et al. [19] reported a case of cervical distraction, presenting as numbness in the roof of the patient's mouth, and the traction had to be discontinued. Bouchoucha et al. [20] found a patient with neurological deficit that existed before traction developed a spastic paraplegia while in halo-gravity traction. However, for the light weight in halo-gravity traction, complications were much less and minor than in halo-pelvic traction or halo-femoral traction. Wilkins et al. demonstrated six patients suffering cranial nerve complications in 70 patients with skeletal traction [21]. Tredwell et al. noted the incidence of apophyseal joint degeneration to be 47.4% in patients with halo-pelvic distraction [22]. Osteoporosis was also noted in patients treated with halo-pelvic or halo-pelvic traction by several authors due to prolonged immobilization, and as much as 76% of patients would sustain fracture due to osteoporosis after traction [23, 24]. In contrast, there was no need of immobilization for patients with halo-gravity traction and osteoporosis could be well evaded. Another advantage of halo-gravity was that it allowed patients to sit or walk freely while traction, making it easy for daily care. It also enabled patients to decrease the weight of traction themselves when they felt discomfort.

REFERENCES

[1] D'Astous, J. L. & Sanders, J. O. (2007). Casting and traction treatment methods for scoliosis. *Orthop Clin North Am*, *38*(4), 477-84, v.

[2] Caubet, J. F. & Emans, J. B. (2011). Halo-gravity traction versus surgical release before implantation of expandable spinal devices: a comparison of results and complications in early-onset spinal deformity. *J Spinal Disord Tech*, *24*(2), 99-104.

[3] Rinella, A., Lenke, L., Whitaker, C., et al. (2005). Perioperative halo-gravity traction in the treatment of severe scoliosis and kyphosis. *Spine* (Phila Pa 1976), *30*(4), 475-82.

[4] Koller, H., Zenner, J., Gajic, V., et al. (2012). The impact of halo-gravity traction on curve rigidity and pulmonary function in the treatment of severe and rigid scoliosis and kyphoscoliosis: a clinical study and narrative review of the literature. *Eur Spine J*, *21*(3), 514-29.

[5] Garabekyan, T., Hosseinzadeh, P., Iwinski, H. J., et al. (2014). The results of preoperative halo-gravity traction in children with severe spinal deformity. *J Pediatr Orthop B*, *23*(1), 1-5.

[6] Sponseller, P. D., Takenaga, R. K., Newton, P., et al. (2008). The use of traction in the treatment of severe spinal deformity. *Spine* (Phila Pa 1976), *33*(21), 2305-9.

[7] Liu, H., Yang, C., Zheng, Z., et al. (2015). Comparison of Smith-Petersen osteotomy and pedicle subtraction osteotomy for the correction of thoracolumbar kyphotic deformity in ankylosing spondylitis: a systematic review and meta-analysis. *Spine*, *40*(8), 570-579.

[8] Yang, C., Zheng, Z., Liu, H., et al. (2016). Posterior vertebral column resection in spinal deformity: a systematic review. *Eur Spine J*, *25*(8), 2368-75.

[9] Watanabe, K., Lenke, L. G., Bridwell, K. H., et al. (2010). Efficacy of perioperative halo-gravity traction for treatment of severe scoliosis (>/= 100 degrees). *J Orthop Sci*, *15*(6), 720-30.

[10] Park, D. K., Braaksma, B., Hammerberg, K. W., et al. (2013). The efficacy of preoperative halo-gravity traction in pediatric spinal deformity the effect of traction duration. *J Spinal Disord Tech*, *26*(3), 146-54.

[11] Nemani, V. M., Kim, H. J., Bjerke-Kroll, B. T., et al. (2015). Preoperative halo-gravity traction for severe spinal deformities at an SRS-GOP site in West Africa: protocols, complications, and results. *Spine* (Phila Pa 1976), *40*(3), 153-61.

[12] Qiu, Y., Liu, Z., Zhu, F., et al. (2007). Comparison of effectiveness of Halo-femoral traction after anterior spinal release in severe idiopathic and congenital scoliosis: a retrospective study. *J Orthop Surg Res*, *2*, 23.

[13] Keeler, K. A., Lenke, L. G., Good, C. R., et al. (2010). Spinal fusion for spastic neuromuscular scoliosis: is anterior releasing necessary when intraoperative halo-femoral traction is used? *Spine* (Phila Pa 1976), *35*(10), E427-33.

[14] Bumpass, D. B., Lenke, L. G., Bridwell, K. H., et al. (2014). Pulmonary function improvement after vertebral column resection for severe spinal deformity. *Spine* (Phila Pa 1976), *39*(7), 587-95.

[15] Sucato, D. J. (2010). Management of severe spinal deformity: scoliosis and kyphosis. *Spine* (Phila Pa 1976), *35*(25), 2186-92.

[16] Dove, J., Hsu, L. C. & Yau, A. C. (1980). The cervical spine after halo-pelvic traction. An analysis of the complications of 83 patients. *J Bone Joint Surg Br*, *62-b*(2), 158-61.

[17] Muheremu, A., Ma, Y., Ma, Y., et al. (2017). Halo-pelvic traction for severe kyphotic deformity secondary to spinal tuberculosis. *Medicine (Baltimore)*, *96*(28), e7491.

[18] Janus, G. J., Finidori, G., Engelbert, R. H., et al. (2000). Operative treatment of severe scoliosis in osteogenesis imperfecta: results of 20 patients after halo traction and posterior spondylodesis with instrumentation. *Eur Spine J*, *9*(6), 486-91.

[19] Sink, E. L., Karol, L. A., Sanders, J., et al. (2001). Efficacy of perioperative halo-gravity traction in the treatment of severe scoliosis in children. *J Pediatr Orthop*, *21*(4), 519-24.

[20] Bouchoucha, S., Khelifi, A., Saied, W., et al. (2011). Progressive correction of severe spinal deformities with halo-gravity traction. *Acta Orthop Belg*, *77*(4), 529-34.

[21] Wilkins, C. & MacEwen, G. D. (1977). Cranial nerve injury from halo traction. *Clin Orthop Relat Res*, (126), 106-10.

[22] Tredwell, S. J. & O'Brien, J. P. (1980). Apophyseal joint degeneration in the cervical spine following halo-pelvic distraction. *Spine* (Phila Pa 1976), *5*(6), 497-501.

[23] Abu Salim, F. & Zielke, K. (1982). Osteoporosis and halo traction in scoliosis patients (author's transl). *Z Orthop Ihre Grenzgeb*, *120*(3), 330-2.

[24] Korovessis, P., Konstantinou, D., Piperos, G., et al. (1994). Spinal bone mineral density changes following halo vest immobilization for cervical trauma. *Eur Spine J*, *3*(4), 206-8.

Chapter 7

EOS AND SURGERY: TECHNIQUES, INDICATIONS AND LIMITATIONS

*Ashok N. Johari**
Children's Orthopaedic Centre, Mumbai, India

ABSTRACT

Background: Early onset scoliosis (EOS) is a challenging group of disorders, the management of which has witnessed a sea of change in the last decade. Recent developments have worked to improve the treatment of children with EOS. This chapter provides the reader with a brief description of the surgical/therapeutic modalities, their indications for use, and clinical results. Current treatment philosophy has been reviewed through recent publications related to the surgical treatment of EOS. Indications for the use of different modalities as also their limitations are discussed. Complication rates for all surgical techniques for treatment of EOS remain high because of the chronic and repetitive nature of lengthening surgeries, the implant bulk, and the stresses placed on any instrumentation in a mobile spine. Surgical decisions are subjective and not reproducible because of the heterogeneity of patients, varying ages and magnitudes of the deformity and short follow-up for surgical interventions. Younger children, neuromuscular and syndromic children, and higher curve magnitude appear to be associated with higher complication rates. Dual growing rods seem to have better initial correction, maintenance of correction, increased T1-S1 length gain, and decreased implant-related problems such as rod breakage and hook. Newer hybrid fixation techniques have developed in the recent years for growth sparing reporting greater success.

Keywords: early onset scoliosis, surgery, growth, infantile deformity, complications

---

* Corresponding Author Email: drashokjohari@hotmail.com (Ashok N. Johari, Consultant)

EARLY ONSET SCOLIOSIS - A BRIEF INTRODUCTION

The Scoliosis Research Society defines Early Onset Scoliosis as "Scoliosis with onset less than the age of 10 years, regardless of aetiology." Because of the challenge of maintaining the remaining growth of the spine and because of the potential for progressive increase of the deformity, these group of patients have different treatment methodologies with the common goal of maintaining the spine as anatomically intact as possible and allowing it to reach its full potential for growth.

All distortions secondary to altered spinal growth viz underdeveloped thoracic cage, short trunk and height, disproportionate body habitus, low weight, respiratory and cardiac dysfunctions demand attention [1, 2]. Tachypnea, dyspnea, chronic obstructive pulmonary disease, tracheomalacia, tachycardia and weight loss often prove more worrisome than the deformity of the spine itself. Spinal deformities associated with rib cage anomalies requiring fusion have highest risk of developing restrictive pulmonary disease. Recognizing the importance of pulmonary function, a few developmental principles should be understood. Bronchial tree and alveolar complement are maximally developed by 8 years of age, and the thoracic volume at 10 years of age is 50% of expected adult volume [3]. This has led to a paradigm shift from fusion surgeries to non-fusion/growth friendly surgeries and emergence of numerous growth-friendly surgical options that allow growth of spine and at the same time control curve progression. These fusionless surgeries are not free of complications. Flynn et al. [4] in his growing rod graduates found <50% patient achieved additional corrections, 81% had some areas of auto-fusion, stiff spine, or a completely fused spine.

Surgery – Indications

Surgical indications are not difficult to define:

1. Progressive deformity not amenable to conservative control
2. Unacceptable deformity, increasing decompensation
3. Rarely, neurological deterioration

The surgeons' experience and expertise, patient's age, etiological factors, comorbidities etc. may all influence decision making for surgery. In general, a worsening deformity associated with increasing cardiorespiratory deterioration may signal the need for surgical intervention. Idiopathic, syndromic and neuromuscular scoliosis are best treated with growth rod techniques. At what exact point should surgery be offered remains a subjective decision based on the age of the patient, magnitude of the deformity, co-morbidities present and the experience and expertise of the treating surgeon.

Contra-Indications

Children below the age of 3 years and within the lower percentiles for weight should be managed with other alternative modalities as the risk of implant related complications is high.

Untreated spinal dysraphism is a contraindication to any form of distraction treatment. A tethered low lying cord, syringomyelia, fatty filum terminale, Arnold Chiari malformation, split cord malformation [5] etc. may need neurosurgical intervention prior to the scoliosis treatment as distraction can lead to neurological deterioration.

Syndromic children with significant medical co-morbidities may not be suitable candidates for repeated procedures. A thorough evaluation for other systemic co-morbidities must be conducted prior to starting treatment. Short angular curves of a congenital or neurofibromatosis aetiology are best treated with an early definitive fusion and correction of deformity if necessary.

Surgical Techniques in EOS: Author's Experience

A number of surgical techniques form the repertoire in managing EOS. Historically, the Harrington distraction rod was used as a growth rod. With better understanding of spinal deformities the sagittal contour was recognized but the major problem of derotation of the spine still remains unresolved for early onset scoliosis. The single growing rod evolved into double rods. The inconvenience of repeat distractions led to the design of the magnetic expansion rods which are now in use. The Shilla technique [6] involves apical fusion and proximal and distal elongation of the spine by the design of the screw rod interface.

Newer techniques involved extraspinal distraction with use of VEPTR (vertical expandable prosthetic titanium rib) [7] and related devices developed for thoracic expansion and indirect correction of the spine. Hybrid versions fix to the spine and rib cage. Growth modulation and stapling devices [8] are also being used for well selected cases.

The authors experience is largely with growth rods and hence their use is detailed below with a brief description of the other devices.

GROWTH RODS

Growth rods are ideally suited for long curves of a moderate magnitude of around 50 degrees. Predominantly kyphotic deformities do not respond well to GR treatment as posterior distraction is kyphogenic and the incidence of implant related complications increase.

Growth rods allow for placement of the implant at the ends of the curve and serial expansion (Figure 1). Because of the fear of auto fusion, the spine is not exposed and the rods are tunneled in the submuscular/subcutaneous planes. Serial expansions are carried out at a frequency mutually agreeable to the patient and the surgeon. Ideally 2 expansions are recommended annually but these involve repeat hospitalizations and surgery though the surgery is not major.

The largest clinical series involving dual growing rods was published by Akbarnia et al. [9] in 2005. The mean curve magnitude improved from 82 degrees pre-operatively to 38 degrees after the first surgery and 36 degrees at final follow-up. Patients were lengthened a mean of 6.6 times for a mean T1-S1 length increase of 1.2 cm/y and an increase in lung space ratio from 0.87 to 1. There were a total of 13 complications (56%) in 11 patients. Another, more recent series, showed a slightly better curve correction and more length gained when lengthenings were performed at intervals of 6 months [10]. Paloski et al. [11] studied the timing of distraction using the multicenter Growing Spine Study Group (GSSG) cohort of 46 patients with 16 patients who had lengthening at less than 9 months intervals and 30 patients who had lengthening at more than 9 months intervals. There were no significant differences in the Cobb angle, T1-S1 height and instrumented segment length gain at last distraction or final fusion.

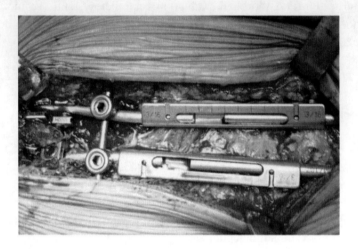

Figure 1. Growth rods.

Complications are frequent and related to the prolonged treatment required of distraction-based techniques. A comprehensive analysis of complications from single and dual rod constructs reports 58% of the 140 patients evaluated had at least 1 complication [12]. The complication rate increased by 24% for each additional procedure performed, and complication rate decreased by 13% for each year of increased patient age at treatment initiation. There were less instrumentation complications in dual as opposed to single rods, and patients with subcutaneous rods had more wound complications, prominent implants, and unplanned procedures than those with submuscular rods. Wound complications are more common when lengthenings were performed at more frequent intervals, whereas implant-related complications occur more often when lengthenings were performed at longer intervals [13].

Regarding neurological safety, the insertion and lengthening of both single and dual growing rods appears to be extremely safe with an overall incidence [13] of neuromonitoring changes of 0.9%, and only 1 reported clinically detectable transient neurological deficit (0.1%) in a patient with a known intradural tumor.

Sankar et al. [12], reported a "Law of Diminishing Returns" for repeated lengthenings of growing rods. Their study on 38 patients, noted the mean T1-S1 length gain from the first lengthening was 1.04 cm and progressively less with subsequent procedures. This is important in deciding the right age when lengthening should be initiated as the maximum T1-S1 length gain will be achieved in the first one or two years. Optimizing the timing of the initial procedure is important for length gain and deformity correction.

His study also mentions that fusion of the upper thorax, as is performed for the upper anchors of growing rods, has been shown to adversely affect pulmonary function. Hybrid systems utilizing standard hooks avoid this fusion by using ribs as the upper anchor. He also showed that in similar patient populations, the hybrid instrumentation had a complication rate of 0.86/patient, the dual growing rods 2.3/patient, and the VEPTR 2.37/patient.

Skaggs et al. [14] in their multi-center study have shown bilateral hybrid growing rods produce on average 1.2 cm/y of T1-S1 growth which is comparable with that found with dual growing rods and superior to that of VEPTR.

Suken et al. [15] showed that growth rods had a positive effect on sagittal vertical axis, which returned patients to a more neutral alignment through the course of treatment.

Growth rod management of a case of idiopathic scoliosis in a 10 year old is presented. (Figures 2 – 5b.)

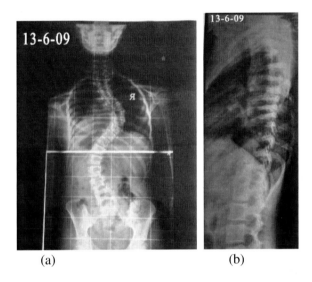

Figure 2. Anterior-posterior (a) and lateral (b) preoperative radiographs.

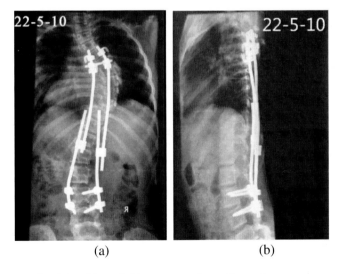

Figure 3. Anterior-posterior (a) and lateral (b) postoperative radiographs.

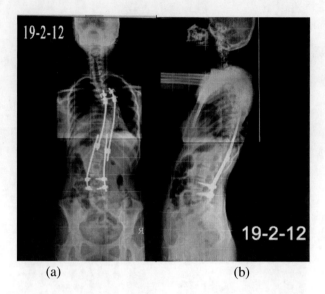

Figure 4. Anterior-posterior (a) and lateral radiographs following 4th distraction.

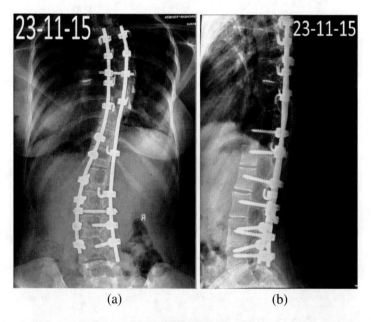

Figure 5. Anterior-posterior (a) and lateral (b) radiographs following posterior instrumented fusion. Conversion to the final posterior instrumented fusion was done 5 years after the index procedure.

SHILLA

In the Shilla procedure, multi-planar correction is obtained by pedicle fixation at the apex of the deformity. This usually involves instrumentation and fusion of 3 to 4 segments. Four to 6 gliding pedicle screws are then placed at each end of the construct. The rods are left long at the ends to allow the sliding screws to move along the rods with spinal growth. Normal sagittal contours are maintained and the anchor screw slide cranially and caudally on the dual rods as the patient grows. With correction and stabilization of the most deformed apical segment there is theoretically less stress on the end anchor points. The patients are placed in a thoracic-lumbar spinal orthosis for 3 months after the surgery.

A retrospective study [6] of the original forty patients treated with the Shilla method for a severe deformity of a growing spine was performed to determine the efficacy of the procedure. Average age at the index surgery was six years and eleven months, and the average duration of follow-up for the thirty-three eligible patients was seven years. The curves averaged 69° (range, 40° to 115°) preoperatively and 38.4° (range, 16° to 74°) at the time of the most recent follow-up or prior to definitive spinal instrumentation and fusion. Complications included secondary infections (six patients), alignment issues (eight patients), and implant-related problems (twenty-four patients), with some patients experiencing more than one complication.

Andras et al. [16] in a retrospective multicenter case matched comparison of 36 patients treated with dual GRs versus 36 patients treated with the Shilla procedure reported better improvement in coronal Cobb angle correction (36° versus 23°) and T1-S1 length gain (8.8 cm versus 6.4 cm) at 4.3 years follow-up in patients that underwent treatment with traditional GRs. The complication rates were similar between the two groups. Although the Shilla patients had fewer surgeries than GR patients, the unplanned revision rates for implant complications were higher in the Shilla group with no significant differences between the groups for number of procedures for implant complications.

MAGNETIC GROWTH RODS

The very first report of a magnetic rod is from 2004 when Jean Dubousset and Arnaud developed and used the Phoenix device. The first multicenter study of 33 patients by Akbarnia et al. [17] documented results in 14 cases of EOS (idiopathic, neuromuscular, congenital and neurofibromatosis) treated with MAGEC rod instrumentation (Figure 6). The mean age was 8 year and 10 mo. They compared the results of single *vs* dual rods. The mean improvement in Cobb angles was 46% and 48% respectively in single and dual rods respectively. There was no significant difference in both groups in the average T1-T12 growth but the difference was significant in T1-S1 growth. Partial loss of distraction was the most common complication after 11 of 68 distractions (2 in dual and 9 in single rods). The loss was regained and maintained in subsequent distractions. No other implant related complications were noted. In none of the cases proximal junctional kyphosis was seen [17].

Dannawi et al. [10] reported on 34 children (mean age 8 years) of EOS with mean Cobb's angle of 69 degrees. At mean follow up of 15 months both groups single and dual rods had a statistically significant improvement in mean pre-operative, immediate postoperative and final Cobb angles and also significant increase in the mean T1-S1 distance. No patient developed a post-operative fusion. The complications met were: superficial infection and rod breakage in 2 (one in each group), loss of distraction in 2 patients with single rod (rectified subsequently) and hook pull out in one patient with dual rod. Trimming of rod was done in one with hardware prominence. Overall complications were fewer as compared to conventional growth rods.

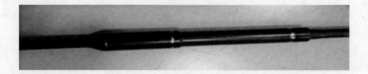

Figure 6. Magnetic growth rod.

A linear decline in the length gained is also seen after serial distractions with MCGR [23]. In older children reduced distraction ratio is observed in the concave rod. Gilday et al. have shown that the observed increase in rod length was lower than programmed and the lengthening was inversely proportional to tissue depth, so that deeper the rod is placed, lesser is the distraction achieved [19].

Keskinen et al. (20) compared the efficacy of using MdGR in primary versus conversion from previously operated TGR and found that scoliosis can be equally controlled after conversion from TGR to MdGR, but the growth from baseline is less in conversion group.

Teoh et al. [21] with a long follow up study could get a 43% correction of scoliosis in primary cases whereas it was only 2% in the conversion case, but the curves were maintained till the last follow up. They reported 75% (6/8) patients required revision surgeries, 4 of which were for rod problems and one for proximal junctional kyphosis.

Choi et al. [22] in a retrospective multi-centric study of MCGR proposed a classification of complications related to the procedure. Of the 115 operated patients, 54 had a minimum 1-year follow-up and were analyzed. They classified complications as wound/implant related and early (< 6 months) or late > 6 months. Implant related: (1) rod breakage; (2) failure of lengthening requiring revision surgery; and (3) anchor pull outs. Wound related complications: Surgical site infection (deep) requiring additional surgical intervention.

They summarized complications as: (1) 42% had at-least 1 complication; (2) 15% revision surgery, at least one; (3) 11% rod breakage (33% early, 66% late); (4) 11% (6 pts.) failure of lengthening, 4 distracted in subsequent visits, 2 rods were exchanged; (5) 13% anchor point problems; and (6) 3.7% (2 pts.) deep infection, one each early (drainage and antibiotic) and late (rod penetration, requiring removal of one of the dual rods).

Another concern with the Magnet driven rods is the cost as they are expensive. Recent evidence however points out the cost effectiveness of these devices and the relative psychological advantage of avoidance of repeat surgeries. Charroin et al. [23] compared the expenses in TGR *vs* MCGR over a period of 4 years based on a simulation model using assumptions obtained from literature search or their local experience. They found that MCGR procedure induces a strong expense at start, then costs evolve gradually because of the difference of TGR strategy. Despite its major unit cost, their results show that the use of MCGR could lead to lower direct costs with a time horizon of 4 years. Also improvement of quality of life could be indirectly evaluated considering that about 2 surgeries and hospital stays per patient-year could be avoided using MCGR. The limitations of the study included: (1) the basis of estimation of costs, i.e., a simulation model; (2) not taking into account outpatient direct costs and indirect costs such as parent's time off work; and (3) assumptions of long term results of MCGR based on the short term, few published series. Jenks et al. [24] found equal efficacy of both but the added advantage of MAGEC being a robust cost saving at the end of 6 years. Thus NICE issued a positive recommendation for the use of MAGEC for EOS. Similar recommendations were made by Rolton et al. [25] and Armoiry et al. [26], with a significant cost saving at the end of 5 years.

Indian Experience

The author (ANJ) has reported the results of MCGRs in 10 patients largely with congenital scoliosis, with a mean age at surgery of 10.6 years (8-13 years) and a mean pre-operative Cobb angle of 83°. Distraction was performed at 3 monthly intervals. At a mean 14.3 months follow-up (Range: 7 to 21 months), the Cobb angle was reported to be 65° (mean correction 21.62%). An average of 3.4 distractions were performed per patient with 73.25% distraction achieved in-situ [27]. There were no significant complications. A case example from this series is presented (Figures 7a – 10b).

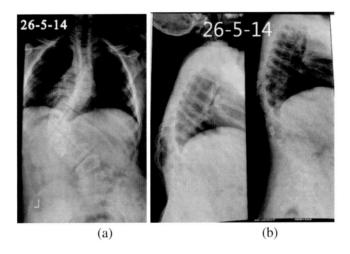

Figure 7. Anterio-posterior (a) and lateral (b) preoperative radiographs.

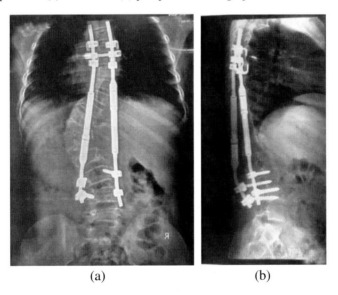

Figure 8. Anterior-posterior (a) and lateral (b) postoperative radiographs following magnetic growth rod insertion (26-11-2014).

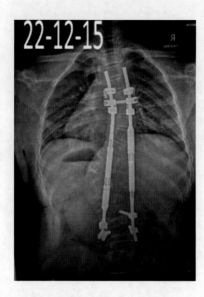

Figure 9. Anterior-posterior (a) and lateral (b) radiographs following magnetic growth rod insertion.

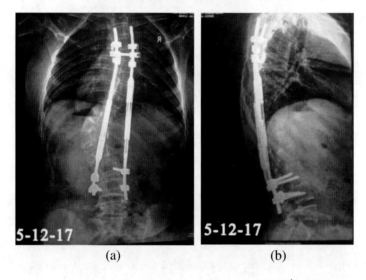

(a) (b)

Figure 10. Anterior-posterior (a) and lateral (b) radiographs following 10th distraction of magnetic growth rod.

GROWTH ROD GRADUATES AND DEFINITIVE SURGERY

Jain et al. evaluated 167 patients from the GSSG database who were treated with GRs. Thirty children did not undergo final fusion, of which 26 had retained GRs while 4 had them removed due to infection. 137 children underwent final fusion. Patients were followed up for a minimum follow-up of two years after the last surgery [28]. No significant differences were observed in the final curve magnitude and trunk height between the groups. They concluded that as there is significant autofusion, final fusion may be avoided if the final alignment and trunk height is satisfactory and there are no implant related issues.

Kocyigit et al. [29] prospectively studied 26 children where GR treatment was initiated before 10 years of age. At the age of 14 years, the children underwent one of three procedures- removal of GR instrumentation alone, removal of the GRs along with instrumented fusion, or continuation of GR lengthening. Nine of the 10 cases where the GRs were removed and not replaced with new instrumentation developed worsening of the deformity clinically and underwent fusion with instrumentation. They concluded that removal of the GRs without inserting new instrumentation was not advisable. Implants should either be retained or extended to additional levels along with fusion in patients where there is an extension of the curve cephalad or caudad to the originally instrumented segments.

Flynn et al. (4) evaluated 99 patients treated with either definitive fusion or by retaining GRs and subsequently followed-up until they were 14 years or later (until skeletal maturity). In 55% of the patients, the fused levels were the same as growth rod levels. Of the 62 patients regarding whom information was available, minimal correction was noted in 11, moderate correction in 30, substantial correction in 9 and worsening in 12 patients. The spine was observed to be stiff in 62% patients, with 22 children needing spinal osteotomies.

Poe-Kochert et al. [30] reported that 20% of 119 patients who underwent a definitive fusion at the end of GR treatment developed 30 complications requiring 57 additional procedures over a follow-up duration of 4.3 years. These included infection, instrumentation failure, prominent instrumentation, pseudarthrosis, and coronal or sagittal deformity. There is a possibility of further revision surgery after the definitive fusion for growth rod graduates and long-term follow-up was recommended.

VEPTR (VERTICAL EXPANDABLE PROSTHETIC TITANIUM RIB)

VEPTR is indicated for the treatment of skeletally immature patients with thoracic insufficiency syndrome (TIS). Approved anatomic diagnoses of TIS include flail chest syndrome, constrictive chest wall syndrome that includes rib fusion and scoliosis, hypoplastic thorax syndrome, which includes Jeune's syndrome, Achondroplasia, Jarcho-Levin syndrome and Ellis Van Creveld syndrome, and progressive scoliosis of congenital or neurogenic origin without rib anomaly. Campbell et al. (7) studied 27 children with congenital scoliosis associated with fused ribs and found a mean correction of the scoliosis from 74 to 49 degrees, and thoracic spine height increased by a mean of 7.1 mm/y. There were 52 complications (193%) in 22 patients. The most common complication was "asymptomatic" proximal migration of the device through ribs in 7 patients. Hasler et al. [31] studied 23 children with non-congenital EOS. Cobb correction was from 68 degrees preoperatively to 54 degrees at the final follow-up. Although space available for the lung (SAL) significantly increased, the percentage predicted pulmonary values were not reported. There were 23 complications (100%) of which 16 were wound complications and 7 implant-related complications. In children older than 10 years comparable correction and a lower complication rates have been documented

Nelson et al. [32] studied application of VEPTR in 10 patients with AMC with mean follow-up of 4.2 years and found 17% correction in scoliosis and 8% correction in kyphosis. They had 6 complications in 4 patients: 3 infections, 2 rib failures, and 1 implant failure. Six patients had proximal junctional kyphosis.

STAPLES AND ANTERIOR TETHER, GROWTH MODULATION OF THE SPINE

Patients considered for this procedure should have at least 1 year of growth remaining and a deformity that could also be considered for bracing. According to Betz and colleagues (8), the thoracic and lumbar curves should be <45 degrees with minimal rotation and flexible to <20 degrees. The sagittal thoracic curve should be <40 degrees. Betz et al. followed [33] children with thoracic curves and 15 with lumbar curves who were treated at mean age of 9. In the thoracic curvatures, 78% either stabilized or improved when the curves were <35 degrees at staple insertion. Larger curves demonstrated a 75% progression rate past 50 degrees. In patients less than age 10 with thoracic curves of all curve magnitudes, there was a 75% success rate. The stapling also appeared to have a positive effect on sagittal contour in patients with hypo-kyphosis. Lumbar curves demonstrated an 87% success rate overall and 100% success rate in patients under the age of 10. Complications included rupture of a previously unrecognized diaphragmatic hernia, overcorrection of 1 curve, atelectasis, and superior mesenteric artery syndrome.

Tethers, like staples, produce correction by convex growth inhibition, but use flexible connections between the vertebral anchor points. Both tethers and staples do produce chemical, cellular, and vascular changes in the disk and end plate, although the significance of these changes is unknown. Samdani et al. [34] reviewed 32 patients who underwent thoracic vertebral body tethering with a minimum one-year follow-up. Mean age at surgery was 12 years, the mean pre- operative thoracic curve magnitude was average of 46° which corrected to average of 25° on first erect and 18° at most recent. One patient experienced prolonged atelectasis, which required a bronchoscopy; otherwise, no major complications were observed.

LIMITATIONS IN EOS SURGERY

There are still many challenges to be overcome in the management of EOS. Frail patients with comorbidities, implant bulk and sometimes the difficulties in contouring implants all add to complication rates.

Complications are common in both conventional GR and MCGR systems. Apart from the complications related to repeat surgeries and anesthesia, others in conventional GR are psychological issues, anxiety and depression [35]. Other complications including unplanned trips to the operating room are similar [36].

Risk factors for complications are curve magnitude, younger age at initiation of growth rod treatment (<5 years), syndromic etiology, and hyperkyphosis [37]. As the amount of force needed increases with each distraction and the length gain decreases due to the stiffness, the distraction forces exerted are increased leading to possible implant failures.

Both conventional GR and MCGR release titanium and aluminum ions with MCGR additionally releasing vanadium ions leading to metallosis within the tissues [38].

Kwan et al. reported unplanned reoperation rates of 46.7% in 30 EOS patients treated with MCGR with a mean follow-up of 3 years [39]. Causes were distraction failure, proximal anchor failure, rod breakage and infection. Risk factors for distraction failure are larger patients, magnet proximity to each other and magnets close to the apex. Proximal junctional kyphosis continues to remain a concern.

With newer long-term studies coming up, we are now coming across specific complications of growing rods *viz*: (1) failure of distraction; (2) fatigue failure of implant; (3) proximal junctional kyphosis; (4) loss of sagittal balance due to non-contourable long actuator for magnetic rods; (5) less reliable results on conversion from traditional growth rods to MCGR; and (6) more reliability on dual rods.

In a study on sagittal profile following MCGR in EOS, Akbarnia et al. [40] showed that the thoracic kyphosis was reduced in cases with pre-existing thoracic kyphosis more than 40 degrees and had no effect on other regional sagittal parameters.

Inaparthy et al. [41] reported incidence of proximal junctional kyphosis (PJK) in 28% cases of EOS operated with MCGR. It was common in males, all the cases were syndromic in etiology and 50% of them were conversion from traditional growth rods. But the presence of PJK was not an indication for further surgery.

DISCUSSION

There has been an expansion of treatment options for the young child with scoliosis. No single algorithm for treating EOS has been proposed. Numerous obstacles, including small, heterogeneous patient populations and regulatory challenges in prospectively studying off-label devices, make rigorous clinical research challenging in this area. In part for these reasons, the comparative effectiveness of various treatment strategies is not well elucidated.

Potential adverse outcomes of GR or VEPTR treatment of EOS include failure to prevent progressive deformity or thoracic insufficiency syndrome, an unacceptably short or stiff spine or deformed thorax, increased family burden of care, and potentially negative psychological consequences from repeated surgical interventions. Neither technique reliably controls all deformity over the entirety of growth period. Infections are common to both GR and VEPTR. Rod breakage and spontaneous premature spinal fusion beneath rods are troublesome complications in GR, whereas drift of rib attachments and chest wall scarring are anticipated complications in VEPTR treatment. Indications for GR and VEPTR overlap, but thoracogenic scoliosis and severe upper thoracic kyphosis are best treated by VEPTR and GR, respectively.

In the first case matched study between traditional growth rods (TGR) and MCGR in 2014 by Akbarnia et al. [42], they compared 12 MCGR patients to 12 case matched TGR patients. The average follow up for TGR was 1.6 year more as compared to MCGR who had 2.5-year mean follow up. Major curve correction, annual T1-T12 and T1-S1 growth was similar in both groups. Incidences of unplanned surgical revisions were similar in both groups but the MCGR patients had 57 fewer surgical procedures. Most of the complications were related to implant failure. In the MCGR group loss of distraction was commonest (63%), and in the TGR (90%).

Jenks et al. in a meta-analysis of the published literature made provisional recommendations for NICE (National Institute for Health and Care Excellence). These were:

1. MAGEC would avoid repeat surgeries and reduce complications and have benefit for physical and psychological aspects of patient and family
2. Indicated for use in children between ages of 2 to 11

3. The system is cost saving as compared to conventional growth rods from about three years after the index procedure.

Figueiredo et al. [43] based on a systematic review of 6 papers found MCGR to be a safe and effective technique and an alternative to traditional growth rods. There were limitations due to the limitations of existing literature and potential bias in literature due to this novel technique being in early phases. Yoon et.al. [44] evaluated 6 patients with early-onset NMS treated with MGRs, with a mean follow-up of 2.5 years. They found significant postoperative improvements in coronal deformity (P = 0.028), forced vital capacity (P = 0.028), and forced expiratory volumes (P = 0.027). Given the risk of infection in this population, technology like MGRs, allowing distraction without multiple surgeries, may decrease complication rates.

Michael et al. [45] presented 12 clinical and radiographic vignettes about patients with early-onset scoliosis to 13 experienced spine surgeons who were members of the Chest Wall and Spine Deformity Study Group. The reviewers were asked to choose type of treatment, type of construct, construct location, and whether a thoracotomy should be performed. They found that although most surgeons agreed about the indication for surgery, they found wide variability in choice of construct type, number of constructs, and level of instrumentation.

CONCLUSION

Rigid indications for surgical interventions currently do not exist for this patient population. Treatment options made by the group of surgeons experienced in treating EOS reflect individual preferences and opinions. There is difficulty in choosing among treatment options in children with EOS as there are several priority areas where better evidence needs to be developed to help surgeons formulate optimal strategies. Additional research is needed to develop and validate classification systems that can guide operative indications. Casting in curves less than 60° till the child is older for surgery and growing rods either conventional or MCGR are the current standard of care but long-term data will determine if MCGR will be the better bet of the two?

REFERENCES

[1] Johari AN, Maheshwari SK, Nemade AS, Maheshwari RS. Management of Early onset Scoliosis. *Current Orthopaedic Practice* 2017; 28: 31-37.
[2] Dimeglio A, Canavese F. The growing spine: how spinal deformities influence normal spine and thoracic cage growth. *Eur Spine J* 2012; 21: 64-70.
[3] Zeltner TB, Burri PH. The postnatal development and growth of the human lung. II. Morphology. *Respir Physiol.* 1987;67:269–282.
[4] Flynn JM, Tomlinson LA, Pawelek J, Thompson GH, McCarthy R, Akbarnia BA, the Growing Spine Study Group. Growing_rod graduates: Lessons learned from ninety-nine patients who completed lengthening. *J Bone Joint Surg Am.* 2013;95:1745-50.

[5] Johari AN, Nemade AS, Andar U. *Congenital Spinal Deformity and Occult Spinal Dysraphism in Current Progress in Orthopedics*, Vol. 2, 2017, 128-158, Tree Life Media ISBN: 978-93-83989-16-4

[6] McCarthy RE, McCullough FL. Shilla Growth Guidance for Early-Onset Scoliosis Results After a Minimum of Five Years of Follow-up. *J Bone Joint Surg Am.* 2015;97:1578-84

[7] Campbell RM Jr, Smith MD, Mayes TC, et al. The effect of opening wedge thoracostomy on thoracic insufficiency syndrome associated with fused ribs and congenital scoliosis. *J Bone Joint Surg Am.* 2004;86-A:1659–1674.

[8] Betz R, Ashgar J, Samdani AF. Non-fusion anterior stapling. In: Akbarnia BA, Yazici M, Thompson GH, eds. *The Growing Spine: Management of Spinal Disorders in Young Children.* New York: Springer; 2010:568–577.

[9] Keskinen H, Helenius I, Nnadi C, Cheung K, Ferguson J, Mundis G, Pawelek J, Akbarnia BA. Preliminary comparison of primary and conversion surgery with magnetically controlled growing rods in children with early onset scoliosis. *Eur Spine J.* 2016.

[10] Dannawi Z, Altaf F, Harshavardhana NS, Sebaie HE, Noordeen H. Early results of a remotely-operated magnetic growth rod in early-onset scoliosis. *Bone Joint J.* 2013; 95-B: 75-80.

[11] Paloski MD, Sponseller PD, Akbarnia BA, Thompson GH, Skaggs DL, Pawelek JB, Nguyen PT, Odum SM; Growing Spine Study Group. Is There an Optimal Time to Distract Dual Growing Rods? *Spine Deform.* 2014;2(6):467-470.

[12] Sankar WN, Acevedo DC, Skaggs DL. Comparison of complications among growing spinal implants. *Annual Meeting of the Pediatric Orthopaedic Society of North America.* Las Vegas, NV: 2009.

[13] Akbarnia BA, Asher MA, Bagheri R, et al. Complications of dual growing rod technique in early onset scoliosis: can we identify risk factors. *41st Annual Meeting of the Scoliosis Research Society.* Miami, FL: 2006.

[14] Skaggs DL, Myung KS, Yazici M, et al. Hybrid growth rods using spinal implants on ribs. *The 4th International Congress on Early Onset Scoliosis and Growing Spine.* Toronto, Canada: 2010.

[15] Shah SA, et al. The Effect of Serial Growing Rod Lengthening on the Sagittal Profile and Pelvic Parameters in Early-Onset Scoliosis.; *SPINE* Volume 39, Number 22, pp E1311-E1317.

[16] Andras LM, Joiner ER, McCarthy RE, McCullough L, Luhmann SJ, Sponseller PD, Emans JB, Barrett KK, Skaggs DL; Growing Spine Study Group. Growing Rods Versus Shilla Growth Guidance: Better Cobb Angle Correction and T1-S1 Length Increase But More Surgeries. *Spine Deform.* 2015 May;3(3):246-252.

[17] Akbarnia BA, Cheung K, Noordeen H, Elsebaie H, Yazici M, Dannawi Z, Kabirian N. Next generation of growth-sparing techniques: preliminary clinical results of a magnetically controlled growing rod in 14 patients with early-onset scoliosis. *Spine* (Phila Pa 1976) 2013; 38: 665-670 [PMID: 23060057 DOI: 10.1097/BRS. 0b013e3182773560].

[18] Ahmad A, Subramanian T, Panteliadis P, Wilson-Macdonald J, Rothenfluh DA, Nnadi C. Quantifying the 'law of diminishing returns' in magnetically controlled growing rods. *Bone Joint J.* 2017;99-B(12):1658-1664.

[19] Gilday SE, Schwartz MS, Bylski-Austrow DI, Glos DL, Schultz L, O'Hara S, Jain VV, Sturm PF. Observed Length Increases of Magnetically Controlled Growing Rods are Lower Than Programmed. *J Pediatr Orthop.* 2018 Mar;38(3):e133-e137.

[20] Keskinen H, Helenius I, Nnadi C, Cheung K, Ferguson J, Mundis G, Pawelek J, Akbarnia BA. Preliminary comparison of primary and conversion surgery with magnetically controlled growing rods in children with early onset scoliosis. *Eur Spine J* 2016; 25: 3294-3300 [PMID: 27160822 DOI: 10.1007/s00586-016-4597-y].

[21] Teoh KH, Winson DM, James SH, Jones A, Howes J, Davies PR, Ahuja S. Do magnetic growing rods have lower complication rates compared with conventional growing rods? *Spine J* 2016; 16: S40-S44 [PMID: 26850175 DOI: 10.1016/j.spinee.2015.12.099].

[22] Choi E, Yaszay B, Mundis G, Hosseini P, Pawelek J, Alanay A, Berk H, Cheung K, Demirkiran G, Ferguson J, Greggi T, Helenius I, La Rosa G, Senkoylu A, Akbarnia BA. Implant Complications After Magnetically Controlled Growing Rods for Early Onset Scoliosis: A Multicenter Retrospective Review. *J Pediatr Orthop.* 2017;37(8):e588-e592.

[23] Charroin C, Abelin-Genevois K, Cunin V, Berthiller J, Constant H, Kohler R, Aulagner G, Serrier H, Armoiry X. Direct costs associated with the management of progressive early onset scoliosis: estimations based on gold standard technique or with magnetically controlled growing rods. *Orthop Traumatol Surg Res* 2014; 100: 469-474 [PMID: 25128440 DOI: 10.1016/j.otsr.2014.05.006].

[24] Jenks M, Craig J, Higgins J, Willits I, Barata T, Wood H, Kimpton C, Sims A. The MAGEC system for spinal lengthening in children with scoliosis: A NICE Medical Technology Guidance. *Appl Health Econ Health Policy* 2014; 12: 587-599 [PMID: 25172432 DOI: 10.1007/s40258-014-0127-4].

[25] Rolton D, Richards J, Nnadi C. Magnetic controlled growth rods versus conventional growing rod systems in the treatment of early onset scoliosis: a cost comparison. *Eur Spine J* 2015; 24: 1457-1461 [PMID: 25433541 DOI: 10.1007/s00586-014-3699-7].

[26] Armoiry X, Abelin-Genevois K, Charroin C, Aulagner G, Cunin V. Magnetically controlled growing rods for scoliosis in children. *Lancet* 2012; 380: 1229 [PMID: 23040859 DOI: 10.1016/S0140-6736(12)61713-9].

[27] Johari AN, Nemade AS. Growing spine deformities: Are magnetic rods the final answer? *World J Orthop* 2017. 18; 8(4): 290-363.

[28] Jain A, Sponseller PD, Flynn JM, Shah SA, Thompson GH, Emans JB, Pawelek JB, Akbarnia BA; Growing Spine Study Group. Avoidance of "Final" Surgical Fusion After Growing-Rod Treatment for Early-Onset Scoliosis. *J Bone Joint Surg Am.* 2016. 6;98(13):1073-8.

[29] Kocyigit IA, Olgun ZD, Demirkiran HG, Ayvaz M, Yazici M. Graduation Protocol After Growing-Rod Treatment: Removal of Implants without New Instrumentation Is Not a Realistic Approach. *J Bone Joint Surg Am.* 2017, 20;99(18):1554-1564.

[30] Poe-Kochert C, Shannon C, Pawelek JB, Thompson GH, Hardesty CK, Marks DS, Akbarnia BA, McCarthy RE, Emans JB. Final Fusion After Growing-Rod Treatment for Early Onset Scoliosis: Is It Really Final? *J Bone Joint Surg Am.* 2016;98(22):1913-1917.

[31] Hasler CC, Mehrkens A, Hefti F. Efficacy and safety of VEPTR instrumentation for progressive spine deformities in young children without rib fusions. *Eur Spine J.* 2010;19:400–408.

[32] Nelson et al. The Efficacy of Rib-based Distraction With VEPTR in the Treatment of Early-Onset Scoliosis in Patients With Arthrogryposis. *J Pediatr Orthop* 2014;34:8–13.

[33] Betz RR, Ranade A, Samdani AF, et al. Vertebral body stapling: a fusionless treatment option for a growing child with moderate idiopathic scoliosis. *Spine*. 2010;35:169–176.

[34] Samdani AF et al. Anterior vertebral body tethering for immature adolescent idiopathic scoliosis: one year results on first 32 patients: *Eur Spine J* (2015) 24:1533–1539.

[35] Aslan C, Olgun ZD, Ertas ES, Ozusta S, Demirkiran G, Unal F, Yazici M. Psychological Profile of Children Who Require Repetitive Surgical Procedures for Early Onset Scoliosis: Is a Poorer Quality of Life the Cost of a Straighter Spine? *Spine Deform*. 2017;5(5):334-341.

[36] Akbarnia BA, Pawelek JB, Cheung KM, Demirkiran G, Elsebaie H, Emans JB, Johnston CE, Mundis GM, Noordeen H, Skaggs DL, Sponseller PD, Thompson GH, Yaszay B, Yazici M; Growing Spine Study Group. Traditional Growing Rods versus Magnetically Controlled Growing Rods for the Surgical Treatment of Early-Onset Scoliosis: A Case-Matched 2-Year Study. *Spine Deform*. 2014 Nov;2(6):493-497.

[37] Upasani VV, Parvaresh KC, Pawelek JB, Miller PE, Thompson GH, Skaggs DL, Emans JB, Glotzbecker MP; Growing Spine Study Group. Age at Initiation and Deformity Magnitude Influence Complication Rates of Surgical Treatment with Traditional Growing Rods in Early-Onset Scoliosis. *Spine Deform*. 2016;4(5):344-350.

[38] Yilgor C, Efendiyev A, Akbiyik F, Demirkiran G, Senkoylu A, Alanay A, Yazici M. Metal Ion Release During Growth-Friendly Instrumentation for Early-Onset Scoliosis: A Preliminary Study. *Spine Deform*. 2018;6(1):48-53.

[39] Kwan KYH, Alanay A, Yazici M, Demirkiran G, Helenius I, Nnadi C, Ferguson J, Akbarnia BA, Cheung JPY, Cheung KMC. Unplanned Reoperations in Magnetically Controlled Growing Rod Surgery for Early Onset Scoliosis with a Minimum of Two-Year Follow-Up. *Spine* (Phila Pa 1976). 2017 15;42(24):E1410-E1414.

[40] Akbarnia BA, Cheung KMC, Kwan K, Samartzis D, Ferguson J, Tkakar Chrishan, Panteliadis P, Nnadi C, Helenius I, Yazici M, Demirkiran GH, Alanay A. The effect of magnetically controlled growing rod on the sagittal profile in early onset scoliosis patients. Posters. *Spine J* 2016; 16: S72-S93 [DOI: 10.1016/j.spinee. 2016.01.112].

[41] Inaparthy P, Queruz JC, Bhagawati D, Thakar C, Subramanian T, Nnadi C. Incidence of proximal junctional kyphosis with magnetic expansion control rods in early onset scoliosis. *Eur Spine J* 2016; 25: 3308-3315 [PMID: 27435487 DOI: 10.1007/s00586-016-4693-z].

[42] Akbarnia BA, Pawelek JB, Cheung KMC, Demirkiran G, Elsebaie H, Emans JB, Johnston CE, Mundis GM, Noordeen H, Skaggs DL, Sponseller PD, Thompson GH, Yaszay B, Yazici M, Growing Spine Study Group. Traditional Growth Rods vs magnetically controlled growing rods for the surgical treatment of early-onset scoliosis: a case matched 2 year study. *Spine Deformity* 2014; 2: 493-497 [DOI: 10.1016/j.jspd.2014.09.050].

[43] Figueiredo N, Kananeh SF, Siqueira HH, Figueiredo RC, Al Sebai MW. The use of magnetically controlled growing rod device for pediatric scoliosis. *Neurosciences* (Riyadh) 2016; 21: 17-25 [PMID: 26818162 DOI: 10.17712/nsj.2016.1.20150266].

[44] Yoon WW, Sedra F, Shah S, et al. Improvement of pulmonary function in children with early-onset scoliosis using magnetic growth rods. *Spine*. 2014;39:1196–1202.

[45] Michael G. Vitale MD, MPH, Jaime A. Gomez MD, Hiroko Matsumoto MA, David P. Roye Jr MD; Variability of Expert Opinion in Treatment of Early-onset Scoliosis. *Clin Orthop Relat Res* (2011) 469:1317–1322 DOI 10.1007/s11999-010-1540-0.

In: Scoliosis: Diagnosis, Classification and Management Options ISBN: 978-1-53614-464-2
Editors: F. Canavese, A. Andreacchio and H. Xu © 2018 Nova Science Publishers, Inc.

Chapter 8

GROWTH FRIENDLY IMPLANTS WITH RIB ANCHORS IN EARLY ONSET SCOLIOSIS

Alaaeldin A. Ahmad[1,*], *Loai J. Aker*[2] *and Yahia B. Hanbali*[2]

[1]Pediatric Orthopedic Surgeon, Palestine Polytechnic University, Palestine,
Adjunct Faculty – The Medical Of University South Carolina (MUSC), US
[2]Faculty of Medicine and Health Sciences, An-Najah National University,
Nablus, Palestine

INTRODUCTION

Early Onset Scoliosis (EOS) is a complex pathology that covers a variety of etiologies including idiopathic, neuromuscular, syndromic, and congenital types, with onset before the age of 10 years. Its natural history is associated with progressive deterioration in pulmonary function and poor quality of life. Also, EOS patients may have associated pathological cardiopulmonary and gastrointestinal conditions which may exacerbate the burden of spinal deformity on pulmonary function. However, Spinal fusion in young children is not preferred anymore in treating EOS due to catastrophic consequences on spinal growth and long-term pulmonary compromise. (Skaggs et al. 2014, Odent et al. 2015, Bess et al. 2010).

Surgical treatment of EOS should have the objectives of fulfilling maximum pulmonary function, spine length, with minimal hospitalizations, complications and family burden (Bess et al. 2010).

EOS growth-friendly surgical treatment with Harington system utilized a stainless-steel rod-and-hook system. The system was promising, but had high rate of hook dislodgement, rod breakage, and flat back. Moe et al. introduced modifications to the systems which allowed contouring the rod along the lumbar lordosis, and decreased rates of post op flat back, and fusion rates (Matsumoto et al. 2014).

Technological advances significantly improved the growth-friendly spinal implants. These implants aim to correct the abnormal curvature while maintaining the growth of the spine and the thorax. The safety and efficacy of Growth-friendly techniques in the treatment of EOS in

---

[*] Corresponding Author Email: alaaahmad@hotmail.com (Alaaeldin A. Ahmad, Associate Professor)

addition to improvements in the quality of life in EOS patients was documented in the literature. (Akbarnia et al. 2008, Akbarnia et al. 2005, Arandi et al. 2014, Skaggs et al. 2014).

The growth friendly techniques can be classified into 3 main categories:

Compression Based Systems

Like vertebral staples and tethers, based on The Hueter-Volkmann law which indicates that physis growth rate can be increased by distractive forces, and decreased by compression forces. (Skaggs et al. 2014).

This technique is advantageous as it allows a fusionless, reversible control of the curvature while maintaining disk viability. However, implants are at risk of failure, and the growth limiting mechanism makes the system non-ideal in the immature spine. (Newton et al. 2008, Skaggs et al. 2014).

Distraction Based Systems

Growing Rods, VEPTR, and MAGEC rods are examples of distraction based systems. With anchors located proximal and distal to the apex of the deformed vertebrae. These anchors, which can be applied on the ribs, spine or pelvis, are implemented to exert mechanical distractive forces across the deformed segment. These distraction forces are supposed to help correct the spinal deformity while maintaining the vertebral and pulmonary growth. MAGEC rods has an advantage of distraction in the outpatient clinic with no need for surgery. (Skaggs et al. 2014).

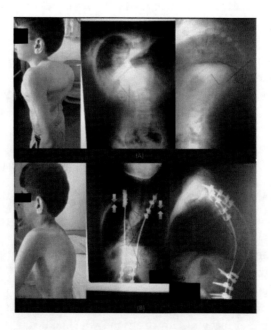

Figure 1. A 9-year-old patient with EOS and kyphosis with AP and lateral x-rays preop (A), and showing curve correction grossly and on x-rays after index surgery (B).

Guided Growth Systems

McCarthy and colleagues developed the Shilla technique to incorporate rods and pedicle screw–based guided growth system. A limited fusion for few vertebrae is applied to the apex of the curve where the dual rods are fixed through pedicle screws. Pedicle screws in the cephalad and caudal vertebrae are not rigidly attached to the rods so that vertical growth can occur. (McCarthy and McCullough 2015).

In this Chapter, the Author's demonstrates his experience in the treatment of EOS through a fusionless surgical construct that involved the use of distractive based system of dual rods attached to proximal rib-hooks anchors, and distal spine/pelvic screws. Also, surgical outcomes and biomechanical features reported in other studies about growing rods construct with spine-based and rib-based proximal anchors are discussed. The modifications demonstrated by the author suggest improvement of construct stability, correction of coronal scoliosis curve, with minimal complications in addition to its unique role in correcting kyphotic deformities.

CONSTRUCTS BIOMECHANICAL FEATURES

The Hybrid Growing Rods system introduced the usage of rib-hooks as proximal anchors, and a distal spinal anchor through pedicle screws or supralaminar hook in distraction based systems. The use of rib anchors allows better soft tissue coverage, more motion at rib-hook interface and so less probability of autofusion. Also, utilizing rib anchors abandoned the need for fusion in upper thoracic segment (T1-3) done in traditional growing rods systems, which may lead to autofusion of uninstrumented levels and pulmonary function compromise in the long term (Karol et al. 2008, Skaggs et al. 2014, Miller and Vitale 2016). It was also found that rib anchors had less than one fourth the risk of rod breakage compared to spine anchors. This might be due to the less rigid system of rib hooks and the allowed ''slop'' at hook-rib interface with the normal motion of the costovertebral joint. (Yamaguchi et al. 2014). These features make rib anchors a convenient tool since anchors in fusionless implants bear the entire mechanical load during the treatment period which increases the risk of implant failure, compared to spinal fusion in adolescent idiopathic scoliosis. (Miller and Vitale 2016).

Practically, Rib hooks are relatively easier to apply without the need for fluoroscopy, and are neurologically-safer since they are far away from the spinal canal.

On the other hand, applying pedicle screws in proximal thoracic vertebrae can be very challenging with abnormal morphology in these vertebrae. (Miller and Vitale 2016), in addition to concerns about pedicle screws use in young children owing to their smaller pedicular anatomy, and suboptimal bone quality(Myung et al. 2014) (Figure 2).

Vitale et al. reported no significant difference among patients with rib based anchors and those with spinal based anchors regarding curve correction, proximal anchor migration or quality of life. (Miller and Vitale 2016).

In a study concerning the failure load of constructs by Akbarnia et al. (Akbarnia et al. 2014), this study dealt with 4 types of construct on immature porcine spines: (SS) bilateral screw on T5-T6, (HH) T5-T6 laminar hooks, (TPL) included a T5, T6 hook construct between the transverse process (TP) and lamina, (RR) hooks facing down on T5 and hooks facing up on T6 just lateral to transverse process, axial pull force was applied to all specimens, ultimate load and displacement at failure were observed. The ultimate load was found greatest in RR group followed by SS group then HH group and lowest in TPL, statistically significant differences among RR and HH, RR and TPL, and SS and TPL pairs. There was no statistically significant difference between: RR and SS, SS and HH, and HH and TPL. On the other hand, no failure found in instruments. (Myung et al. 2010).

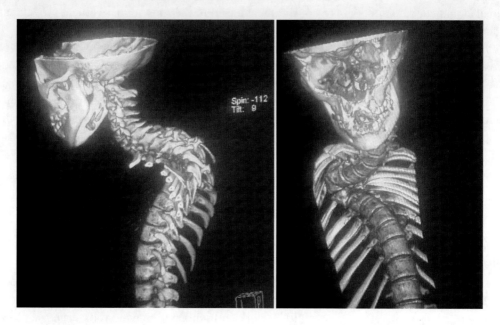

Figure 2. An example of severe upper thoracic kyphoscoliosis in a 3 years old female. 3 rib construct might be the only choice as proximal anchor.

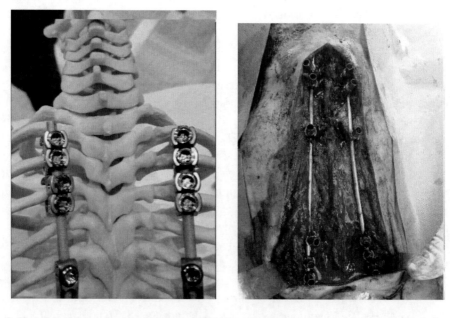

Figure 3. Examples of proximal 3 rib (right) and 4 rib anchors (left) beginning from the 2nd rib.

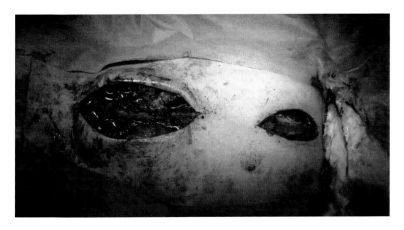

Figure 4. An approach with 2 separate incisions; used mainly for myelomeningocele.

SURGICAL TECHNIQUE

The fusionless surgical management is indicated in EOS when the deformity is severe (often, curve greater than 50 degrees) or rapidly progressive, with significant potential for the spine to grow. Surgery is contraindicated if the patient is medically unfit, has an active infection, with soft tissue compromise, inadequate bone stock or those whose care giver is unable to provide appropriate clinical follow-up. (Miller and Vitale 2016).

Preoperatively, multidisciplinary involvement to address associated potential medical and surgical problems, in addition to optimizing nutritional status are vital. Also full AP and lateral x-rays preop views are needed for surgical planning, with Spine MRI to evaluate the presence of neuroaxial pathology. (Miller and Vitale 2016).

The operation is performed under general anesthesia, with the patient in the prone position. A straight longitudinal midline incision was performed from T2 downwards. Afterwards, the attached edge of the trapezius and rhomboidus major is dissected extraperiosteally and distracted laterally. Erector spinae muscles are also distracted laterally and exposed to the rib extraperiosteally.

Laminar hooks are used as anchors preferably beginning from 2nd rib putting at least 5 hooks according to Vitale for better stability of the anchors proximally (Miller and Vitale 2016, Vitale et al.)

The hooks are either put all facing upwards (Skaggs et al. 2014), or putting them in clawing fashion with 2 proximal hooks facing downwards and one or two distal hooks facing upwards which would increase the stability proximally specially with thoracic kyphosis (Gross 2012)

Distally, screws were put in the lumbar spinal segment or the iliac part. An appropriately determined length, 4.5 titanium rod, is selected, contoured to maintain the adequate sagittal planes in the thoracic and lumbar regions locked with all the anchors. Correction is maintained through the cantilever effect mainly specially in kyphosis which prevents the possibility of hook dislodgment. Two centimeters of the rod is preserved and locked distal to the distal anchors for future lengthening. C-arm and neuromonitoring need to be used in all cases. Mobilization is not restricted postoperatively. Postoperative lengthening was performed every 6–9 months. The procedure includes the following steps: the rods are lengthened by unlocking and distracting the distal screws distally (through the previously preserved 2 cm), which usually takes one or two lengthening times. Then, the rods are changed distally and the proximal rod was engaged with the distal one by domino for lengthening. The incorporation of dominos is done in lengthening surgeries but not in the first "index" surgery because we think that correction is best done in the 1st surgery by using the rod without dominos. The patients need full-length spine radiographs in the coronal and the sagittal views standing or sitting preoperatively, postoperatively, and on follow-up sessions.

According to the literature, the proximal and distal anchor sites should be considered wisely to withstand mechanical forces over a long course of treatment efficiently. For rib-based anchors, it is advised to use multiple rib anchors (e.g., ≥ 5) at the T2-T4 segment to decrease the risk of rib fracture or implant related complications. The first rib is avoided to decrease the risk of brachial plexus palsy. (Miller and Vitale 2016).

During instrumentation of lowest vertebrae, the Cobb should be spanned with least amount of instrumented spine. In idiopathic cases, the lumbar Spine is very suitable. However, many patients with syndromic or neuromuscular scoliosis need stabilization of the pelvis due to early-onset pelvic obliquity (Miller and Vitale 2016).

The Authors recommend to:

1. Use the 4.5 rod system for small children
2. Do always extraperiosteal dissection when exploring the spine
3. Try to put the rib hooks as near as possible to the transverse process

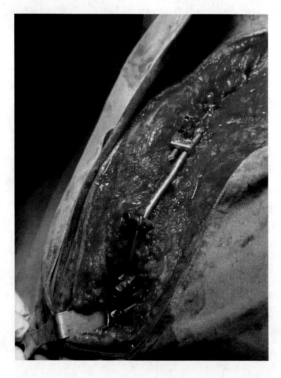

Figure 5. A 3 rib construct successfully implemented in EOS patient with proximal kyphosis.

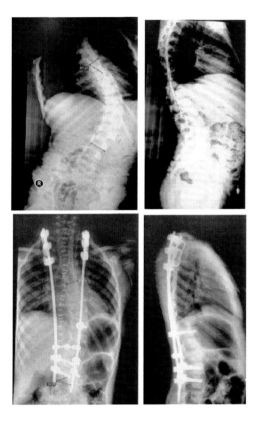

Figure 6. A 7 year-old patient with syndromic Early Onset Scoliosis, with AP, and lateral x-rays preop (up), and after the index surgery with 3rib construct (below).

4. Moderate compression of the hooks for the clawing to avoid rib fusion in the future
5. Depend mainly on the cantilever effect to correct kyphosis.
6. Remove the cross link during the 1st lengthening process
7. Put the anchors in the appropriate distal level to avoid the DJK

SURGICAL OUTCOMES

Appropriate surgical treatment of EOS is vital to prevent catastrophic consequences related to cardiopulmonary functions in addition to correcting the spinal deformity. With the evolution of fusionless surgical techniques, many constructs were introduced which are classically classified into distraction based systems, compression based systems, or growth guided systems. These systems traditionally relied on spinal fixation proximally and distally. Hybrid constructs, where rib based proximal anchors were implemented, have brought many theoretical and practical advantages into EOS surgical treatment. In this section, surgical outcomes of rib based growing rod surgeries will be illustrated and compared to other spinal based constructs in terms of curve correction and rate of complications.

Vitale et al. reported a comparison between 73 EOS patients who had rib-based proximal anchors and 33 who had spine-based proximal anchors with average follow up of 1.16 years.

No significant difference in spinal curve correction (29% vs. 36% correction) was found between rib and spine anchor groups (Vitale et al.).

As for spinal based Growing rods studies, Akbarnia et al. reported on dual growing rods used in 23 EOS patients for at least 2 years treatment period, the curve corrected from a mean of 82 degrees preoperatively, to 36 degrees at the last follow-up or post-final fusion. There was also an increase in T1-S1 length from 23.01 cm to 32.65 cm at last follow-up or post-final fusion with a meanT1-S1 length increase of 1.21 cm per year. In This study, a total of 13 complications occurred in 11 patients (48%). (Akbarnia et al. 2005).

In another study, the outcomes of growing rods surgeries between 175 patients with thoracic and thoracolumbar/lumbar curves were demonstrated. The lumbar spine showed inherently greater flexibility, and more initial correction than thoracic curves. However, both groups had similar correction rate in their curves (thoracic of 46%, thracolumbar/lumbar of 39%) at the last follow up. Also, there was no significant difference in implant complication rate (45% and 47%, respectively). Also, at the latest follow up, both groups had T1-S1 spinal height values similar to predicted values for normal children (up to 10 years of age) according to Dimeglio (Arandi et al. 2014).

With the improvements mentioned in correction of the curve, and spine growth by distraction based system, it is worth mentioning that lung-related changes are still inconclusive (Skaggs et al. 2014). A report on utilizing VEPTR for treating 24 patients with spondylothoracic dysplasia for a mean follow-up of 3 years, the forced vital capacity had an increase of 11%/year, but a 56% decline in the respiratory system compliance, which indicates more stiffness occurred. Yet, over the course of treatment by Growing Rods, patients were found to gain more weight, indicating better nutritional status which is considered a pulmonary function proxy. (Motoyama, Yang, and Deeney 2009, Noordeen et al. 2011, Skaggs et al. 2014).

In the Author's experience, which utilized a hybrid rib construct surgery with serial lengthening for the treatment of 71 EOS, 64 had scoliosis or kyphoscoliosis, 7 had kyphosis with a mean of 43.9 months of follow-up, and mean age at index surgery was 66.6 months. Forty patients underwent 4rib construct, 28 had 3rib construct. 3 patients had 2rib construct. In patients who had scoliosis/kyphoscoliosis deformity, preoperatively, the coronal Cobb angle was 63.1 and became 51.6 in last follow up. (16.8% correction) P value < 0.005. Coronal balance preoperatively was 22.8 and became 22.3 in the last follow up. Apical Vertebral Translation (AVT) was 33.4mm preoperatively and became 34.7 in the last follow up. Both coronal balance and AVT changes were not significant statistically. For T1-S1 spine height of all patients, it was 248.7 mm preop, and became 282.4 in the last follow up. With a mean change by 1.13 cm in T1-S1 height per year. For kyphosis Cobb angle in patients with kyphosis or kyphoscoliosis, the angle was 66.7 and became 38 in the last follow up (42.6% correction). P value < 0.005. Sagittal balance was 35.4 mm and became 24.39 in the last follow up. P value was 0.019 (significant).

To conclude, a survey characterizing the surgical practice in Growing Spine Study Group database of 265 growing rod patients, demonstrated that most growing rods surgeries were used for curves > 60 degrees, for all scoliosis types, in patients who are younger than 10 old. The index surgery was accomplished at a mean age of 6 years and for curves with a mean Cobb angle of 73 degrees. (Yang et al. 2010).

COMPLICATIONS

Although surgical management aims to improve the natural history and quality of life of EOS patients, surgeons and patients' families should also consider the difficulties during the treatment course including potential complications. Spinal fusion, a previously-used protocol to treat EOS, results in short trunk and underdeveloped lungs if the fusion is done before growth is completed. Also, crankshaft phenomenon is a potential complication as the spinal deformity deteriorates in the unfused segments (Bess et al. 2010, Akbarnia and Emans 2010).

In this section, we will demonstrate a group of complications that may occur after non-fusion spine surgeries for EOS, and demonstrate some of the available literature data about complications related to proximal rib-based and spine based constructs.

Growth friendly surgery entails a diverse group of complications. General complications may occur including those due to anesthesia, hospitalization, failure to control the spine deformity, ending growth with a short or stiff spine, or stiff chest (Akbarnia and Emans 2010).

Implant-related complications, like rod fracture, anchor failure, or prominence, represent the most common complications in growing rods surgeries. Rod fractures are the most common problem. With a rate of 15% as reported by Yang et al. They also found that rod fracture risk increases with single rods, previous fracture history, stainless steel rod, rods of small diameter rods, stainless steel rods, and in ambulatory patients (Akbarnia and Emans 2010).

If implant failure is asymptomatic, it may be revised at the time of planned lengthening. If one rod is broken in a dual-rod construct, both rods should be changed to prevent 2nd rod fracture.

Alignment complications may occur and include proximal junctional kyphosis. To decrease its risk, interspinal ligaments should be preserved, and the rods to be contoured into kyphosis proximal to the construct, and extending the upper foundation to T2 or higher (Akbarnia and Emans 2010). In case of thoracic hyperkyphosis, it is advised to contour the rods into kyphosis without excessive correction to prevent implant failure, and to apply connectors at thoracolumbar junction (Akbarnia and Emans 2010).

Also, growing rod surgeries entail fusion related complications since the proximal and distal spinal anchors involve limited fusion at 2-3 adjacent levels at each end of the construct. These complications include fusion nonunion, anchor loosening, and undesired fusion in adjacent levels due to extensive subperiosteal exposures.

Skin-related complications are likely to occur due to performing multiple surgeries on the same incision location, impaired nutritional status in EOS patients. To minimize skin related complication, surgeons are advised to minimize skin retraction and tension, provide skin flaps for full thickness complications, post op padding to decrease pressure on skin, and use submuscular rods (Akbarnia and Emans 2010).

Wound infection can be problematic as deep wound infection may need implant removal. However, superficial infections can be treated with debridement and IV antibiotics if detected early (Akbarnia and Emans 2010).

One of the rare complications in Patient with early onset scoliosis undergoing distraction based surgery is injuring the brachial plexus. The injury may occur when the first rib is pushed superiorly via rib-anchor instrumentation, or by the superior pole of the retracted scapula, or during inferior movement of the scapula while simultaneously correcting a springer deformity. To decrease the risk of brachial plexus injury, it is advised to avoid simultaneous Sprengel reconstruction with insertion of distraction based implants on ribs, and keeping the arm adducted during neuromonitoring of the upper extremities in suspected patients (Joiner, Andras, and Skaggs 2013).

In multiple studies in the literature utilizing growing rods technique with spine-based proximal anchors, the complication rate ranged from 24-58% (Akbarnia et al. 2008, Akbarnia et al. 2005, Arandi et al. 2014, Blakemore et al. 2001, Bess et al. 2010).

Bess et al. analyzed the complications related to EOS growing rods surgeries over 140 patients with spinal based proximal anchors, and reported a complication rate of 19% per procedure, and 58% of patients had minimum of one complication (mean of 1.2 complications per patient). Complication rates was found to increase with increasing the number of surgeries. (Bess et al. 2010)

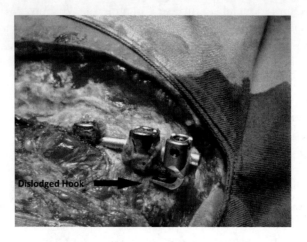

Figure 7. Example of hook dislodgment.

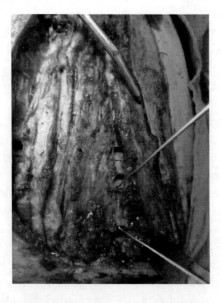

Figure 8. Intraoperative finding of rib autofusion in a patient with EOS.

In Vitale et al. study which compared the outcomes of spine-based and rib based proximal anchors in 106 patients, 11% (8/73) of patients with rib based proximal anchors and 6% (2/33) of patients with spine-based proximal anchors had proximal device migration, with no statistical significance. Five or more proximal anchors were recommended for more protection against proximal device migration (Vitale et al.).

Of the 176 subjects treated by growing rods in a multicenter study, 5.8% with rib anchored Implants had at least 1 rod breakage event, while 28.9% of patients with spine anchored implants had at least 1 rod breakage event. The difference between both groups was significant. However, 26 patients out of 176 had at least 1 anchor pullout with no significance difference between spine and rib anchored groups. The coronal Cobb angle is an influential predictor of rod breakage (Yamaguchi et al. 2014). In another study, having higher upper thoracic curve was found to be associated with increased risk of postoperative complications. These findings might be attributed to more asymmetrical stress on the construct in the presence of higher Cobb angles.(Watanabe et al. 2013, Yamaguchi et al. 2014). Also, Watanabe et al. concluded that 57% of their patients treated with growing rods experienced complications, including implant-related failures (72%), infections (16%), and neurological impairments (3%). Risk factors for complications included a larger upper-thoracic scoliotic curve, thoracic kyphosis, and the number of lengthening surgeries (Watanabe et al. 2013).

In Liang et al. (Liang et al. 2015) study on EOS patients treated by growing rods, postoperative complications affected 23 patients (42%). 66% of Complications were implant-related failures (mostly dislodgement of implants at proximal foundation), alignment complications (11%), infections (11%), 1 neurological impairment, 3 respiratory problems, 2 gastrointestinal problems, 1 urinary problem, and 1 dural tear. The probability of post op complication was found related to curve magnitude in last follow-up and duration between lengthening surgeries. (Liang et al. 2015). Dual growing rods were found to decrease risk of complication in comparison to single rods, which might be due to dissipation of stress on two rods. Also, in dual rods case, the failure of one rod will not affect the stability because of the presence of another intact rod (Liang et al. 2015).

A dilemma is present with markedly progressing thoracic curves, as early surgery may improve the curve and decrease the risk of postop complications. However, this will increase the number lengthening procedures in the long term, and worsen the rate of complications. So surgeons must weigh the need number of procedures during the treatment period to provide adequate spinal and thoracic growth with minimal complications. Interestingly, Liang et al. (Liang et al. 2015) found that doing lengthening procedures at interval of ≥ 9 months showed a higher complications rate compared to an interval of 6 months. From another point of view, lengthening schedules may vary according to the extent of the spine instrumentation and growth rate; lengthening may be done every 4 months in very small children, at 6 month intervals in most children, or every 9 months when only a short segment of spine is spanned. (Akbarnia and Emans 2010), but more research is needed about this aspect.

The placement of the growing rod is another controversial aspect. Although located away from subperiosteal exposure, subcutaneous growing rods placement showed more complications and unplanned surgeries than submuscular rod placement. Due to more soft tissue coverage, submuscular rod placement is currently advocated (Bess et al. 2010, Liang et al. 2015, Akbarnia and Emans 2010).

In the Author's experience with rib-based proximal anchors, out of 71 EOS patients studied over a mean follow-up of 43.9 months, 24 patients (33%) had 44 complications: 2 incidents of broken rod, one UTI, one Domino movement, 9 incidents of dislodgement of distal screw, 6 incident of superficial skin infection post op, 6 proximal hook dislodgements, 5 screw or rod protrusion through skin, 1 dislodgement of proximal screw after fusion, one rib fracture, one shoulder bursitis, one SMA syndrome. 10 patients had PJK. The angle in all of them was < 17 degrees. Out of the 40 patients who had 4 rib construct, 6 had PJK. Out of the 28 patients who had 3rib construct, 3 had PJK, 3 patients had 2 rib construct, and out of them, 1 patient had PJK. 5 out of the 10 patients who had PJK were found to have their proximal anchor in the 2nd rib.

CONCLUSION

We believe that 3 clawing rib construct technique has advantages in the early onset scoliosis especially when associated with kyphosis due to:

1. Easy application
2. Strong anchor proximally
3. Avoid kyphogenic effect during rod lengthening
4. Adjustment of the rod to control the apex
5. Long lever arm without fusion
6. No need for post-operative brace with the dual rod

REFERENCES

Akbarnia, B. A., Breakwell, L. M., Marks, D. S., McCarthy, R. E., Thompson, A. G., Canale, S. K., Kostial, P. N., Tambe, A. & Asher, M. A. (2008). "Dual growing rod technique followed for three to eleven years until final fusion: the effect of frequency of lengthening." *Spine (Phila Pa 1976)*, *33* (9), 984-90. doi: 10.1097/BRS.0b013 e31816c8b4e.

Akbarnia, B. A., Marks, D. S., Boachie-Adjei, O., Thompson, A. G. & Asher, M. A. (2005). "Dual growing rod technique for the treatment of progressive early-onset scoliosis: a multicenter study." *Spine (Phila Pa 1976)*, *30*, (17 Suppl), S46-57.

Akbarnia, B. A., Yaszay, B., Yazici, M., Kabirian, N., Blakemore, L. C., Strauss, K. R., Glaser, D. & Group Complex Spine Study. (2014). "Biomechanical Evaluation of 4 Different Foundation Constructs Commonly Used in Growing Spine Surgery: Are Rib Anchors Comparable to Spine Anchors?" *Spine Deform*, *2* (6), 437-443. doi: 10.1016/j.jspd.2014.04.001.

Akbarnia, Behrooz A. & John, B. Emans. (2010). "Complications of Growth-Sparing Surgery in Early Onset Scoliosis." *Spine*, *35* (25), 2193-2204. doi: 10.1097/BRS.0b013 e3181f070b5.

Arandi, N. R., Pawelek, J. B., Kabirian, N., Thompson, G. H., Emans, J. B., Flynn, J. M., Dormans, J. P. & Akbarnia, B. A. (2014). "Do Thoracolumbar/lumbar Curves Respond Differently to Growing Rod Surgery Compared With Thoracic Curves?" *Spine Deform*, *2* (6), 475-480. doi: 10.1016/j.jspd.2014.04.002.

Bess, S., Akbarnia, B. A., Thompson, G. H., Sponseller, P. D., Shah, S. A., El Sebaie, H., Boachie-Adjei, O., Karlin, L. I., Canale, S., Poe-Kochert, C. & Skaggs, D. L. (2010). "Complications of growing-rod treatment for early-onset scoliosis: analysis of one hundred and forty patients." *J Bone Joint Surg Am*, 92 (15), 2533-43. doi: 10.2106/ jbjs.i.01471.

Blakemore, L. C., Scoles, P. V., Poe-Kochert, C. & Thompson, G. H. (2001). "Submuscular Isola rod with or without limited apical fusion in the management of severe spinal deformities in young children: preliminary report." *Spine (Phila Pa 1976)*, 26 (18), 2044-8.

Gross, R. H. (2012). "An alternate method of fixation for management of early-onset deformity with thoracic kyphosis." *J Pediatr Orthop*, 32 (6), e30-4. doi: 10.1097/BPO.0b013e31824b2826.

Joiner, E. R., Andras, L. M. & Skaggs, D. L. (2013). "Mechanisms and risk factors of brachial plexus injury in the treatment of early-onset scoliosis with distraction-based growing implants." *J Bone Joint Surg Am*, 95 (21), e161. doi: 10.2106/jbjs.m.00222.

Karol, L. A., Johnston, C., Mladenov, K., Schochet, P., Walters, P. & Browne, R. H. (2008). "Pulmonary function following early thoracic fusion in non-neuromuscular scoliosis." *J Bone Joint Surg Am*, 90 (6), 1272-81. doi: 10.2106/jbjs.g.00184.

Liang, J., Li, S., Xu, D., Zhuang, Q., Ren, Z., Chen, X. & Gao, N. (2015). "Risk factors for predicting complications associated with growing rod surgery for early-onset scoliosis." *Clin Neurol Neurosurg*, 136, 15-9. doi: 10.1016/j.clineuro.2015.05.026.

Matsumoto, M., Watanabe, K., Hosogane, N. & Toyama, Y. (2014). "Updates on surgical treatments for pediatric scoliosis." *J Orthop Sci*, 19 (1), 6-14. doi: 10.1007/s00776-013-0474-2.

McCarthy, R. E. & McCullough, F. L. (2015). "Shilla Growth Guidance for Early-Onset Scoliosis: Results After a Minimum of Five Years of Follow-up." *J Bone Joint Surg Am*, 97 (19), 1578-84. doi: 10.2106/jbjs.n.01083.

Miller, Daniel J. & Michael, G. Vitale. (2016). "Rib-Based Anchors for Growing Rods in the Treatment of Early-Onset Scoliosis." *Operative Techniques in Orthopaedics*, 26 (4), 241-246. doi: https://doi.org/10.1053/j.oto.2016.09.006.

Motoyama, E. K., Yang, C. I. & Deeney, V. F. (2009). "Thoracic malformation with early-onset scoliosis: effect of serial VEPTR expansion thoracoplasty on lung growth and function in children." *Paediatr Respir Rev*, 10 (1), 12-7. doi: 10.1016/j.prrv.2008.10.004.

Myung, K. S., Skaggs, D. L., Johnston, C. E. & Akbarnia, B. A. (2014). "The Use of Pedicle Screws in Children 10 Years of Age and Younger With Growing Rods." *Spine Deform*, 2 (6), 471-474. doi: 10.1016/j.jspd.2014.07.002.

Myung, Karen S., David, L. Skaggs., Muharrem, Yazici., Mohammad, Diab., Hilali, H. Noordeen., Michael, G. Vitale. & Charles, E Johnston. (2010). "Hybrid Growth Rods Using Spinal Implants on Ribs: Paper #85." *Spine Journal Meeting Abstracts*, 105-106.

Newton, P. O., Farnsworth, C. L., Faro, F. D., Mahar, A. T., Odell, T. R., Mohamad, F., Breisch, E., Fricka, K., Upasani, V. V. & Amiel, D. (2008). "Spinal growth modulation with an anterolateral flexible tether in an immature bovine model: disc health and motion preservation." *Spine (Phila Pa 1976)*, 33 (7), 724-33. doi: 10.1097/BRS.0b013e31816950a0.

Noordeen, H. M., Shah, S. A., Elsebaie, H. B., Garrido, E., Farooq, N. & Al-Mukhtar, M. (2011). "*In vivo* distraction force and length measurements of growing rods: which factors influence the ability to lengthen?" *Spine (Phila Pa 1976)*, *36* (26), 2299-303. doi: 10.1097/BRS.0b013e31821b8e16.

Odent, T., Ilharreborde, B., Miladi, L., Khouri, N., Violas, P., Ouellet, J., Cunin, V., Kieffer, J., Kharrat, K. & Accadbled, F. (2015). "Fusionless surgery in early-onset scoliosis." *Orthop Traumatol Surg Res*, *101* (6 Suppl), S281-8. doi: 10.1016/j.otsr.2015.07.004.

Skaggs, D. L., Akbarnia, B. A., Flynn, J. M., Myung, K. S., Sponseller, P. D. & Vitale, M. G. (2014). "A classification of growth friendly spine implants." *J Pediatr Orthop*, *34* (3), 260-74. doi: 10.1097/bpo.0000000000000073.

Vitale, Michael G., Hiroko, Matsumoto., Nicholas, Feinberg., Stephen, Maier., Evan, P. Trupia., Shay, Warren., Matthew, Shirley., Sumeet, Garg., John, Flynn., Peter, F. Sturm., Francisco, Sanchez Perez-Grueso., David, P. Roye. & David, L. Skaggs. Proximal Rib vs Proximal Spine Anchors in Growing Rods: A Multicenter Prospective Cohort Study." *Spine Deformity*, *3* (6), 626-627. doi: 10.1016/ j.jspd.2015.09.039.

Watanabe, K., Uno, K., Suzuki, T., Kawakami, N., Tsuji, T., Yanagida, H., Ito, M., Hirano, T., Yamazaki, K., Minami, S., Kotani, T., Taneichi, H., Imagama, S., Takeshita, K., Yamamoto, T. & Matsumoto, M. (2013). "Risk factors for complications associated with growing-rod surgery for early-onset scoliosis." *Spine (Phila Pa 1976)*, *38* (8), E464-8. doi: 10.1097/BRS.0b013e318288671a.

Yamaguchi, K. T., Jr. Skaggs, D. L., Mansour, S., Myung, K. S., Yazici, M., Johnston, C., Thompson, G., Sponseller, P., Akbarnia, B. A. & Vitale, M. G. (2014). "Are Rib Versus Spine Anchors Protective Against Breakage of Growing Rods?" *Spine Deform*, *2* (6), 489-492. doi: 10.1016/j.jspd.2014.08.007.

Yang, J. S., McElroy, M. J., Akbarnia, B. A., Salari, P., Oliveira, D., Thompson, G. H., Emans, J. B., Yazici, M., Skaggs, D. L., Shah, S. A., Kostial, P. N. & Sponseller, P. D. (2010). "Growing rods for spinal deformity: characterizing consensus and variation in current use." *J Pediatr Orthop*, *30* (3), 264-70. doi: 10.1097/BPO.0b013e3181d40f94.

Chapter 9

GROWTH AND ADOLESCENT IDIOPATHIC SCOLIOSIS

Ismat Ghanem[1,2], MD and Maroun Rizkallah[1,], MD*

[1]Faculty of Medicine, Saint-Joseph University, Beirut, Lebanon
[2]Hôtel-Dieu de France University Hospital, Saint-Joseph University, Beirut, Lebanon

ABSTRACT

Idiopathic scoliosis is a disease of the growing spine. Remaining growth and curve magnitude are highly correlated to the risk of progression and aggravation of the disease. Remaining growth can be estimated by repeated biometric measurements, tanner sign and bone age estimation. Puberty is the turning point in the natural history of this disease. The first two years following puberty are a phase of acceleration where 90% of growth occurs. Lateral olecranon radiograph is effective for estimating bone age during this phase. Acceleration segment is followed by a deceleration phase of three years where menarche occurs. Bone age during this phase is evaluated by hand x-rays and the Risser sign. Estimation of idiopathic scoliosis curve progression showed that a 30° curve at the beginning of puberty together with 20°to 30° curves with more than 10° of annual curve progression has a 100% risk of progression towards the 45° surgical threshold. In these severe curves, anticipation may be the key for effective treatment strategy. Treating these curves at the appropriate moment before increased stiffness and severity would lead to a better outcome.

Keywords: idiopathic scoliosis, bone age, puberty, growth spurt, anticipation

INTRODUCTION

Idiopathic scoliosis is a disorder of the growing spine (Alain Dimeglio and Canavese 2013). It is a highly heterogeneous condition with some patients presenting with rapidly progressive curves and others progressing indolently (Newton Ede and Jones 2016). Risk factors for curve progression include sex, initial curve severity, location of the deformity, and

---

[*] Corresponding Author Email: maroun.rizkallah@gmail.com.

particularly the remaining growth (Lonstein and Carlson 1984). Therefore, progression of idiopathic scoliosis correlates with skeletal growth, peaking during adolescent growth spurt and slowing or even stopping at skeletal maturity (Little et al. 2000). Remaining growth and maturity are major parameters that should be taken into account when assessing a patient presenting with scoliosis (DiMeglio et al. n.d.; James O Sanders et al. 2007; James O Sanders 2007). One should keep in mind that growth is not a monotonous process, and that it has periods of acceleration and deceleration; with puberty being the major turning point (Duval-Beaupère and Lamireau 1985). Maturity indicators include chronological age, biometric variables, menarche, secondary sexual characteristics development and skeletal maturity (bone age) (Sitoula et al. 2015). A spine surgeon should know these parameters and how to measure them in order to plan the best treatment at the right moment (Alain Dimeglio and Canavese 2013). Of note, surgery is recommended in adolescents with a curve magnitude of more than 45 to 50 degrees (Altaf et al. 2013), and is indicated for clinically significant deformities or deformities that are more likely to progress (Altaf et al. 2013). Therefore, anticipating the progression of curves by analyzing the risk factors is an essential step in the treatment strategy. This would sometimes lead to an early spinal fusion in order to avoid a guaranteed curve progression and insure a better correction (Charles et al. 2006).

PUBERTY, THE MAJOR TURNING POINT OF GROWTH

Puberty is defined as the transitional period from childhood through the secondary sexual characteristics development to the achievement of final height (Shim 2015). During this period, a rapid increase in height, known as pubertal growth spurt, causes an increase in spinal deformity (Busscher, Wapstra, and Veldhuizen 2010; Charles et al. 2006; Cheung et al. 2004; Yrjönen and Ylikoski 2006; Ylikoski 2003; Wever, Tonseth, and Veldhuizen 2002). The years preceding puberty are characterized by a constant decline in height velocity (Holmgren et al. 2017). Predicting timing and magnitude of growth spurt is of paramount importance to predict scoliosis curve progression, and therefore to propose timely treatment (Busscher, Wapstra, and Veldhuizen 2010). Children should be closely followed up during this period, knowing that puberty starts insidiously and that it is not a sudden event (Alain Dimeglio and Canavese 2013). Puberty is a bi-phased process. The first phase, the acceleration phase, starts at bone age of 11 in girls and 13 in boys (DiMeglio et al. n.d.). Its first stigmata is the increase in growth velocity (standing height) to greater than 0.5 cm per month, or greater than 6 and 7 cms/year in girls and boys respectively (Little et al. 2000; Song and Little, n.d.). Another stigmata signing the beginning of puberty is the appearance of secondary sexual characteristics with the first appearance of pubic hair, the swelling of the testicles and the budding of the nipples (tanner stage 2) (Tanner and Whitehouse 1976; Karlberg et al. 2003). This phase, lasting for 2 years and characterized by rapid growth is followed by a steady decrease in growth rate (DiMeglio et al. n.d.). This deceleration phase lasts 3 more years (Alain Dimeglio and Canavese 2013). Menarche occurs in this phase (DiMeglio et al. n.d.). The lower limbs stop growing after menarche, and no growth at all is noted 2 years following menarche (DiMeglio et al. n.d.). Therefore, once the beginning of puberty is confirmed, the children should be examined at 6 months regular intervals where measurements should be repeated, noted and analyzed. Each visit should include a thorough interrogatory with a detailed physical exam: Biometric measurements for growth monitoring, assessment of secondary sexual characteristics, bone age evaluation for estimation of remaining growth. All these are necessary steps to assess curve progression and the patient's scoliotic risk (Table 1).

Table 1. A checklist with 11 questions a spine surgeon should ask to have a complete assessment of the growth status of a patient presenting with idiopathic scoliosis

	Questions that the spine surgeon should ask while assessing a children with idiopathic scoliosis
	How tall is the child?
	What is the child's sitting height?
	How long is the subischial leg length?
	How much has the child grown in a single year?
	What is the child's chronologic age?
	What is the bone age?
	How much growth does the child have left in the trunk and in the lower limbs?
	Exactly what point has the child reached on his or her developmental peak?
	Where is the child in relation to puberty and the pubertal peak?
	What about the Tanner signs?
	How much does the child weigh?

Biometric Measurements: Objective Way to Monitor Growth

Different body length dimensions have their own typical growth pattern but follow all the distal to proximal growth maturity gradient: body parts that are more distal will have their pubertal growth spurt earlier, following the same sequence in all children (James O Sanders 2007; A Dimeglio, n.d.; Rao, Joshi, and Kanade, n.d.; Iuliano-Burns, Mirwald, and Bailey, n.d.). Foot length is the body dimension with the earliest pubertal growth spurt (Busscher, Wapstra, and Veldhuizen 2010). This is important on the first visit as patients' parents may easily recall the change of the shoe size of their child (Ford, Khoury, and Biro 2009).

However, the four most important biometric measurements for growth monitoring are:

- Standing height: This marker constitutes the sum of two sub-markers: sitting height and sub-ischial height. Both regions grow at different velocities. Therefore, standing height cannot easily account for the loss of trunk height in children with severe spinal deformity (Alain Dimeglio and Canavese 2013; DiMeglio et al. n.d.). Standing height is preferably measured in centimeters with the patient standing on a stadiometer with shoes and socks off. The children are encouraged to stretch out to the maximum height with the application of a gentle upward pressure under the mastoid processes, with the examiner watching to confirm that the heels were not off the ground (James O Sanders et al. 2007).
- Sitting height: correlates strictly with trunk height. This is measured in centimeters, using a rigid wooden stool sufficiently high that the feet of the child could not reach the floor (James O Sanders et al. 2007). When spinal deformity is diagnosed, a loss of sitting height is correlated to the severity of this deformity. A gain in sitting height of 12 to 13 cm occurs in puberty (DiMeglio et al. n.d.; A Dimeglio, n.d.).

- Arm span: Being relatively constantly correlated to standing height, (arm span = 97% of standing height throughout puberty and into adulthood) this measurement is helpful in estimating standing height in non-ambulatory children. This is measured in cm from the ends of the middle finger in one hand to the other with arms maximally outstretched (James O Sanders et al. 2007). The rule is that arm span divided by 2 gives an idea of sitting height, and divided by 4 gives an idea of T1 S1 segment (Alain Dimeglio and Canavese 2013; Alain Dimeglio and Canavese 2012).
- Weight: During pubertal spurt, weight usually doubles. The gain is estimated to be 5 kg by year of puberty. Weight has to be at least 40 kg for the pubertal spurt to be normal (Alain Dimeglio and Canavese 2012; DiMeglio et al. n.d.).

These measures should be performed twice annually, with one measurements preferably performed near the child's birthday, and during the same period of the day (Busscher, Wapstra, and Veldhuizen 2010). The maximum growth rate is called peak height velocity (PHV), and the corresponding age called the peak growth age (PGA) (James O Sanders 2007). Girls have PHV of 8 cm/year +/- 1 cm and boys have a PHV of 9 cm/year +/-1.5 (Beunen et al. n.d.; James O Sanders 2007).

Bone Age, the Tool to Estimate Remaining Bone Growth

Around half of children have bone age that is different from chronological age. With bone age being a significant factor estimating remaining bone growth, and therefore estimating spine deformity evolution, accurate determination of this variable becomes a must (Charles et al. 2008; Charles et al. 2006; DiMeglio et al. n.d.).

Accelerating phase of growth starts at bone age 11 in girls and 13 in boys (Alain Dimeglio and Canavese 2013). One of the first signs clearly visible on anteroposterior radiographs is the ossification of the sesamoid bone of the thumb (Alain Dimeglio and Canavese 2013). Ossification of the triradiate cartilage occurs at 12 and 14 years of bone age in girls and in boys, respectively (A Dimeglio, n.d.). This corresponds to the mid-point of the acceleration phase (A Dimeglio, n.d.). The acceleration phase ends at the aged of 13 and 15 in girls and boys respectively (Alain Dimeglio and Canavese 2013). This relates with the elbow physis closure (Sauvegrain, Nahum, and Bronstein 1962).

Any skeletal region with consistent physeal markers can be used to determine skeletal age (Busscher, Wapstra, and Veldhuizen 2010). The most commonly used markers of skeletal age in patients with adolescent idiopathic scoliosis are the hand, the wrist the elbow and the iliac apophysis (Figure 2) (Busscher, Wapstra, and Veldhuizen 2010).

The Risser sign, evaluating the stage of ossification of the iliac apophysis, is the most commonly used method to determine skeletal maturity in patients with adolescent idiopathic scoliosis (James O Sanders et al. 2007). It was originally described in 1958 (RISSER 1958). However, Risser sign was shown to be poorly correlated to the acceleration phase of growth in puberty (James O Sanders et al. 2007). Iliac apophysis begins to show ossification around 18 to 24 months following the beginning of puberty, therefore two-third of puberty, i.e., most of the growth and subsequently any curve progression, occur before Risser 1 (James O Sanders et al. 2007; James O Sanders et al. 2008; Charles et al. 2007). Furthermore, posteroanterior pelvis

X-ray used to reduce breast irradiation in patients does not show the iliac apophysis ossification as good as the anteroposterior x-ray does (Izumi 1995).

The Greulich and Pyle index is also widely used for determination of bone age and maturity (Greulich, W. W., & Pyle 1959). It is limited by being widely spaced in time during the critical period of growth spurt (James O Sanders et al. 2007). Furthermore, hand and wrist X-rays are difficult to assess in the acceleration phase of puberty (Alain Dimeglio and Canavese 2013).

The Tanner-Whitehouse III RUS score based on hand and wrist x-rays was shown to strongly predict the acceleration phase of growth (James O Sanders et al. 2007). The Sanders method for assessment of bone age introduced in 2008 is derived from it (James O Sanders et al. 2008). It is based on radiographic analysis of fingers and metacarpals (James O Sanders et al. 2008). Eight stages are identified. Stages 1 and 2 correspond to prepubertal period, stages 3 and 4 correspond to the growth acceleration phase (Risser grade 0), and stages 5 to 8 cover Risser 1 to 5 until full skeletal maturity (James O Sanders et al. 2008; Neal, Shirley, and Kiebzak 2017). This method was shown to be reliable and to correlate more strongly with idiopathic scoliosis curve behavior than Risser sign and Greulish and Pyle atlas (Alain Dimeglio and Canavese 2013).

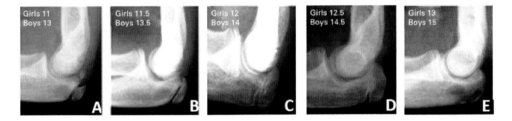

Figure 1. Figure showing the simplified Dimeglio's method of skeletal age assessment: A: two ossification nuclei (11 years in girls and 13 years in boys), B: half-moon image (11.5 years in girls and 13.5 years in boys), C: rectangular aspect (12 years in girls and 14 years in boys), D: beginning fusion (12.5 years in girls and 14.5 years in boys), E: complete fusion (13 years in girls and 15 years in boys).

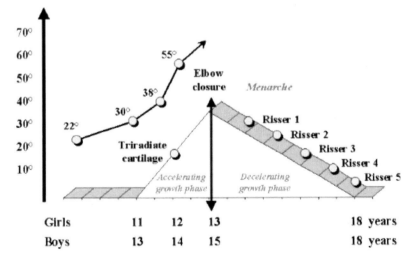

Figure 2. Figure showing the pubertal diagram in girls and boys, adopted from Charles et al. 2006. (Charles et al. 2006).

Sauvegrain et al. developed in 1962 a method to assess skeletal maturity using anteroposterior and lateral radiographs of the left elbow (Sauvegrain, Nahum, and Bronstein 1962). Elbow radiographs provide useful information from bone age 10 to 13 years and 12 to 15 years in girls and boys respectively (Diméglio et al. 2005; Sauvegrain, Nahum, and Bronstein 1962). This method was simplified by Dimeglio et al. in 2005 who showed that the morphology of the olecranon apophysis on lateral elbow radiographs goes through five distinct appearances at 6 months intervals (Figure 1) (Diméglio et al. 2005; DiMeglio et al. n.d.; Canavese et al. 2014). This is clinically significant because it happens between 11 and 12.5 years of bone age in girls and 13 and 15.5 years of bone age in boys, when the Risser sign is still 0 (Alain Dimeglio and Canavese 2013).

Both Dimeglio and Sanders methods were shown to have a modest learning curve and an ease of clinical application. Both methods, when compared, were equally reliable with a correlation that was equally strong for boys and girls (Canavese et al. 2014). Therefore, lateral elbow radiograph is effective when assessing skeletal maturity during the pubertal growth spurt. A hand radiograph is preferable prior to puberty and from Risser grade 1 to 5. A combination of both methods adequately covers the gap between elbow fusion and Risser grade 1, as one complements the other (Canavese et al. 2014).

THE SCOLIOTIC RISK, THE ART OF ANTICIPATION

One main predictor for scoliotic curve progression in patients with adolescent idiopathic scoliosis is the onset of the pubertal growth spurt (Duval-Beaupere et al. 1970; Lonstein and Carlson 1984; Alain Dimeglio and Canavese 2013; DiMeglio et al. n.d.; Little et al. 2000). Growth remaining, estimated via biometric measurements, secondary sexual characteristics evaluation and bone skeletal maturity assessment, helps the spine surgeon predict the main scoliotic curve progression (Duval-Beaupere et al. 1970; Lonstein and Carlson 1984; Alain Dimeglio and Canavese 2013; DiMeglio et al. n.d.). Risk of progression is high during acceleration phase, and then decreases progressively from Risser 1 to Risser 5 (Alain Dimeglio and Canavese 2013). Another main predictor is the curve magnitude (Sitoula et al. 2015; Tan et al. 2009; Charles et al. 2006; Charles, Canavese, and Diméglio 2017; Duval-Beaupère and Lamireau 1985). The more severe the main curve is at the beginning of the growth spurt, the more important is the predicted progression (Sitoula et al. 2015; Tan et al. 2009; Charles et al. 2006; Charles, Canavese, and Diméglio 2017; Duval-Beaupère and Lamireau 1985). Different studies led to different cut points of main curves Cobb angles predicting progression; mainly, a curve greater than 25 to 30 degrees is at significant risk of progression (Sitoula et al. 2015; Tan et al. 2009; Charles et al. 2006; Charles, Canavese, and Diméglio 2017; Duval-Beaupère and Lamireau 1985). Other predictors shown to influence curve progression in idiopathic scoliosis patients are sex and curve location, with thoracic curves being at higher risk of progression than lumbar curves (Charles et al. 2006).

It is important to predict curve progression as surgery is indicated when the progressing deformity reaches 45 degrees. Therefore, taking the two major risk factors of curve progression into consideration, during the acceleration phase of puberty a 5° curve is associated with a 10% risk of progression for surgery, a 10° curve with a 20% risk of progression, a 20° curve with a 30% risk of progression, and a 30° curve raises the risk to virtually 100% (Duval-Beaupere et al. 1970; Charles et al. 2006; Charles et al. 2007; Charles, Canavese, and Diméglio 2017; DiMeglio et al. n.d.). During the deceleration phase, the risk of progression is lower. At Risser sign I there is a 10% risk of progression for a 20° curve and a 60% risk for a 30° curve; at Risser sign II there is a 2% risk for a 20° curve and 30% risk for a 30° curve; at Risser III there is a 12% risk of progression for a curve of ≥20°; at Risser sign IV the risk of progression is markedly decreased; at Risser sign V skeletal maturation has ended (Alain Dimeglio and Canavese 2013; DiMeglio et al. n.d.).

Charles et al. showed that in patients with scoliotic curves, especially main thoracic ones, exceeding 30° at the beginning of puberty, the risk of progression to surgery is nearly 100%. In patients with curves ranging between 21° and 30°, the risk of progression to surgery varies from 30 to 75%. Patients in this section need to be closely monitored in the ascending accelerating phase of puberty, and their annual curve progression velocity should be calculated. An increase of less than 6° per year is reassuring. An increase of 6° to 10° per year is associated to 70% of evolution to surgery. An increase of more than 10° per years or more than 1° per month represents a 100% risk of evolution towards surgery (Charles et al. 2006; Charles, Canavese, and Diméglio 2017; Alain Dimeglio and Canavese 2013; DiMeglio et al. n.d.).

These results led to the concept of anticipation (Charles, Canavese, and Diméglio 2017; Charles et al. 2006; Alain Dimeglio and Canavese 2013; DiMeglio et al. n.d.). Waiting for the patient with idiopathic scoliosis to reach and exceed the surgical threshold may lead to stiff and severe curves (Charles, Canavese, and Diméglio 2017; Charles et al. 2006; Alain Dimeglio and Canavese 2013; DiMeglio et al. n.d.). These curves would be difficult to correct, leading to only partial curve reduction (Charles, Canavese, and Diméglio 2017; Charles et al. 2006; Alain Dimeglio and Canavese 2013; DiMeglio et al. n.d.). Therefore, an earlier intervention at earlier stages could be more advantageous, allowing an easier curve reduction (Charles, Canavese, and Diméglio 2017; Charles et al. 2006; Alain Dimeglio and Canavese 2013; DiMeglio et al. n.d.). This is still a theoretical conclusion based on retrospective studies as no higher level studies have been performed on this subject (Charles et al. 2006; Charles, Canavese, and Diméglio 2017). The risks of operating patients in their growth spurt are the crankshaft phenomenon and the deficit of trunk growth (DiMeglio et al. n.d.). Crankshaft phenomenon can be avoided in waiting for the closure of the triradiate cartilage that usually happens in the year that follows the beginning of puberty (Roberto et al. n.d.; J O Sanders, Herring, and Browne 1995). Also, a curve reduction to 0° reduces significantly the risk of the crankshaft phenomenon (DiMeglio et al. n.d.). The deficit on the trunk growth will be balanced by the correction of the deformity as the remaining growth on the thoracic spine in 3.6 cm and 3.9 cm in girls and boys respectively and the remaining growth on the lumbar spine in 2.1 cm and 2.3 cm in girls and boys respectively (DiMeglio et al. n.d.).

CONCLUSION

Idiopathic scoliosis is a dynamic disease of the spine strongly correlated to the remaining growth potential. Predicting progression of the deformity, when possible, is important and would intervene in the treatment strategy. Besides the curve magnitude, remaining growth is essential for analyzing possible curve progression. Remaining growth may be estimated through assessment of bone age (skeletal maturity), of secondary sexual characteristics, and of regular biannual biometric measures. Acceleration phase of puberty starts at 11 and 13 years of bone age in girls and boys respectively. It lasts for 2 years during which the majority of growth, and 90% of curve progression occur. In this phase, lateral elbow radiograph is the best to assess bone age. This phase is followed by the descending phase lasting 3 years in which Risser sign and hand X-rays are preferable for bone age assessment. Curves of more than 30° at the beginning of the growth spurt and those between 20° and 30° with more than 10° of annual curve progression are at nearly 100% risk of progression to surgery. In these patients, anticipation is the key for an effective treatment strategy, where aggressive scoliosis should be treated before it is too late to get the best outcome.

Conflict of Interest

No conflict of interest and no funding.

REFERENCES

Altaf, Farhaan, Alexander Gibson, Zaher Dannawi, and Hilali Noordeen. 2013. "Adolescent Idiopathic Scoliosis." *BMJ (Clinical Research Ed.)* 346 (April): f2508. http://www.ncbi.nlm.nih.gov/pubmed/23633006.

Beunen, G, M Thomis, H H Maes, R Loos, R M Malina, A L Claessens, and R Vlietinck. n.d. "Genetic Variance of Adolescent Growth in Stature." *Annals of Human Biology* 27 (2): 173–86. http://www.ncbi.nlm.nih.gov/pubmed/10768422.

Busscher, Iris, Frits Hein Wapstra, and Albert G Veldhuizen. 2010. "Predicting Growth and Curve Progression in the Individual Patient with Adolescent Idiopathic Scoliosis: Design of a Prospective Longitudinal Cohort Study." *BMC Musculoskeletal Disorders* 11 (May): 93. doi:10.1186/1471-2474-11-93.

Canavese, F, Y P Charles, A Dimeglio, S Schuller, M Rousset, A Samba, B Pereira, and J-P Steib. 2014. "A Comparison of the Simplified Olecranon and Digital Methods of Assessment of Skeletal Maturity during the Pubertal Growth Spurt." *The Bone & Joint Journal* 96–B (11): 1556–60. doi:10.1302/0301-620X.96B11.33995.

Charles, Yann Philippe, Federico Canavese, and Alain Diméglio. 2017. "Curve Progression Risk in a Mixed Series of Braced and Nonbraced Patients with Idiopathic Scoliosis Related to Skeletal Maturity Assessment on the Olecranon." *Journal of Pediatric Orthopedics. Part B* 26 (3): 240–44. doi:10.1097/BPB.0000000000000410.

Charles, Yann Philippe, Jean-Pierre Daures, Vincenzo de Rosa, and Alain Diméglio. 2006. "Progression Risk of Idiopathic Juvenile Scoliosis during Pubertal Growth." *Spine* 31 (17): 1933–42. doi:10.1097/01.brs.0000229230.68870.97.

Charles, Yann Philippe, Alain Diméglio, Federico Canavese, and Jean-Pierre Daures. 2007. "Skeletal Age Assessment from the Olecranon for Idiopathic Scoliosis at Risser Grade 0." *The Journal of Bone and Joint Surgery. American Volume* 89 (12): 2737–44. doi:10.2106/JBJS.G.00124.

Charles, Yann Philippe, Alain Diméglio, Michel Marcoul, Jean-François Bourgin, Amélie Marcoul, and Marie-Cécile Bozonnat. 2008. "Influence of Idiopathic Scoliosis on Three-

Dimensional Thoracic Growth." *Spine* 33 (11): 1209–18. doi:10.1097/BRS.0b013e31 81715272.

Cheung, John, Albert G Veldhuizen, Jan P K Halbertsma, Natasha M Maurits, Wim J Sluiter, Jan C Cool, and Jim R Van Horn. 2004. "The Relation between Electromyography and Growth Velocity of the Spine in the Evaluation of Curve Progression in Idiopathic Scoliosis." *Spine* 29 (9): 1011–16. http://www.ncbi.nlm.nih.gov/pubmed/15105674.

Dimeglio, A. n.d. "Growth in Pediatric Orthopaedics." *Journal of Pediatric Orthopedics* 21 (4): 549–55. http://www.ncbi.nlm.nih.gov/pubmed/11433174.

Dimeglio, Alain, and Federico Canavese. 2012. "The Growing Spine: How Spinal Deformities Influence Normal Spine and Thoracic Cage Growth." *European Spine Journal : Official Publication of the European Spine Society, the European Spinal Deformity Society, and the European Section of the Cervical Spine Research Society* 21 (1): 64–70. doi:10.1007/s00586-011-1983-3.

———. 2013. "Progression or Not Progression? How to Deal with Adolescent Idiopathic Scoliosis during Puberty." *Journal of Children's Orthopaedics* 7 (1): 43–49. doi:10.1007/s11832-012-0463-6.

Diméglio, Alain, Yann Philippe Charles, Jean-Pierre Daures, Vincenzo de Rosa, and Boniface Kaboré. 2005. "Accuracy of the Sauvegrain Method in Determining Skeletal Age during Puberty." *The Journal of Bone and Joint Surgery. American Volume* 87 (8): 1689–96. doi:10.2106/JBJS.D.02418.

DiMeglio, Alain, Alain Dimeglio, Federico Canavese, Yann Philippe Charles, and Philippe Charles. n.d. "Growth and Adolescent Idiopathic Scoliosis: When and How Much?" *Journal of Pediatric Orthopedics* 31 (1 Suppl): S28-36. doi:10.1097/BPO.0b013 e318202c25d.

Duval-Beaupere, G, J Dubousset, P Queneau, and A Grossiord. 1970. "[A Unique Theory on the Course of Scoliosis]." *La Presse Medicale* 78 (25): 1141–6 passim. http://www.ncbi.nlm.nih.gov/pubmed/5429561.

Duval-Beaupère, G, and T Lamireau. 1985. "Scoliosis at Less than 30 Degrees. Properties of the Evolutivity (Risk of Progression)." *Spine* 10 (5): 421–24. http://www.ncbi.nlm.nih.gov/pubmed/4049108.

Ford, Kanti R, Jane C Khoury, and Frank M Biro. 2009. "Early Markers of Pubertal Onset: Height and Foot Size." *The Journal of Adolescent Health : Official Publication of the Society for Adolescent Medicine* 44 (5): 500–501. doi:10.1016/j.jadohealth.2008.10.004.

Greulich, W. W., & Pyle, S. I. 1959. "Radiographic Atlas of Skeletal Development of the Hand and Wrist." *The American Journal of the Medical Sciences* 238 (3): 393.

Holmgren, Anton, Aimon Niklasson, Lars Gelander, A Stefan Aronson, Andreas F M Nierop, and Kerstin Albertsson-Wikland. 2017. "Insight into Human Pubertal Growth by Applying the QEPS Growth Model." *BMC Pediatrics* 17 (1): 107. doi:10.1186/s12887-017-0857-1.

Iuliano-Burns, S, R L Mirwald, and D A Bailey. n.d. "Timing and Magnitude of Peak Height Velocity and Peak Tissue Velocities for Early, Average, and Late Maturing Boys and Girls." *American Journal of Human Biology : The Official Journal of the Human Biology Council* 13 (1): 1–8. doi:10.1002/1520-6300 (200101/02)13:1<1::AID-AJHB1000 >3.0.CO;2-S.

Izumi, Y. 1995. "The Accuracy of Risser Staging." *Spine* 20 (17): 1868–71. http://www.ncbi.nlm.nih.gov/pubmed/8560333.

Karlberg, Johan, Chi-Wai Kwan, Lars Gelander, and Kerstin Albertsson-Wikland. 2003. "Pubertal Growth Assessment." *Hormone Research* 60 (Suppl 1): 27–35. doi:10.1159/000071223.

Little, D G, K M Song, D Katz, and J A Herring. 2000. "Relationship of Peak Height Velocity to Other Maturity Indicators in Idiopathic Scoliosis in Girls." *The Journal of Bone and Joint Surgery. American Volume* 82 (5): 685–93. http://www.ncbi.nlm.nih.gov/pubmed/10819279.

Lonstein, J E, and J M Carlson. 1984. "The Prediction of Curve Progression in Untreated Idiopathic Scoliosis during Growth." *The Journal of Bone and Joint Surgery. American Volume* 66 (7): 1061–71. http://www.ncbi.nlm.nih.gov/pubmed/6480635.

Neal, Kevin M, Eric D Shirley, and Gary M Kiebzak. 2017. "Maturity Indicators and Adolescent Idiopathic Scoliosis: Evaluation of the Sanders Maturity Scale." *Spine*, November. doi:10.1097/BRS.0000000000002483.

Newton Ede, Matthew M P, and Simon W Jones. 2016. "Adolescent Idiopathic Scoliosis: Evidence for Intrinsic Factors Driving Aetiology and Progression." *International Orthopaedics* 40 (10): 2075–80. doi:10.1007/s00264-016-3132-4.

Rao, S, S Joshi, and A Kanade. n.d. "Growth in Some Physical Dimensions in Relation to Adolescent Growth Spurt among Rural Indian Children." *Annals of Human Biology* 27 (2): 127–38. http://www.ncbi.nlm.nih.gov/pubmed/10768418.

Risser, J C. 1958. "The Iliac Apophysis; an Invaluable Sign in the Management of Scoliosis." *Clinical Orthopaedics* 11: 111–19. http://www.ncbi.nlm.nih.gov/pubmed/13561591.

Roberto, R F, J E Lonstein, R B Winter, and F Denis. n.d. "Curve Progression in Risser Stage 0 or 1 Patients after Posterior Spinal Fusion for Idiopathic Scoliosis." *Journal of Pediatric Orthopedics* 17 (6): 718–25. http://www.ncbi.nlm.nih.gov/pubmed/9591972.

Sanders, James O. 2007. "Maturity Indicators in Spinal Deformity." *The Journal of Bone and Joint Surgery. American Volume* 89 Suppl 1 (February): 14–20. doi:10.2106/JBJS.F.00318.

Sanders, James O, Richard H Browne, Sharon J McConnell, Susan A Margraf, Timothy E Cooney, and David N Finegold. 2007. "Maturity Assessment and Curve Progression in Girls with Idiopathic Scoliosis." *The Journal of Bone and Joint Surgery. American Volume* 89 (1): 64–73. doi:10.2106/JBJS.F.00067.

Sanders, James O, Joseph G Khoury, Shyam Kishan, Richard H Browne, James F Mooney, Kali D Arnold, Sharon J McConnell, Jeanne A Bauman, and David N Finegold. 2008. "Predicting Scoliosis Progression from Skeletal Maturity: A Simplified Classification during Adolescence." *The Journal of Bone and Joint Surgery. American Volume* 90 (3): 540–53. doi:10.2106/JBJS.G.00004.

Sanders, J O, J A Herring, and R H Browne. 1995. "Posterior Arthrodesis and Instrumentation in the Immature (Risser-Grade-0) Spine in Idiopathic Scoliosis." *The Journal of Bone and Joint Surgery. American Volume* 77 (1): 39–45. http://www.ncbi.nlm.nih.gov/pubmed/7822354.

Sauvegrain, J, H Nahum, and H Bronstein. 1962. "[Study of Bone Maturation of the Elbow]." *Annales de Radiologie* 5: 542–50. http://www.ncbi.nlm.nih.gov/pubmed/13986863.

Shim, Kye Shik. 2015. "Pubertal Growth and Epiphyseal Fusion." *Annals of Pediatric Endocrinology & Metabolism* 20 (1): 8–12. doi:10.6065/apem.2015.20.1.8.

Sitoula, Prakash, Kushagra Verma, Laurens Holmes, Peter G Gabos, James O Sanders, Petya Yorgova, Geraldine Neiss, Kenneth Rogers, and Suken A Shah. 2015. "Prediction of Curve

Progression in Idiopathic Scoliosis: Validation of the Sanders Skeletal Maturity Staging System." *Spine* 40 (13): 1006–13. doi:10.1097/BRS.0000000000000952.

Song, K M, and D G Little. n.d. "Peak Height Velocity as a Maturity Indicator for Males with Idiopathic Scoliosis." *Journal of Pediatric Orthopedics* 20 (3): 286–88. http://www.ncbi.nlm.nih.gov/pubmed/10823591.

Tan, Ken-Jin, Maung Maung Moe, Rose Vaithinathan, and Hee-Kit Wong. 2009. "Curve Progression in Idiopathic Scoliosis: Follow-up Study to Skeletal Maturity." *Spine* 34 (7): 697–700. doi:10.1097/BRS.0b013e31819c9431.

Tanner, J M, and R H Whitehouse. 1976. "Clinical Longitudinal Standards for Height, Weight, Height Velocity, Weight Velocity, and Stages of Puberty." *Archives of Disease in Childhood* 51 (3): 170–79. http://www.ncbi.nlm.nih.gov/pubmed/952550.

Wever, D J, K A Tonseth, and A G Veldhuizen. 2002. "Curve Progression and Spinal Growth in Brace Treated Idiopathic Scoliosis." *Studies in Health Technology and Informatics* 91: 387–92. http://www.ncbi.nlm.nih.gov/pubmed/15457762.

Ylikoski, Mauno. 2003. "Height of Girls with Adolescent Idiopathic Scoliosis." *European Spine Journal : Official Publication of the European Spine Society, the European Spinal Deformity Society, and the European Section of the Cervical Spine Research Society* 12 (3): 288–91. doi:10.1007/s00586-003-0527-x.

Yrjönen, Timo, and Mauno Ylikoski. 2006. "Effect of Growth Velocity on the Progression of Adolescent Idiopathic Scoliosis in Boys." *Journal of Pediatric Orthopedics. Part B* 15 (5): 311–15. http://www.ncbi.nlm.nih.gov/pubmed/16891955.

In: Scoliosis: Diagnosis, Classification and Management Options ISBN: 978-1-53614-464-2
Editors: F. Canavese, A. Andreacchio and H. Xu   © 2018 Nova Science Publishers, Inc.

Chapter 10

PHYSIOTHERAPY AND SCOLIOSIS: WHAT TO DO AND WHAT TO REASONABLY EXPECT FROM IT

Jacques Deslandes[*]
Department of Orthopedics and Rehabilitation, Polyclinique St. Odilon, Moulins, France

ABSTRACT

The role of the spine, apart from the fact that it protects the spinal cord and nerve roots, is to provide a human being with a stable upright position, despite gravity, whilst enabling mobility when walking, performing movements and doing sports. Several systems manage these functions. First of all is the osteoarticular system, which generates movements, is capable of powerful, and responsible for synergic action of muscles coupled with their aponeuroses, structures which store and restitute the energy produced by muscle fascicles. The spine follows complex biomechanical laws which involve the osteoarticular and muscular system but, by itself, the vertebral column is incapable of establishing and maintaining static or dynamic states of equilibrium. Spine motricity depends on the spinal cord and cerebral centers where instructions are formulated, which are constantly being adjusted by feedback loops to ensure that actions performed match the expected motor task while also controlling the spine's stability and that of the individual. Scoliosis perturbs this static and particularly the dynamic three-dimensional equilibrium, disrupting the harmony necessary to the spine's good function at all times.

Physical Therapy (PT) programs aim to have an effect on several elements through dynamic interaction or on these elements' organization in order to attempt to stop or correct scoliosis deformities as early as possible, before they become very structured. Generalized physiotherapy (which is not curve-specific) has, to date, not proven to be effective, and therefore other better structured programs dedicated to scoliotic pathology Physiotherapeutic Scoliosis Specific Exercises (PSSE) have emerged initially in Europe. They use exercises that are specific to the deformity being treated and that are as tailor-made as possible to the patient. The latter is carefully assessed medically and in terms of rehabilitation, and learns exercises initially in a specialized scoliosis treatment unit. Even if there are differences between the programs, all of these involve corrective exercises to loosen the scoliosis-affected spine, sustained muscular consolidation work but, above all,

---

[*] Corresponding Author Email: ja.desl@orange.fr (Polyclinique St. Odilon, Department of Orthopedics and Rehabilitation, Av. du Prof. E. Sorel, 03000 Moulins, France).

active correction of curvatures, work on the equilibrium of the spine and of the patient, tying this in with the optimization of his/her own proprioception. Regular work done at home or in the scoliosis patient's living environment is then implemented and monitored. Those in favor of these programs put forward positive clinical studies that are most often for mild curvatures, with a lack of side effects – notwithstanding the risk of evolution – and, finally but probably most importantly, quoting the patient's commitment in an active program. The detractors, on the other hand, highlight the low quality of publications, the waste of time and money and, above all, the lack of any studies demonstrating that, like with bracing, there may be a reduction in the risk of progression to a need for surgery. So, even if recent PSSE studies have better arguments and methodology to support them than the earlier ones that were carried out in more undifferentiated forms of rehabilitation, the level of scientific evidence demonstrating their capacity to even stop the progression of scoliosis remain insufficient. These methods may be used as an initial approach to scoliosis, through motivational active participation, be used to improve muscle capacity, physical condition, and the comfort and quality of life linked to the patient's health. They must, however, not be a substitute for orthopedic treatment, should it be required, nor should it replace the time a growing child or adolescent spends doing fun or sports activities which are indispensable to his/her physical and psychological well-being.

Keywords: spine, physical therapy, PSSE, scoliosis, assessment

INTRODUCTION

Idiopathic scoliosis is a complex three-dimensional deformity of the spine, the causes of which are still partly to be clarified. As early as 1950, it was defined by I. Ponsetti and B. Friedman [1] according to zones of deformity. Thus, for decades now, one refers to thoracic, double thoracic, lumbar, double major (thoracic and lumbar), triple curve scoliosis to designates the area(s) affected. The scoliosis process can be further complicated during adult life with cardio-respiratory conditions – the risk of which increases with certain thoracic curves of more than 50° Cobb angle at the end of growth –, with degenerative processes, particularly lumbar due to disc disease, and more insidiously, with progressive contamination through the stiffening and deformation process of adjacent areas. Topographic classification has the advantage of being simple but is as important as the topography of the actual scoliosis, the age at which the process began, the equilibrium or lack of it of the spine, the harmonious repartition or not of body masses subjected to the scoliosis process, the lever effect of active and passive forces acting on the spine which generate moments of deformation as this deformation progressively worsens, and finally, the dynamics of the human body which is preserved or altered by the scoliosis process.

Beyond the simple descriptive aspect of the curb using the Cobb method, the loss of flexibility defines the structurality of the scoliosis curve; inversely, a curve which is sufficiently flexible to disappear with active posture modifications is considered to be non-structural and often remains within the limits of normal movement. By definition, a functional curve straightens with no particular residual twisting remaining when the patient is lying down or leaning laterally. Similarly, a complete deformation corrected with a shoe lift which compensates for the unequal length in lower limbs is a functional deformation or scoliotic attitude rather than actual scoliosis.

It seems logical that exercises to improve both the flexibility and the active control of the spine should be used to treat and/or prevent the aggravation of moderate scoliotic curves, particularly as the parents of a child suffering from scoliosis don't necessarily easily understand a simple wait-and-see monitoring approach once scoliosis has been diagnosed. The defenders of this type of treatment subscribe to this kind of logic.

According to detractors, studies regarding a Physical Therapy (PT) based treatment mainly concern populations with non-severe scoliosis, heterogeneous in terms of age and risk of spontaneous aggravation, that are rarely taken into account: the result being that a lack of aggravation could be attributed to the treatment when in fact the natural progression would have had the same result.

It is, therefore, important that the rehabilitative methods currently used for idiopathic scoliosis during the pubertal growth phase be reviewed. Arguments for and against the use of PT alone or in combination with bracing should also be reviewed and any complementary rehabilitation should be targeted pre- or post-operatively in scoliosis surgery.

Problems linked to congenital and neuromuscular scoliosis are not addressed in this document as they are of a different nature. Very early onset scoliosis has other treatment needs as PT programs cannot apply to very young children.

PHYSIOTHERAPY AND SCOLIOSIS GENERALITIES

Conservative therapeutic standards for scoliosis vary from country to country, according to schools of thought and even according to the differing health professionals involved. Using physiotherapy is not a universally established or recognized as being useful. Even if it is rather difficult to explain how isolated exercises can help correct a complex three-dimensional structural deformity like scoliosis, several physiotherapy teams have developed treatment protocols for patients who have deformities that are not yet very pronounced, and over the last few years, have worked on getting these validated.

The exercises used to treat moderate scoliosis curves which do not yet require bracing aim to combine the maintenance or restoration of flexibility of the scoliotic zones, muscular work for active stabilization of the spine, posture correction and sometimes respiratory development in thoracic scoliosis cases. The frequency, intensity and duration of therapy sessions are very variable, according to the protocols.

As far back as scientific publications on scoliosis and the surgical treatment of the latter have been published, and with the advent of increasingly precise indications for severe cases of scoliosis, no reference literature has ever really supported isolated rehabilitative management of scoliosis. With regard to conservative treatments, only bracing has been the subject of lively debates between the proponents of its efficacy and the sceptics.

In 1988, John Lonstein [2] wrote: "from before the dawn of orthopedics in the 18th century, physicians [...] have attempted to treat idiopathic scoliosis with exercises. There has never been a single scientific article documenting the value of exercise. Conversely, there have been publications comparing the results of exercise treatment with a simultaneous control group. No differences have been shown."

In 1999, another renowned orthopedic surgeon, Robert A. Dickson [3], on the subject of conservative treatment of scoliosis declared: "time and common sense prevent me from discussing any other conservative treatment modality than bracing."

Yet as early as 1976, before these publications, during experimental work on mice, the man considered to be the father of scoliotic spinal surgery, Paul Randal Harrington [4], raised questions regarding the possible reversibility of scoliosis, under certain conditions. Harrington was a visionary and was passionate about researching the etiology of the so-called idiopathic scoliosis and the pathogenic distortion process. Several works suggest that scoliosis may have the capacity to correct itself if the underlying cause of its progressive development is eliminated.

With this vision of a possible reversibility or aggravation control in mind, attempts to treat scoliotic curves through exercise programs are not new in Europe. But since the early 2000s, the desire to rationalize and clarify practices which were hitherto fairly undocumented, supporting them with scientific evidence has begun to emerge, driven in particular by a group of international therapists from the International *Society on Scoliosis Orthopaedic and Rehabilitation Treatment* (SOSORT), created in 2004.

The objective of these targeted treatments – Physiotherapy Scoliosis Specific Exercises (PSSE) – are the prevention and reduction of scoliosis aggravation, of discomfort in the back, prevention of respiratory disorders and, finally, the improvement of the esthetic aspect of the back though active and postural correction. Throughout a treatment, therapists must keep in mind that one is not trying to replace bracing when the progression of the scoliosis makes it clearly necessary. These so-called specific therapeutic modalities have bit by bit spread throughout Europe, with variations being developed by different schools and different countries, to eventually extend to the Anglo-Saxon world [5].

REHABILITATION METHODS

The Lyon Method

Historically, Charles Gabriel Pravaz – French orthopedic surgeon and inventor of the hypodermic syringe – in the orthopedic and pneumatic institute he created in Bellevue, Lyon, around 1830, came up with: "a new approach based on a comprehensive series of therapeutic agents to treat the curvatures of the spine."

The current therapeutic method known as the *Lyon approach* began under the impulse of Pierre Stagnara who, while he developed spinal surgery, also opened an orthopedic treatment and scoliosis rehabilitation center. In this center, physiotherapy is often carried out in preparation for, and mainly in addition to the wearing of corrective casting and/or bracing, not as a standard protocol, but rather, having to be adapted to each individual child. It aims to have an early effect on the spine in order to eliminate the asymmetrical constraints that the growing zones of a scoliotic spine usually undergo. Exercises in extension of the thoracic scoliosis zones are contraindicated, whereas kyphosis movements are encouraged while maintaining lumbar lordosis. Segmented corrective passive mobilization of the different curvatures, overall active muscular stabilization through deep spinal muscle action if possible to target a reduction in gibbosity, and proprioception and respiratory work are all regularly used here. Sports is also strongly advised and adapted according to the scoliosis patient's age.

The Schroth Method

Katarina Schroth, who suffered from scoliosis herself, based her first work in 1921 on her own case and developed an intensive functional treatment of scoliosis, in her own institute in Meissen in Germany. Over the last few years it has regained notoriety in many countries, and lately, especially so in the Anglo-Saxon countries.

The analysis of defects and corrections that results from the *Schroth method* (Figure 1) is based on the concept of body blocks that undergo deviation and rotation during the scoliosis process. Active exercises use dynamic 3D postural correction lying down, sitting and standing up in order to restore a normal position to these body blocks. Many tools may be used to carry out these exercises: rehabilitation wall bars, working with rigid or elastic harnesses, cushions, balls.

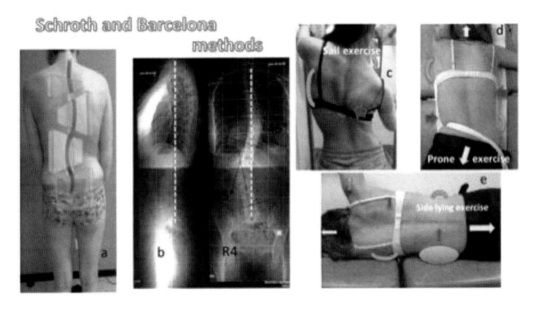

Figure 1. Schroth and Barcelona methods. Assessment using the Barcelona Scoliosis Physical Therapy School system: every type of scoliosis is classified using the so-called block pattern as per K. Schroth's initial work, which was then modified by M. Rigo in 2010. Each block illustrates the shift and rotation of the different scoliosis and pelvic curvatures. This allows the physical therapist to clearly visualize the different elements that need correcting. A correction well taught to the patient imposes three dimensional postural control of his/her spine. During exercise, the patient must produce intense self-correcting force from their own musculoskeletal system, including complete respiratory work, to work on thoracic concavities and convexities. a: illustration of blocks on a patient; b: X-rays; c: sail exercise – to open up the concavity of the thoracic curvature; d: prone exercise – aiming for correction of thoracic and lumbar curvatures; e: side lying exercise – aiming for correction with possibility of adjusting activity with cushions, a lower limb support and asymmetric pelvic traction.

Assessment using the Barcelona Scoliosis Physical Therapy School system: every type of scoliosis is classified using the so-called block pattern as per K. Schroth's initial work, which was then modified by M. Rigo in 2010. Each block illustrates the shift and rotation of the different scoliosis and pelvic curvatures. This allows the physical therapist to clearly visualize the different elements that need correcting. A correction well taught to the patient imposes three dimensional postural control of his/her spine. During exercise, the patient must produce intense self-correcting force from their own musculoskeletal system, including complete respiratory work, to work on thoracic concavities and convexities.

- Exercises performed lying down suppress gravity and help achieve a correction of scoliotic deviations that is more precise and better felt by the patient. The patient who is lying prone uses active axial elongation to achieve detorsion with a localization of the active recruitment of muscles which is as precise as possible, aiming to actively obtain a reduction of gibbosities and an expansion of concave zones. Exercises performed lying on the side are done with foam blocks, in order to have better support of the convex zones and better correction of the spine.
- When standing up or sitting down, one is mindful of the posture, of active correction and of exercises performed with muscle control in maximum intensity in order to try to correct scoliosis curvatures as best as possible.
- Additional correction on these diverse curvatures can be obtained by the therapist with passive guided mobilization.
- It is essential, in this technique, to teach the patient progressively to carry out his exercises by himself. The cumulative daily amount recommended by the program is significant: every day, 10 minutes warmup, supervised group work exercises for 1.5 hours in the morning and the same again in the afternoon, individual physical training of 15 minutes between the two sessions. Additionally, patients carry out their exercises without the therapist's control this time, 1.5 hours twice daily. To that one adds massages and relaxation twice a week, respiratory work aimed at thoracic curvatures in particular; finally, there is a psychological support session.

After a stay, usually at the center, given the density of attention given (6 to 8 hours of daily exercises over 4 to 6 weeks), scoliosis patients have to carry on practicing the specific rehabilitative work they have learned at the center at least 30 minutes every day.

The patient will regularly be seen thereafter in order to update the program and to organize the scoliosis monitoring.

Variations of this program have then been developed in different countries:

- In Germany, under the guidance of Hans-Rudolf Weiss and Axel Hennes [6]: *Integrated Scoliosis Rehabilitation Best Practice Program* – this is a multifaceted program combining: a specific attempt to normalize the sagittal plane, simple exercises to correct scoliosis, if possible 3D, carried out by the patient in their own natural environment, finally, shift exercises inspired by Minn Metha's side-shift exercises.
- In Spain: *the Barcelona Scoliosis Physical Therapy School (BSPTS)* takes up the Schroth approach with active exercises under sensory-motor control and physiotherapist control so that the patient can learn to improve his/her posture

depending not only on the spine's anatomy but also on the quality of the neuro-motor control. The protocol often works together with a bracing treatment where the brace is made according to the orthopedic treatment's therapeutic objective specifications, according to Manuel Rigo [7].

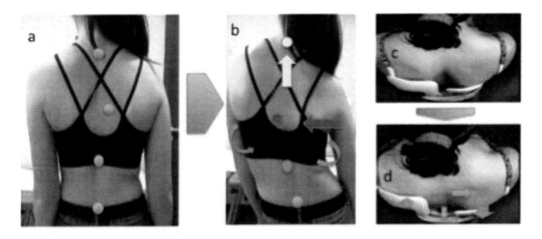

Figure 2. Side shift method. a, b: Patient with a right thoracic curvature - sequence of side shift exercises in the standing position. The arrows illustrate the corrective movement of the spine during side shift exercise. The patient actively shifts her trunk away from the convexity of the curvature while sitting or standing (here standing) and holds the position for ten seconds. c, d: top view of a patient wearing a 3D brace showing the role of breathing coupled with the use of a brace and that of shifts on the shape of the scoliotic trunk and the rebalancing of the spine towards a correction of curvatures on the coronal plane (blue arrow), the sagittal plane (green arrow) and the horizontal plane (orange arrows).

The SEAS Approach

In the early 60s, in Italy, a PSSE-type rehabilitative method was developed with the aim of providing scientific evidence to treatment objectives and their modalities. It resulted in the *SEAS approach*, under the direction of Antonio Negrini, then Stefano Negrini and his collaborators [8]: in close partnership with the Lyon Method on which it based itself to begin with to formalize its own program which aims for:

- active 3D self-correction instead of simple self-elongation which could aggravate the risk of flat back
- muscular stabilization of the spine through active exercise
- calling on self-correction reflexes that can be used in daily activities by the individual
- better patient understanding of the disease and techniques used to help him/her take ownership of them and therefore better comply with the treatment
- individual diversification of exercises to avoid the weariness effect which comes with very repetitive exercises

In the SEAS method, improvement of spinal stability through active self-correction is the main objective. The asymmetric constraint of the growing scoliotic spine results in unbalanced development of the spine, and therefore progressive aggravation of the scoliosis. For Ian Stokes [9] different scoliosis patients adopt different muscular strategies; some of these strategies involve asymmetrical constraints that lead to a progression of the scoliosis during growth while other muscular strategies don't. It was therefore logical for the Negrini team to drawn on this hypothesis in order to try to get the patient who was in a very active rehabilitative mode to draw on his/her virtuous muscular actions.

Moreover, the authors consider that sensitive feedback and exercises could at least contribute to slowing down the scoliosis process. Within this framework, the brace is not only a biomechanical corrective device but also a sensitive stimulation device that can help in the understanding of the misalignment and therefore engage in its correction.

The Side Shift Method

In 1985, Minn Mehta, a well-known personality in the world of scoliosis, described a technique which is still used nowadays: the *side shift* [10]. The method (Figure 2) consists in having the patient carry out an active lateral translation toward the concave scoliotic curve; the lateral movement at the lower extremity of the curvature is reduced or inversed and the curve is then corrected; once the correction is done, patients must hold the position 10 seconds then return to the neutral position and repeat the exercise at least 30 times daily, then as often as possible, particularly when they have been sitting down, which are periods during which they must maintain the corrected position as long as possible. Then, T. Maruyama [11] added the hitch exercise to the side shift to treat lumbar and thoracolumbar curvatures: when standing, patients have to raise their heel on the convex side while maintaining their hip and knee in an anatomical position in order to actively correct the scoliosis curve by reducing the convex zone; the correction must be maintained for 10 seconds and this should be repeated at least 30 times daily.

REHABILITATION AND SCOLIOSIS: THEORETICAL AND EXPERIMENTAL CONCEPTS

Cerebral Control in Scoliosis

The spinal engine is a 3D/4D (space and time) structure which requires precise and constant coordination between the central nervous system and the combination of spine and bone structures, muscles, discs, ligament elements and other supportive tissues. It is logical that any change or aggression which modifies this precise, well-constructed structure, particularly in a growing organism, may lead to a deforming pathology, such as spinal scoliosis.

In clinical practice, one easily links the risk of the advent of scoliosis with preliminary central neurological damage such as cerebral palsy in children or a progressive loss of active muscle control and postural tone in patients suffering from myopathy. In another register, the change in discal structures and vertebral arthrosis in older subjects generates scoliosis, particularly the group of lumbar scolioses known as De Novo. This kind of scoliosis is linked to a collapse of the anatomical elements subjected to kyphosis and torsion, leading bit by bit to an evolving discogenic degenerative cascade.

In the field of primary research, experimental data in mice that are genetically melatonin deficient shows that scoliosis develops in these mice if they are made to be bipedal; restoring normal levels of melatonin prevents the development of scoliosis; the topographic target of the dysfunction linked to a lack of melatonin seems to be located in the thalamus paraventricular nucleus. This is in keeping with the fact that most recent studies on the pathogenesis of scoliosis converge toward one or several problems in the central nervous system. But the indispensable condition for this is bipedalism as this deficiency has no effect in quadruped mice [12, 13].

The control of posture, of walking, depends on multiple sources of somato and sensory-motor, visual, vestibular information that act through several connections in the brain. The programs in the motor areas of the brain act to enable anticipatory postural adjustments, to restore balance or to carry out very specific movements [14].

The study of postural instability in scoliosis patients, even at small angles, shows significant alteration with lower postural performance in AIS, this being linked with the deformities even if all these patients have a Cobb angle of less than 25°; even if in simple studies of static posturography differences already exists, studies in dynamic mode show a loss of efficiency in the information processing system, particularly the proprioceptive system; subjects also have huge difficulties in using anticipatory strategies when faced with provoked imbalances and rely more to reactive strategies [15].

Scoliosis and the Spine Muscles

Muscles, aponeuroses and fascia represent the often forgotten parts of the spine, yet, they make-up half of the mass of the entire rachis. Muscles are an essential component of the spine biomechanics because they help regulate moments of flexion – extension, of lateral inflexion and torsion, and counteract shearing forces. Their functional failure is increasingly highlighted among the etiological causes of a loss of alignment of the spine, particularly on the sagittal plane. The anatomy of spine muscles should be reviewed, starting with fundamental functional concept based on muscle-aponeuroses-tendon synergy. The works of Zajac, Ettema and Huijing have provided a new vision of the internal morphology of muscles with a notion of muscle pennation and a better understanding of the significance of the aponeurosis function (Figure 3).

The essential role in maintaining the spine's attitude is attributed to the postural muscle tone, particularly with permanent contractions of the paravertebral muscles; their numerous neuromuscular spindles assimilate them, their mechanical role aside, to tension regulator captors. The muscle must not be seen as a simple set of muscle fascicles; the aponeurosis is the intrinsic complementary element of the muscle which ensures functional continuity from the endomysium collagen tissue to the tendon structure with which it attaches to the bone. The aponeurosis has a mechanical purpose: it plays the role of a rubber band which, when under tension beyond its relaxed length, stores strength (which requires energy expenditure to be placed under tension) and when tension ends, it recovers its initial length and therefore restores the stored energy. A parallel should be drawn between muscle action, the flexibility or rigidity of muscle chains and the notion that the spine is a tensegrity structure made-up of vertebral bodies separated by discs and held together by ligaments, fascia and muscles. The mechanical stability of the spine heavily depends on the balance between spine compression and the tension in the musculoligamentous structures: without pre-tension, the spine becomes unstable and collapses, with too much tension it buckles. According to the tensegrity principle, balanced tension is what provides stability.

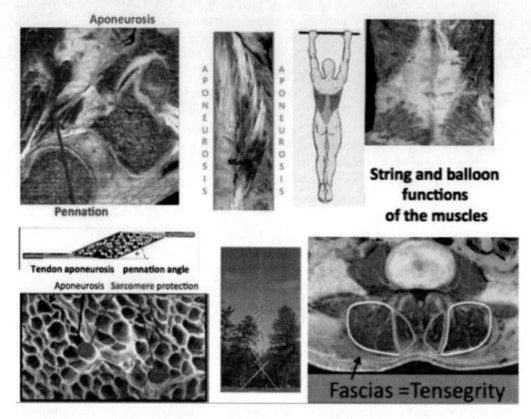

Figure 3. Action of muscles and aponeurosis on the spine. Muscle power is provided by the sarcomere (red structure), modulated by the pennation angle of muscle fibers but all around the aponeurosis structures (white structures), while fascias participate in the mechanics of the spine. These elements are integrated into one complete functional unit that links muscles – aponeurosis – tendons. Tensegrity is the stabilization that is enabled by the dynamics of tension and compression (vertebral bone structures, discs, aponeurosis, ligaments, fascias, muscles). Spine muscles have two activities: elongation-contraction which is completed by the energy release of aponeurosis tensioning during contraction and by their fascias, a "balloon" function providing stability to the spine.

Joris Crijns et al. [16] modeled how growth under the effect of posterior and anterior tensions that limit the spine's freedom might, by following the tensegrity principle, lead to a scoliotic spine model. Several animal studies manage to obtain scoliotic spines in immature animals by implanting tethers. The histological examination of these scoliotic zones shows asymmetrical vertebral growth and a remodeling of the discs whereas under conditions of modulated constraint the growth zones remain active [17]. In the animal experimental models, tethering is the key to developing scoliosis. When the tether is removed, the spine deformity no longer increases even if growth still occurs in the young test animal.

Modeling the muscles also helps to move forward in the understanding of their biomechanical action. Muscles that act on the spine seem to use two different kinds of mechanisms: the first is the activity of muscles in elongation–contraction with motor action and also restitution of energy with the help of their internal aponeurotic structures – an integral part of the muscular apparatus; the second, works through the contraction of muscles encased in their peripheral aponeurotic compartment and their fascia encasing spine muscles: that "balloon" effect gives the spine its stability. Beyond modification measures of CSAs (cross sectional areas) of the target muscles (erector spinae, multifidus, psoas major) and the quantification of fatty infiltration of these muscles, related to ageing and/or degenerative damage to the spine, current research exploits ultrasound and MRI data in order to obtain quantitative calculations of muscle volumes. Mathematical modeling methods progressively integrate posture control to the anatomy, working from proprioceptive information [18] toward personalized global models in order to understand the vicious circles that take place when postural alignment and/or the muscle system is altered in order to try and prevent the evolution of certain spinal pathologies.

Several works by a team in Kansas City have found an asymmetry in the quality and histology of paravertebral muscles between the concave and convex sides of the scoliotic spines. The study of muscle strength in isometric rotation movements in scoliosis patients (Biodex balance assessment; Shirley, NY) also shows an asymmetry in the performance between concave and convex rotation muscles [19]. The results of tests seem significantly lower when in contraction toward the concavity of the main curb compared with contractions toward convexity. This same team tried to implement an intensive muscular program during a pilot study, aiming to correct this asymmetry of rotation muscle strength with 4-month long intensive work using a torso rotation machine (32 training sessions, each lasting about 25 minutes). After 4 months, strength gained during the tests was of 28% to 50%, thus demonstrating the possibility of regaining strength, and above all, of normalizing the imbalance that was initially seen in scoliosis patients. The analysis of results also seemed to show a short term stabilization of the Cobb angle of scoliosis curvatures, but it was not confirmed in the longer term [20].

Scoliosis and Its Vicious Cycle

In his vicious cycle theory, Ian Stokes [21] proposed (Figure 4) that scoliosis imposes asymmetrical constraints to vertebral growth zones: unbalanced growth of vertebrae and disc remodeling are the responses to these non-symmetrical forces. The progression of scoliosis occurs when rapid growth of the spine is added to these biomechanical phenomena. In an experimental study on muscles strategies [9], the simulation creates corrective muscle activations that could, at least in experimental theory, inverse the vicious cycle. According to this simulation, the probability of progression of the scoliosis would depend on the individual strategy used to activate the muscles of the spine; this might lead one to believe that conservative management (PT and bracing) generally might, at least theoretically, influence the progression of scoliosis

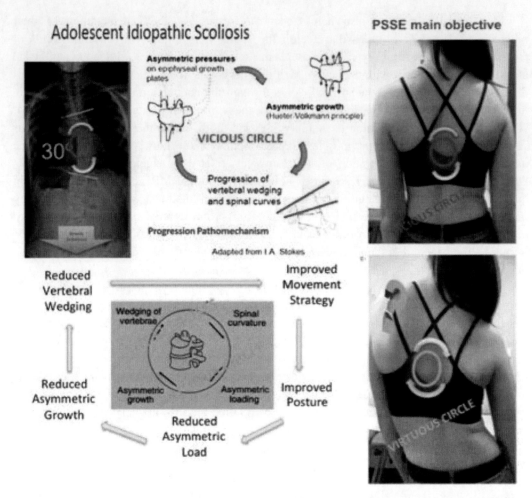

Figure 4. Mechanobiology of treatment. Vertebral growth is modulated by loading according to the Huetter Volkmann principle. After the onset of scoliosis, the orientations of the vertebrae were modified in all three planes, and as a result, the spine became mechanically unstable. As a result of this mechanical instability, intervertebral pressures no longer were distributed equally. Osseous growth was perturbed and the vertebrae became deformed. These asymmetrical constraints produce – through a vicious cycle mechanism (Ian Stokes) – spine deformation (vertebrae, discs, musculo-ligamentous structures) which in turn increases the asymmetrical constraints on the growth zones. If the onset of the scoliotic process is the result of impaired dynamic balance, its correction (virtuous cycle) can – before a vicious cycle process is established – hope to counteract the deformation mechanism.

ASSESSMENT OF PHYSIOTHERAPY IN THE TREATMENT OF SCOLIOSIS

According to SRS guidelines, rational indications for PSSEs (Figure 5) might be low angle progressive curves in not yet mature AIS patients, in order to:

- Reduce deformity and/or prevent progression
- Limit the need to eventually require bracing for the less marked curves
- Limit in conjunction with bracing the eventual need for surgery for the more marked curves

What assessment data is available in literature?

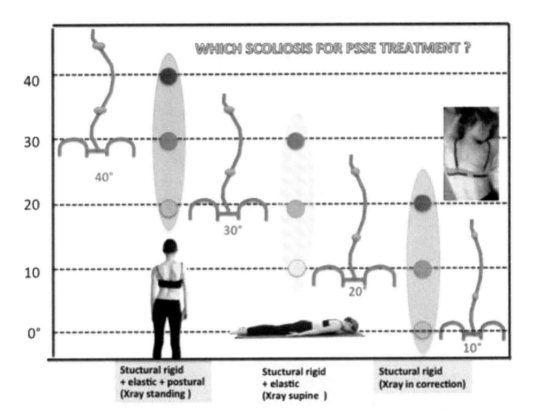

Figure 5. Indication for PSSE treatment according to the severity of a scoliosis. PSS treatments are based on the acknowledgement of deformation, on three-dimensional self-correction to ensure normal spine alignment is restored, on learning muscle stabilization exercises and regularly carrying these out as a daily routine. Scoliotic curvatures include three components that accumulate when the subject is standing; when in supine position, the postural element disappears; when in bending correction posture, or with other reduction techniques, only the rigid structural element remains. A severe scoliotic curvature (red circles) will not respond favorably to rehabilitation techniques alone, as they will not sufficiently correct the significantly rigid element; reduction and permanent bracing are usually indicated. A more moderate and particularly flexible curvature (yellow circles) will stand a greater chance of responding to PSSE treatment. As for intermediary forms (green circles), a PSSE program is usually complementary to orthopedic treatment, sometimes in the form of nighttime hyper-corrective bracing.

- *Simon Mordecai* [22] reviewed the *Centre of Evidence Based Medicine* studies published in English according to their level of evidence: he noted that patient inclusion criteria are often missing, measurements of scoliosis severity are variable, treatment compliance is rarely taken into account and results at the end of a program are assessed in a very disparate fashion. Several studies speak of significant results regarding the Cobb angle post treatment but, in most cases, the differences noted remains below any kind of normal variability and the so-called positive progressions are not reviewed on the longer term to assess if they are maintained in time and with the rest of growth. All in all, for Mordecai, the quality

of the studies is poor and there is no real scientific evidence to support the use of isolated rehabilitation, be it conventional or within a PSSE program.
- In a Cochrane systematic review of 2012 [23], *Michele Romano* has also concluded to a lack of quality scientific studies that might recommend the isolated use of PSSE in cases of AIS.
- Wishing to qualify the issue of whether rehabilitation is effective or not, *Stefano Negrini* asked the question in a 2014 RCT[24] as to how many patients at risk of progression one should treat before reaching the point of bracing implementation fixed at 30°: the answer given is a *number needed to treat* (NNT) of 6. For Negrini, one must treat 6 patients to avoid one of them having an aggravation that leads to bracing. This still requires confirmation because the trial deals with low grade Cobb angle curves that have not yet reached orthopedic treatment stage and whose risk of spontaneous progression is not constant, therefore it is hard to draw a conclusion regarding the real preventive role of the treatment.

It is useful that there should be research that attempts to validate PT – PSSE and their capacity to improve on natural progression, but currently, in order to assess a treatment, one must from the start take into account that the significance of the deformity and patient maturity may be very variable [25, 26]. What's more, it would appear that in progressive scoliosis there is a specific 3D phenotype which appears early on for curves that are still at a very low Cobb angle, but from the start they appear to be engaged in a significant torsional process. Developing a reliable index of severity would be extremely useful in order to be able to guide these types of scolioses toward active modes of therapy if the risk of progression is virtually confirmed [27].

Rehabilitation treatments, just like bracing, are a constraint for the patient as well as representing a significant cost to society. They should not be implemented without an argument for their usefulness or at the expense of educational and sporting activities. It's up to treatments to demonstrate with enough scientific evidence – perhaps with the help of new noninvasive modes of exploration – their efficacy per se, as well as to what degree this efficacy works.

PHYSIOTHERAPY AND BRACING

Rehabilitation Programs

PT exercises – whether alone or in addition to bracing – are commonly used in a number of countries for AIS patients. The exercises that are more specifically targeted for brace wearers have very varied objectives, according to the different schools specialized in scoliosis. For some, these must be carried out independently from the brace – that is, the PT protocol would be identical whether the patient wears a brace or not. For others, specific exercises for device wearers are useful in working toward a synergy of action with bracing. Sometimes exercises are also used in preparation for the implementation of a brace. For exercises that are carried out when the brace is worn, the objective is to maximize the reduction force exerted by both bracing and exercises carried out at once.

Fabio Zaina [28] has conducted a study on the influence of SEAS (Scientific Exercises Approach to Scoliosis) regarding the loss of angle when bracing was very progressively being stopped, weaning having begun once the patient reached Risser stage 3. At the end of treatment, in control patients (No exercises done: 10 patients) there was a loss of +4° in Cobb angle and in SEAS patients (SEAS: 14 patients) there was no loss of Cobb angle.

Kenny Yat Hong Kwan [29] studied the value of a Schroth-type program when combined with bracing (experimental group) compared to bracing alone (control group). The authors started from the conclusions drawn from the BRAIST Study [30] which certainly demonstrates the therapeutic efficacy of bracing in AIS – under conditions where the brace has been worn long enough – but also shows a significant percentage of patients whose scoliosis continues to worsen despite bracing. It is therefore legitimate to attempt to improve treatment results with a therapeutic complement to bracing. The advantage of the Schroth technique is that it is specific to the type of curvature and once it has been learned it can be practiced in everyday activities enabling the patients to be freer to practice sporting and leisure activities.

The rehabilitation program is carried out over 8 weeks in outpatient care: 4 individual sessions with a therapist, once every two weeks, where exercises are shown and taught, then controlled. Then, a program of home exercises is established, with patients returning for feedback with their physiotherapist every 2 months.

An important observation has been made in this study: patients who diligently carry out the prescribed exercises are often the same ones who are compliant with regard to brace wearing.

The results of the work demonstrated an improvement of at least 6° in Cobb angle for 17% of patients in the experimental group versus 4% for the control group, but with different follow-up period of 39 (+/- 11) months for the control group and 18 (+/-6) months for the SSE group. When closely monitoring the effective implementation of exercises for the experimental group, only the patients who respected the exercise plan improved compared to the control group.

What remains to be seen is if this can be reproduced and confirmed in larger series and what degree of improvement one can observe: beyond the Schroth technique, it is the same for other PSSE rehabilitation methods? What is the optimum frequency of exercises, their total quantity? What are the actual effects of the exercises according to whether there is bracing compliance or not?

Sanja Schreiber [31] conducted a similar study with patients who were predominantly braced (68% of the cohort): two groups with an identical risk of progression (65% risk according to Carlson and Lonstein) follow, in addition to their brace, either a standard PT program (control group) or a Schroth PSSE program (experimental group) involving 1 hour of exercise a week under the supervision of a therapist, plus 30 to 45 minutes of exercise at home, over 6 months.

The radiographic assessment includes two measurements: the Largest Curve (LC) and the Sum of Curves (SOC) according to the Cobb method.

The aim is to define the Number Needed to Treat (NNT), the calculation of which is: $NNT = \frac{1}{CER-EER}$ where CER is Control Event Rate and EER is the Experimental Event Rate. The CER and EER are the proportion of patients in the control and experimental group, respectively, who deteriorated by $> 5°$ for the LC or by $>10°$ for the SOC.

Results show that over a 6 month therapeutic intervention one patient will avoid LC deterioration by > 5° or SOC deterioration by >10°, respectively, for every four participants undergoing Schroth PSSE intervention to standard of care compared to receiving standard of care only.

PT and Quality of Integrated Care

The BRAIST Study [30] demonstrated the efficacy of bracing in reducing surgery rates in AIS but the NNT of subjects to avoid surgery is not always identical: where good compliance was verified with electronic sensors integrated into the brace, the NNT was of 3; where monitoring of brace wearing was less controlled, the NNT rose up to 7.

Another study carried out at the *Texas Scottish Rite Hospital* in Dallas, which is a world renowned orthopedic center [32], results show again that patient compliance is hard to obtain: 31% of them wear their brace for 10 hours or more per 24 hours and only 13% wear it 14 hours or more. For the authors of the study, there are many factors that contribute to adherence difficulties with bracing: the discomfort of wearing the device, the awkwardness of the patient with regard to other teenagers and the change in their image at a time when one is precisely building this image. Certain patients may decide that taking the risk of progressing towards surgery is preferable to wearing a brace as prescribed by caregivers. The study also shows that only 44% of patients who virtually do not wear the brace that was prescribed by an expert center spine specialist end up with an indication for surgery which would seem to demonstrate that the bracing indication in these cases was not useful. It is therefore essential to thoroughly target prescriptions in order not to treat patients where there is no benefit to be gained.

The emerging question in the face of these difficulties with a bracing scoliosis treatment is: why is treatment compliance so low? The simplest overall answer is that it is because the patient feels his/her quality of life is affected too much with bracing. A more in-depth analysis of this observation highlights several challenges: the physical problem of discomfort and sometimes external compression pain, the feeling of overall physical constraint and limitation with regard to taking part in team sports activities. The feeling of functional constraint also plays a part with regard to day-to-day activities, causing emotional problems due to the negative image of oneself and with the others when having to wear visible bracing. Finally, there is also a more social problem: life at school, the common living environment of teenagers, when having to wear a brace.

In order to improve treatment compliance and results, one should consider all these difficulties thoroughly, with an often useful monitoring of actual wearing of the brace, with the search for optimization of comfort, with improvement in bracing design as well as the presence of an entire team of caregivers who are attentive to the child's needs. Following the experience of the *Hôspital Sainte Justine* in Montréal [34], the entire team – nurses, physician-surgeon, psychologist, physiotherapist – gets involved when a drop in brace-wearing compliance is observed. According to the particular issues the child faces, remedial actions are targeted, with each specialist acting according to need. The physiotherapists seeing the patient regularly is a key factor in the overall quality of the care.

PHYSIOTHERAPY AND POST-SURGERY SCOLIOSIS

Pulmonary and Lung Function Issues

Bracing has been accused of being responsible for reducing lung function. A Swedish 25 year-long monitoring program [34] of AIS patients with a Cobb angle curves of 28° on average at the start of their bracing treatment, with the brace being worn on average for 4.8 years, resulting in 22° at the end of treatment and 36° at final monitoring, long after the brace ceased to be worn: did not show any significant change in Vital Capacity (VC % predicted according to height and age). Even if during spirometric exploration while wearing a brace, some decrease in lung volume was described, probably due to the external compression of the rib cage, in this very long term study, VC increased from 77% of the VC predicted before treatment to 89% 25 years after the start of treatment, showing no long term difference compared to patients who were not treated who had scoliosis with a Cobb angle which was identical to those who had had been braced, at the time of the final control. Pulmonary and respiratory complications are relatively often documented following spine surgery in AIS: their incidence varies from 0.6 to 3.5%. Even if these complications are often rather poorly described in literature, it seems legitimate to research whether there may be a correlation with preoperative lung function and/or with the severity of the scoliosis curvature. It would appear that the significance of the curvature in AIS does have a correlation, even if only partial, with the risk of postoperative pulmonary complications. The reduction in thoracic lordosis is a particularly strong predictive factor of risk: for the more pronounced hypokyphosis (10° or less kyphosis) the risk is clear. In surgery, that could have an effect on the technique chosen and correction sought, and even be deciding factor as to the usefulness of preoperative respiratory preparation PT [35]. The impact of a non-specific physical lung function rehabilitation program – 10 minutes warm up, aerobic exercises on a mat or on a rehabilitation bike for 40 minutes for a workout at 60-80% maximum heart rate and then 10 minutes of cool down exercises: the entire sequence repeated 3 times a week – on the lung function of a scoliosis surgery candidate (thoracic curve between 45° and 88°) translates as an increased Forced Vital Capacity (the total amount of air that can be forcibly blown out after full inspiration, measured in liters), Inspiratory Capacity, Forced Expiratory Volume 1 (the amount of air that car be forcibly out in 1 second, measured in liters) and of the physical performance assessed with a 6-min walk test. Even if the differences between subjects carrying out the program and the controls are not huge, they are statistically significant [36].

The Role of PT in Early Rehabilitation of an Operated AIS Spine

Rehabilitation may begin, if this is possible, before the operation: around 6 weeks before surgery, patients carry out aerobic exercises 3 times a week, in 30 minute sessions. The intensity of the exercises done is defined depending on the patient's capacity; they also carry out active work on the extensor muscles that provide spine stability, and work on flexibility, if possible twice a day, repeating 20 exercises per set. With the same goal of physical and psychological preparation for the procedure, the patients are, wherever possible, put introduced to a support team where they will meet or contact teens of their age who have already benefited, as they are about to, from scoliosis surgery with the same team, so that they can share their experience and avoid needless fears. In the early postoperative phase, the team must follow the instructions which have been planned preoperatively regarding the first movements out of the bed: at the very start, avoid torsions of the area operated on and show extreme care for the initial trunk bending movements. The patient rapidly gets out of bed: POD 1-2, then begins walking on a flat surface within the limits of his/her tolerance, then, when he/she feels capable, begins bit by bit to walk up and down the stairs. The patient must build up his/her ability to sit up in other places than the bed progressively, working up to 4 daily sequences in a sitting posture. The therapist must teach the patient simple exercises: bending stretches of the cervical spine, working the alignment and head position in the mirror for visual management, pelvis control, particularly in the sagittal plane, progressive work on the gluteal stabilizers and the non-operated bottom part of the lumbosacral region. The program must be well integrated, particularly following the surgeon's recommendations, within a team-based approach, therefore with the nursing staff, the anesthetists who manage pain and monitor the postoperative medical condition, the patient's future caregivers once he/she has left the hospital sector, while also explaining and explaining again to the patient and his/her family that the goal of the instructions is a quick (usually POD 4-5) but safe discharge from hospital. Upon leaving, the patient must be capable of performing – with or without the help of caregivers – a list of physical activities (but in the check list there is also: having controlled and decreasing pain, no clinical sign of infection and/or have a clean dressing, and tolerating oral feeding):

- Being autonomous in his/her bed and for transfers out of the bed
- Being able to remain seated out of the bed at least 1.5 to 2 hours, and this at least twice a day
- Having a near-autonomous ability when moving on a flat surface
- Being able to walk up or down one floor
- Having understood and being able to put into words the precautions he/she must keep in mind during activities until the next visit with the surgeon, often within 3 to 4 weeks, for instance and especially not carrying heavy weights (> 5-6 kgs) without explicitly being allowed to do so, and not engaging in contact sports.

Most often, except in specific cases, a return to school will occur a month after the procedure. Even if these recommendations are personalized according to the type of surgery, surgeon, protocols, usually, dynamic sports involving no major contact is allowed around 6 to 12 months after surgery.

Working toward an Accelerated Discharge Protocol

These protocols are increasingly used following major orthopedic surgery, essentially prosthetic, in adults. The standard duration of a surgical stay in AIS is of 5 to 7 or possibly 10 days. In 2016, James O. Sanders [37] sought to determine whether an accelerated program might reduce the hospital stay, and what impact this may have on the risk of postoperative complications and the management of postoperative pain. Rehabilitation through PT succeeds fully in doing so as an accelerated program is the result of a coordinated effort between nursing staff, PT, the pain management team, surgery of course, all aiming to rapidly facilitate the ability to walk and use standardized pain management. For instance, the staff helps the patient to sit on the edge of the bed or on a seat near the bed on the evening of the day surgery took place, then again on the following day (POD 0 and 1). PT should help with walking on the evening of POD1. Then, the nursing staff helps the patient to walk twice a day without any specific precautions to the spine or need for constant physiotherapist supervision. In the end, patients in an accelerated program usually stay 3.7 days compared to the standard 5-6 day program. The incidence of complications does not seem to increase and the overall cost of surgery is reduced by 22% in the fast track program. In another work by Nicholas D. Fletcher comparing fast track vs conventional programs [38], with more than 100 patients in the fast track program, versus 50 in a conventional program, the conclusions are just as positive for the fast track program with a 50% reduction in hospitalization. With no increase in complications, one observes a drop in costs, an earlier return home as well as a rapid return to normal life for the operated children and their families. Of course, these programs are very demanding in terms of quality and they imply that the entire care team – PT included – be coordinated, reactive and follow a strict protocol.

CONCLUSION

The scoliotic spine is a complex universe involving the musculoskeletal system, the nervous system controlling postural balance, genetics, the laws of biomechanics that control the chain of balance of an upright subject in order to maintain him/her in his/her cone of economy. Due to a probable neuromuscular asymmetry linked to genetics and/or metabolic disorders, a deformity of the spine begins as a progressive torsion in the coronal, sagittal and mainly horizontal planes. It is amplified with growth – a real revolution which is dependent on the growth cartilages which run the show – and can worsen in terms of form and quality into a vicious circle of deformity. As a result, alignments will change but dynamics will too, as will the harmonious balance of movement and a normal maturation of the musculoaponeurotic structures which are essential to the future of the spine. Progressive scoliosis implies orthopedic treatment as it is an orthopedic condition but the growing child who is developing physically and psychologically makes it a pediatric condition too. Rehabilitation programs bring with them the hope of being able to influence the risk of progression. Currently, the level of evidence is insufficient to substitute them to the conservative reference bracing treatment, but they may prepare, and above all, complete or even optimize the action of bracing. For the patient at the center of the program, the constraint imposed by the brace can be overcome if there is a strong close knit and attentive team and rehabilitation must be a privileged moment aiming to rapidly identify and treat any problems caused by the treatment.

REFERENCES

[1] Ponseti IV, Friedman B. Prognosis in idiopathic scoliosis. *J Bone Joint Surg Am.* 1950; 32A(2):381-95.
[2] Lonstein, JE, Winter, RB: AIS; nonoperative treatment. *Orthopedic Clinics NA* 1988; 19: 239–245.

[3] Dickson, RA.: Spinal deformity—AIS. Nonoperative treatment. *Spine* 1999; 24: 2601–2606.

[4] Harrington PR. Is scoliosis reversible? In vivo observations of reversible morphological changes in the production of scoliosis in mice. *Clin Orthop Relat Res.* 1976; 116:103-11.

[5] Berdishevsky H, Lebel VA, Bettany-Saltikov J, Rigo M, Lebel A, Hennes A, Romano M, Białek M, M'hango A, Betts T, de Mauroy JC, Durmala J. Physiotherapy scoliosis-specific exercises- a comprehensive review of seven major schools. *Scoliosis Spinal Disord.* 2016; Aug 4; 11:20.

[6] Weiss HR: Influence of an in-patient exercise program on scoliotic curve. Italian *Journal of Orthopedics and Traumatology* 1992; 18:395-406.

[7] Weiss HR, Negrini S, Rigo M, Kotwicki T, Hawes MC, Grivas TB, Maruyama T, Landauer F. Indications for conservative management of scoliosis (guidelines) SOSORT guideline committee. *Stud Health Technol Inform.* 2008;135:164-70.

[8] Negrini S, Antonini G, Carabalona R, Minozzi S: Physical exercises as a treatment for adolescent idiopathic scoliosis. A systematic review. *Ped Rehab* 200; 6:227-235.

[9] Stokes IAF, Gardner-Morse M. Muscle activation strategies and symmetry of spinal loading in the lumbar spine with scoliosis. *Spine* 2004; 29; 19: 2103-2107.

[10] Mehta MH. Active correction by side shift; an alternative treatment for early idiopathic scoliosis. In: *Scoliosis prevention*. New York, Praeger 1985, pp.126-140.

[11] Maramuya T, Kitagawa T, Takeshita K, Nakamura K. Side shift exercise for idiopathic scoliosis after skeletal maturity. In: *Research into Spinal Deformities* 4, IOS Press, 202, pp.361-364.

[12] Machida M, Dubousset J, Yamada T, Kimura J, Saito M, Shiraishi T, Yamagishi M. Experimental scoliosis in melatonin-deficient C57BL/6J mice without pinealectomy. *J Pineal Res.* 2006; 41(1):1-7.

[13] Machida M, Dubousset J, Miyake A, Yagi M, Takemitsu M. *The possible pathogenesis in adolescent idiopathic scoliosis based on experimental model of melatonin-deficient C57BL/6J mice.* Paper presented by Jean Dubousset at the annual meeting of the Scoliosis Research Society 2016, Prague, Tchequoslovaquia September 21-24.

[14] Takakusaki K. Functional neuroanatomy for posture and gait control. *J Mov Disord.* 2017;10(1):1-17.

[15] Haumont T, Gauchard G, Lascombes P, Perrin P. Postural Instability in Early-Stage Idiopathic Scoliosis in Adolescent Girls. *Spine* 2011; 36(13): 847-854.

[16] Crijns TJ, Stadhouder A, Smit, Theodoor H. Restrained Differential Growth: The Initiating Event of Adolescent Idiopathic Scoliosis? *Spine* 2017 42(12):726-732.

[17] Zhang YG, Zheng GQ, Zhang XS, Wang Y, Scoliosis Model Created by Pedicle Screw Tethering in Immature Goats: The Feasibility, Reliability, and Complications. *Spine* 2009; 34(21): 2305-2310.

[18] Pomero V, Lavaste F, Imbert G, Skalli W. A proprioception based regulation model to estimate the trunk muscle forces. *Comput Methods Biomech. Biomed. Engin.* 2004; 7 (6):331-8.

[19] McIntire KL, Asher MA, Burton DC, Liu W. Trunk rotational asymmetry in adolescents with idiopathic scoliosis: an observational study. *Scoliosis* 2007; 2:9.

[20] McIntire KL, Asher MA, Burton DC, Liu W. Treatment of adolescent idiopathic scoliosis with quantified trunk rotational strength training: a pilot study. *Clinical Spine Surgery* 2008; 21 (5): 349-358.

[21] Stokes IAF, Spence H, Aronsson DD, Kilmer N. Mechanical modulation of vertebral body growth. *Spine* 1996; 21 (10): 1162-1167.

[22] Mordecai SC, Dabke HV Efficacy of exercise therapy for the treatment of adolescent idiopathic scoliosis: a review of the literature. *Eur. Spine J.* (2012) 21: 382-389.

[23] Romano M, Minozzi S, Zaina F, Saltikov JB, Chockalingam N, Kotwicki T, Hennes AM, Negrini S. Exercises for adolescent idiopathic scoliosis: a Cochrane systematic review. *Spine* 2013; 38(14): 883-93.

[24] Negrini S, De Mauroy JC, Grivas TB, Knott T, Kotwicki T, Maruyama T, O'Brien JP, Rigo M, Zaina F. Actual evidence in the medical approach to adolescents with idiopathic scoliosis. *Eur. J. Phys. Rehabil. Med.* 2014; 50:87-92.

[25] Lonstein JE, Carlson JM. The prediction of curve progression in untreated idiopathic scoliosis during growth. *J Bone Joint Surg Am.* 1984; 66(7):1061-71.

[26] Sanders JO, Khoury JG, MD, Kishan S, MD, Browne RH, Mooney III JF, Arnold KD, McConnell SJ, Bauman JA, Finegold DN. Predicting Scoliosis Progression from Skeletal Maturity: A Simplified Classification During Adolescence. *J Bone Joint Surg Am.* 2008; 90: 540-53.

[27] Skalli W, Vergari C, Ebermeyer E, Courtois I, Drevelle X, Kohler R, Abelin-Genevois K, Dubousset J. Early detection of progressive adolescent idiopathic scoliosis. *Spine* 2017; 42(11): 823-830.

[28] Zaina F, Negrini S, Atanasio S, Fusco C, Romano M, Negrini A. Specific exercises performed in the period of brace weaning can avoid loss of correction in adolescent idiopathic scoliosis (AIS) patients: Winner of SOSORT's 2008 award for best clinical paper. *Scoliosis* 2009, 4: 1-8.

[29] Yat Hong Kwan K, Cheng ACS, Yu Koh H, Chiu AYY, Man Chee Cheung K. Effectiveness of Schroth exercises during bracing in adolescent idiopathic scoliosis: results from a preliminary study- "SOSORT Award 2017 Winner". *Scoliosis and Spinal Disorders* 2017; 12:32.

[30] Weinstein SL, Dolan LA, Wright JG, Dobbs MB. Effects of bracing in adolescents with idiopathic scoliosis. *N Engl J Med.* 2013; 369(16):1512-21.

[31] Schreiber S, Parent EC, Hill DL, Hedden DM, Moreau MJ, Southon SC Schroth physiotherapeutic scoliosis-specific exercises for adolescent idiopathic scoliosis: how many patients require treatments to prevent one deterioration? – results from a randomized controlled trial – "SOSORT 2017 Award Winner" *Scoliosis and Spinal Disorders* 2017; 12: 26.

[32] Sanders JO, Newton PO, Browne RH, Katz D, Birch JG, Herring JH. Bracing for Idiopathic Scoliosis: How Many Patients Require Treatment to Prevent One Surgery? *J Bone Joint Surg Am.* 2014; 96:649-53.

[33] Labelle H. A new paradigm for optimizing brace treatment in adolescent idiopathic scoliosis. *Society of Orthopaedic and Rehabilitation Treatment 2017,* Lyon, France May 4-6.

[34] Pehrsson K, Danielsson A, Nachemson A. Pulmonary function in adolescent idiopathic scoliosis: a 25 year follow up after surgery or start of brace treatment. *Thorax* 2001; 56:388-93.

[35] Newton PO, Faro FD, Gollogly S, Betz RR, Lenke LG, Lowe TG. Results of preoperative pulmonary function testing of adolescents with idiopathic scoliosis. A study of six hundred and thirty-one patients. *J Bone Joint Surg Am.* 2005 Sep; 87(9):1937-46.

[37] Dos Santos Alves VL, Stirbulov R, Avanzi O. Impact of a physical rehabilitation program on the respiratory function of adolescents with idiopathic scoliosis. *Chest.* 2006; 130(2):500-5.

[37] Sanders AE, Andras LM, Sousa T, Kissinger K, Cucchiaro G, Skaggs DL Accelerated discharge protocol for posterior spinal fusion patients with adolescent idiopathic scoliosis decreases hospital postoperative charges 22%. S*pine* 42 (2): 92-97.

[38] Fletcher ND, Shourbaji N, Mitchell PM, Oswald TS, Devito DP, Bruce RW. Clinical and economic implications of early discharge following posterior spinal fusion for adolescent idiopathic scoliosis. *J Child Orthop.* 2014; 8(3):257-63.

Chapter 11

THE SCOLIOSIS SPECIFIC PHYSICAL ORTHOPEDIC TEST™: CREATING CONSERVATIVE STREAMS OF CARE FOR YOUTH WITH ADOLESCENT IDOPATHIC SCOLIOSIS (AIS) USING EXERCISE, LIFESTYLE AND MAINTENANCE

Suzanne Clements Martin
Pilates Therapeutics, Alameda, California US

ABSTRACT

The diagnosis of an asymmetrical spinal curve, or scoliosis, is a significant event in the life of a youth. Scoliosis affects many bodily systems, requiring a whole-body system of conservative care intervention, such as the Pilates Method. The goal of the system is to provide the youthful patient with lifestyle adaptations and maintenance programs, converging physical and psychosocial goals, setting up a lifelong habit for a lifelong condition. A multi-disciplinary approach includes judicious exercise, whether or not the youth's condition warrants surgical fixation. The approach for both surgery scenarios addresses both the physical aspects of curve correction and the relevant psychological factors of adolescence.

The chapter introduces a structured program of exercise developed by this writer, the SSPOT™ (Scoliosis Specific Physical and Observational Test), adapted from the Pilates Method created by Joseph Hubertus Pilates. Youth benefit from the general principles of the Pilates Method, which include discipline, precision, centering, flow, breathing, and concentration. A structured program is a safe yet challenging experience to provide a somatic, corrective or conditioning enhancement effect upon body, mind and spirit. The qualified Pilates Movement Educator can provide an optimal conservative stream of care as part of a youthful client's multi-disciplinary scoliosis team.

Keywords: exercise, scoliosis, scoliosis and exercise, adolescence, spinal asymmetry, asymmetry, exercise, Pilates, Pilates method, Pilates method exercise

INTRODUCTION

Scoliosis is a particular category of *spinal asymmetry*. The diagnosis of an asymmetrical spinal curve is a significant event in the life of a youth, and its impact can be lifelong.

Scoliosis is both a medical diagnosis, specifically when the Cobb angle measures beyond ten degrees, the expected physiological norm [1], as well as a basic body type condition. The term *scoliosis* includes both structural and functional asymmetry. For the purposes of this chapter, we define *youth* as between twelve and twenty-two years of age. Although the Tanner Stage Two of reproductive growth spurts begin at approximately age twelve, and the conventional age for skeletal closure is sixteen years for females and seventeen for males, soft tissue, such as musculo-tendinous density and girth along with bony prominence development, continues beyond skeletal closure in addition to social and emotional development completion [2, 3].

We always keep in mind that the ultimate functional goal of adolescence is the successful transition into adulthood, empowering youth with the knowledge and skills needed to take control of their lives [4].

The goal of exercise intervention with youth is to help establish the strongest musculo-skeletal structure to possibly diminish impending structural deformities. The SSPOT™ (Scoliosis Specific Physical and Observational Test) is both a test of strength and flexibility and a framework of exercise goal accomplishment. The SSPOT, in two components discussed further in this Chapter, provides spinal stability, bone-building and functional flexibility through a series of modifications of the Pilates Method Mat Series emphasizing weight-bearing exercises. While specifically made for youth, adults benefit and improve from many elements of the SSPOT as well.

Scoliosis manifests in more ways than a mere lateral curvature, an asymmetry, of the spine. Scoliosis affects many systems. Its significant neuro-physiological and biomechanical impact into the ribcage, pelvis, head and limbs, creates the need for a whole body system of intervention such as the Pilates Method.

Table 1. Transitional sub-stages of adolescence

Defining Adolescence

Early Adolescent (11-13)
    Child ---→ Adolescent
     Initial pubertal transition
     Secondary education transition

Adolescent (14-17)
    Continued pubertal transition
    High school (upper secondary education) transition
    Social independence transition

Young Adult (18-25)
    Adolescent ----→ Adult
     Completed pubertal transition
     Vocational/academic transition
     Social accountability transition

Reprinted with permission. Curtis, Alexa C. (2015) "Defining Adolescence." *Journal of Adolescent and Family Health* 7, no. 2: article, page 25.

Studies citing the benefits of the Pilates Method have included mind-body coordination, thoracic mobility and lumbar spine stability, upper and lower extremity functional improvements as well as enhancement of brain activity [5, 6, 7, 8, 9, 10, 11].

CONSERVATIVE CARE FOR SPINAL ASYMMETRY

Conservative medical care (CMC), by definition, is *care that is not extreme or drastic*. This is the norm of care until certain criteria are met for more aggressive measures. CMC's main goals are to restore or preserve function. The International Scientific Society on Scoliosis Orthopaedic and Rehabilitation Treatment (SOSORT) established guidelines for the conservative care of idiopathic scoliosis and revised them in 2012 [12]. The exercises found in this chapter respect the SOSORT guidelines.

The fundamental goal in conservative physical therapy and/or movement-education intervention for scoliosis for both adolescent and adult age groups includes identification of the asymmetry pattern for that individual along with educating the client how to observe it in themselves [13]. Full conservative care extends into education, not only regarding the specific spinal curve manifestations, but also a functional knowledge of body mechanics (Body Skills), nutrition, energy conservation and generation, exercise for daily comfort and corrective control, emotional stability, and even ergonomic considerations concerning footwear, sleep habits and leisure habits. In essence, we need to provide the youthful patient with a lifestyle adaptation and maintenance program, optimizing physical and psychosocial goals, in order to set up a lifelong habit for a lifelong condition [14].

The conventional use of exercise in the conservative care of scoliosis has a controversial history. Exercise was discouraged in the 1940's and 50's. The prevalence of the scoliosis condition at that time occurred in populations affected by the polio and tuberculosis epidemics [15]. Exercise science was not developed to the extent now evidenced.

The trend away from exercise prescription for those newly diagnosed persisted into the current century. Current trends in scoliosis show that the prevalence of scoliosis in youth today is largely due to unknown causes, idiopathic, and not from infectious or neurologic conditions as was in the past century [16]. With this shift in causal elements is a shift in conservative care involving a multi-disciplinary approach such as physical therapy, occupational therapy, and other physical development practices that dovetail with the medical system.

Evidence points to a change in models that supports conservative intervention whether or not the youth's condition declines to the point of needing surgical intervention. In either case, the judicious use of exercise includes skilled intervention and a working knowledge on the part of the exercise instructor, also known as a movement educator, as to the benefits and limitations of the particular individual's physical and psychosocial needs [17].

The term *conservative* used in this Chapter includes exercise for two situations, one where the youth is not severe in spinal instability or severity of Cobb angle so as to warrant surgery, and one where the youth has elected and received spinal surgical intervention yet can benefit from physical training and exercise to optimize function.

Karen Klippinger, PhD, is a well-known author and instructor of certification of the Pilates Method as well as a continuing education provider on the subjects of anatomy study and kinesiological applications of the Pilates Method to scoliosis. She offers,

"My hope would be that movement specialists from different fields including physical therapy, Pilates, and exercise science will work together to continue to build scientific support for the value of various exercise approaches to potentially reduce the rate of progression of scoliosis, decrease the number of clients with scoliosis who require surgery, or improve the quality of life for adults with scoliosis who are at a lower risk of progression. It is essential that proponents of exercise work together to further this cause and help unveil effective parameters for working with scoliosis."[18].

Other conservative physical therapy and exercise paradigms exist along with the Pilates Method to make up a multi-disciplinary approach. Among the most well-known are the Schroth Method® and Yoga.

The Schroth Method® was developed in the 1920's by physiotherapist Katerina Schroth and is proven to either partially or fully correct the adolescent onset of scoliosis, originally performed in an inpatient setting. Its principles were revolutionary in its three-dimensional and block analysis of the spinal scoliosis curve. Ms. Schroth classified a number of curve types and organized treatment around these specific curve patterns. Schroth Method treatment is based upon the specific curve correction. She advocated use of a mirror so that patients could learn possible postural correction and exercise implementation around the curves. Her Method is still employed in Europe and scattered throughout the United States and Asia.

Yoga for scoliosis was developed in the 1980's by Iyengar Faculty Member Elise Miller and is widely accepted as a beneficial isometric stretch technique for those with scoliosis. Ms. Miller also classified several curve types and advocates specific stretches based upon the specific type category [19, 20].

Since Ms. Schroth's time, both the surgical curve classifications and conservative care protocols expanded to include attention to the postural gravitational curves. This shift is seen in the diagnosis classifications of Dr. Lenke and research of Dr. Piet van Loon, among others. Dr. Lenke's analyses expand into the degree of severity or lack of normal sagittal curve degree. The research of Dr. van Loon further corroborates the sagittal gravitational curve issues by highlighting the need for proper sitting ergonomics and avoidance of prolonged sitting in spinally flexed postures [21, 22].

In addition to spinal skeletal irregularities associated with an asymmetrical spine also include elongation of one humerus, elongated length of ribs engaged in the convex lateral prominence, or gibbus of the scoliosis, shortening of the twelfth rib on the concave side, along with anterior rib cartilage mal-alignment on one side in the region of the floating ribs at ribs 7-10 [23, 24].

Functional issues associated with spinal asymmetry include shoulder girdle dysfunction, heightened lateralization, task limb coordination and preference, eye dominance and compensations during tasks such as walking, compensations which may cause stride length and ground impact differences [25, 26, 27, 28].

Other functional issues involve repetitive preferential sidedness in handling of objects, such as electronic devices, ingraining rotational motor patterns along with sitting difficulties. Another affected functional area is breathing. Although most cases of functional respiratory concern occur at severe levels of Cobb angle, such as beyond seventy degrees, fitness breath levels measured at forty-five degrees were found to impact functional capacity in AIS subjects [29, 30].

Psychological impact is also seen in youth with a scoliosis diagnosis. Youth are particularly vulnerable to emotional difficulties brought on by scoliosis diagnosis and may more readily manifest these issues rather than the presence of pain. Both the Schroth Method and the Pilates Method have been studied to ascertain the influence of these methods considering both Cobb angle correction along with psychological influences such as body image, solitary behavior, and positive outlook. Comparable positive effects are found with Pilates Method exercises along with the use of the Schroth Method. Both demonstrate not only beneficial effects upon the physical aspects of curve correction but also upon psychological factors that affect those in pubescence [31].

Table 2. Stages of functional activity

Rehabilitation Stage	
Clinical Goals	Studio Goals
Stage 1 Restricted Stage	
• Reduce Swelling and pain • Active rest • Evaluate kinetic chain for dysfunction • Aerobic conditioning • Restrict tissue loading • Somatics and mental practice • Take floor exercise class or pool class	
Stage 2: Restoration stage	
• Restore ROM and strength • Progress aerobic conditioning • Begin functional weight bearing and basic skills	• Permit limited movement with restricted tissue loading (padding, taping, etc.) • Concentrate on alignment and stability • Take beginner level dance class
Stage 3: Reacquisition stage	
• Progress strength to "supernormal levels" • Bilateral → Unilateral weight bearing • Eyes open → eyes closed • Slow → Fast movement exercise	• Return to original level class • Progress from 1 class/day to more, as tolerated • Limit number of jumps and rehearsals
Stage 4: Refinement stage	
• Build confidence, carriage and control • Complicate skills • Progress cardiovascular drills • Increase speed and loads • Progress dynamic balance • Increase repetitions	• Unrestricted dance movement • Prescribed warm-up • Implementation of injury management and prevention techniques learned in rehabilitation • Understanding of nutritional needs discussed during rehabilitation

Reprinted with permission. Liederbach, Marijeanne (2008) "Dance Medicine: Strategies for the Prevention and Care of Injuries to Dancers "In: Epidemiology of Dance Injuries: Biopsychosocial Considerations in the Management of Dancer Health. Orthopaedic Section Independent Study Courses: 1- 24; January. Accessed March 30, 2018. DOI:10.17832/isc.2008.18.3.1.

The Pilates Method differs from both yoga and general physical therapy methods such as the Schroth Method in its ability to promote functional movement, and concentrate on the coordination of whole body effects of the spinal curves while addressing the stabilization of the seminal curves themselves. The Pilates Method environment integrates components of the physical therapy/yoga complementary systems, while taking physical development beyond the focal treatment of the curves. The highest forms of function are ambulation, child-bearing for women, handling of unwieldy objects such as small children, throwing, kicking, running, jumping, and endurance sitting for school and work life [32].

To establish goals of higher function, the stages of functional activities may be seen as a continuum traveling from a restricted phase to a restoration phase to a reacquisition or acquisition phase to a refinement phase, an example for dancers as shown in Table_2_ above, thus ensuring successful entry or re-entry into larger forms of exercise and fitness. Mr. Pilates himself offered this opinion concerning physical development:

> "It would be a grave error to assume than even Contrology (the original name of the Pilates Method) exercises alone will remake a man or woman into an entirely physically fit person. To understand this statement better, just remember that exercises as such with relation to physical fitness are somewhat similar to the relationship a grindstone or home bears to an axe or razor. For example, how obvious is the answer to the foolish question as to which of two equally expert woodchoppers would cry "Timber" first, the one with the dull axe or saw, of the one who habitually sharpens his tools nightly in preparation for his work the next day" [33].

In this way the Pilates Method offers a gateway to larger physicality.

SSPOT

This chapter offers a glimpse into a structured program of exercise developed by this writer, the SSPOT® (Scoliosis Specific Physical and Observational Test), based upon the Pilates Method created by Joseph Hubertus Pilates. The SSPOT has two components, the SSPOT-1 (a group of analytical assessments) and the SSPOT-2, with which this chapter is primarily concerned. The SSPOT-2 is a program of specific exercise progressions and principles that feature adaptations and concepts from the Pilates Method appropriate for those with AIS.

As in any exercise program taught by certified exercise instructors, caution must be observed not to confuse the use of this program with medical diagnosis or medical direction. It is meant to be used in conjunction with medical approval, determined by appropriate providers.

The Pilates Environment

The Pilates Environment exists to both assist and challenge the individual client. This environment traditionally progresses from the establishment of a stable skeletal base to a dynamic, moving base of support that can withstand external forces that are generated either with one's own weight or the resistance of a spring system. The specific tools of the Pilates Method include imagery, the use of props, and may or may not include the use of the Pilates devices and the classic mat. The exercises highlighted in this Chapter focus on mat exercises.

The Method's toolbox accentuates self-awareness and facilitates intellectual engagement, along with traditional orthopedic therapeutic development of strength, yet also allowing the development of strength throughout an entire range of motion in multiple planes of force and motion. Youth benefit in so many ways from the general principles of the Pilates Method, which include discipline, precision, centering, flow, breathing, and concentration [34].

The Pilates Method includes the use of props to accentuate its principle of precision and individuation of the exercises. The props accommodate both those with and without spinal fixation surgery.

The wedge is one such prop. Its use is different for the two fixation situations mentioned above. Regarding pre-surgery studies, Khosla et al. found changes in the myo-tendinous junction of multifidi by examining biopsies of pre-operative individuals waiting for spinal fixation due to scoliosis. These changes include fatty infiltrates, and increased vasation on the concave side of the spinal curves indicating a lack of nerve stimulation and consequent appropriate recruitment of fibers. In each case, using a wedge prop to access underused or dysfunctional muscularity helped achieve greater musculo-skeletal balance [35].

In either case, whether or not directly involved with fixation surgery, the wedge, used actively, provides orthotic interaction in two ways: by safely assisting the body to engage difficult-to-access musculature, and by allowing more effective feedforward and feedback biomechanical chain engagement due to better skeletal arrangement. The desired effect is in keeping with the goal of exercise, that is, active exercise engagement, rather than the positional release use of manipulative wedges used in manual therapy by physical therapists.

In addition, Burwell et al. established a distinct need for increased proprioception in their study on the neurological implications of scoliosis [26]. Use of the wedge as a corrective asymmetry tool, in combination with the suggested exercises, addresses the neurological deficit by providing proprioceptive feedback to the brain, thereby challenging the neurological pattern of the spinal rotation.

Using the wedge along with guided imagery, the Pilates Method movement educator (the Pilates Movement Educator) is able to create a safe yet challenging experience that provides a somatic, corrective or conditioning enhancement effect.

These effects aid the client in increasing body awareness and coordination so helpful to a client dealing with a daily task of scoliosis management. Breaking down essential movements that integrate core control with appendage use allows time for neurological re-integration that corrects faulty movement patterns of postural muscle motor patterns that comprise daily movements. The use of imagery as a tool enhances the quality and performance aspects of the desired movement. There is, of course, much evidence to support the use of imagery as a sports mental training activity (see, e.g., [37]).

Corrective exercise becomes incorporated in the SSPOT-2 as the movement educator observes and modifies the exercises according to the stage of the exercise acquisition along with giving individual goals and challenges throughout the exercise session.

The conditioning aspect of the Pilates Method and the SSPOT-2 exercises progress as the youth's understanding, tolerance and precision of movement correctives are achieved. To this end, the SSPOT-2 is composed of a multitude of exercises from which trained instructors may select appropriate movement patterns in a stepped, organized fashion [38]. Pilates Movement Educators trained by accredited institutions typically receive over four hundred hours of instruction for certification. Advanced qualification for special population training such as those with spinal asymmetry is available from multiple sources. All certified educators must legally and ethically demonstrate continued learning from reputable sources. Governmental regulations and certifying organizations of the Pilates Method dictate that the Pilates Movement Educators keep pace with new advances of exercise science and therapy science by requiring all certified instructors to complete continuing education. Therefore within all three aspects of the use of the Pilates Method: somatic, corrective and conditioning, with a focus on the special population of youth with spinal asymmetry, a unique management program detailed for the youth is devised [39].

The SSPOT-1 and 2 not only provide a framework of individualized exercise coached by a Pilates Movement Educator, it also provides the educator with the opportunity to create for the youthful client a lifelong system of management and maintenance.

SSPOT-1

The SSPOT-1 involves mostly standing observations with some additional functional tests in sitting and supine. In a series of nineteen observational tests conducted by the movement educator, an asymmetry specific profile of the youth's standing functional posture and also preferential movement patterns. These include full body observations from the head to the feet, taking note of: positioning of the shoulder girdle upon the ribcage, variation of the head over the thorax, screening of the axial trunk rotation with a Scoliometer®, observation of arm length discrepancy in elevation, pelvic obliquity, knee mal-alignment, and foot posture. Also included are preferential tests regarding eye dominance, axial spinal rotation range, supine straight leg raise pelvic stability, vertical seated trunk compression, and femoral-pelvic dysfunction.

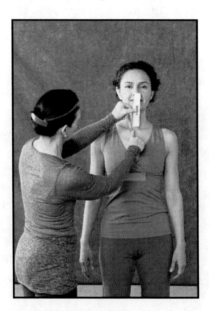

Figure 1. Clinical assessment.

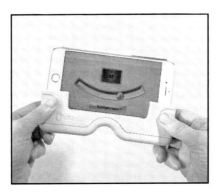

Figure 2. Scoliometer.

Evidence shows the use of the Scoliometer® can alert an exercise instructor or school screening expert to refer a youth into the medical system for monitoring. Surface topography observation with the use of a flat surface such as a book has also been shown to be a valid screening method. The forward spinal flexion test is not meant for those who have already undergone surgical fixation. However, the other standing tests offer insight for those who have had surgical spinal fixation since lateral preference and limb dominance likely perpetuate the internal twist in spite of fixation [40].

The purpose of combining the standing postural findings and the Scoliometer® forward bend test along with notation of the dominance, preference and limb functional strategies in the SSPOT-1 is to create a plan for remediation of sidedness, vestibular balance as well as provide elements to add to the exercises of the SSPOT-2. In addition, attention to motion preference re-patterning may uncover fascial restrictions. Evidence indicates that restriction of motion may also occur from fascial sources of constriction [41].

This recent research into the fascial system provides greater avenues to influence this functional aspect of AIS. The use of combined planes of motion through body-weight-bearing resistive action allows full fascial line use, such as the Spiral Line described in the framework classified by manual therapist and author Tom Myers.

Scoliosis musculo-fascial imbalances often follow Myers' Spiral Line which follows a helical track encompassing "the side of the skull across the neck to the opposite shoulder and ribs, and back across the belly to the front of the hip, the outside of the knee, the inside of the ankle, and under the arch of the foot, and back up the leg and back to the skull" [42].

An important note is that the functional tests of preference and limb strategies applies to both post-operative as well as the non-operated youth population. One issue particular to post-operative youth is one of expectation that the fixation surgery will hold the youth up permanently as an artificial scaffolding throughout the entire body.

As with any surgical procedure, a certain amount of generalized de-conditioning occurs due to the need for immobilization and restricted motion for a period of time. Youth may mistake the abundance of youthful rapid healing as a sign of full recovery. Relief of seeing the spine once again brought into its central vertical line may obscure the need for post-operative rehabilitation and actual full restoration.

For this reason, the qualified Pilates Movement Educator is a great influence in guiding the youth to optimize outcome for a satisfied result [43].

SSPOT-2

The SSPOT-2 is a series of approximately fifteen mat exercise progressions based upon the original thirty-four exercises from *Return to Life* by Joseph H. Pilates.

Not all exercise is appropriate for all people. In an effort to clearly delineate those exercises not indicated for those with spinal fixation, note the indication for each exercise to differentiate those that are fully unsuitable for the youth having undergone spinal fixation. A special section at the end provides additional needs of this sub-group of operative youth. In addition, youth who have been prescribed braces should not wear the brace during the SSPOT-2 exercises unless specifically indicated by the medical team.

Youth of both the operative and non-operative groups respond well to concrete thinking. Full body involvement as in play activities combined with a level of enjoyment, with the potential goal of physical mastery aids full engagement and ensures compliance.

A sampling of the exercises from the SSPOT-2 is presented here. Advanced level special population movement educators receive training in the assessment performance level assignments ranging from fair to good to excellent. The level assignments along with the individual corrective cues from the movement educator provide guideposts to lead the way. The acquisition of the exercises and their appropriate performance provide both a baseline as well as a template of progress for each youth as they are repeated over a period of time.

(A multiple-week program, such as the ten-week program developed by this writer, the Spinal Asymmetry and Scoliosis Program™, is recommended to progress and track these milestones of accomplishment.)

The Pilates Method mat philosophy of using closed kinetic chain connection to the ground highlights the use of eccentric, anti-gravitational lengthening contractions promoting the ability to manipulate one's center of gravity and body weight in spatial orientations. Bodily asymmetry correlates with external spatial boundaries [44].

Each exercise segment gives the opportunity to devote analysis, concentration and focus upon the individual's particular corrective areas such as equal weight into all five toes (Achilles tendon length, flexor hallucis length, lumbo-pelvic dissociation), weakness of one side versus the other, wobbling or inability to balance. Using these exercises in front of a mirror for instant feedback enables the youth to have a goal for the task as well as come to more neutral terms with self-image.

Traditional plank exercises form the foundation to begin. Performed in three spatial orientations, facing downwards, facing sideways and facing upwards accentuates the exploration and need for learning the interplay of the three-dimensional spinal asymmetry influence upon the whole body.

Modified versions proceed into full isometric planks and then proceed into moving versions, challenged by the addition of the movement of the legs. These foundational planks in their beginning modified versions are appropriate for youth who have undergone spinal fixation since the spine is held in essentially a neutral position throughout an isometric exercise.

Beginning with half-planks, a foundation is set to activate the essential center of gravity stabilization process, accessing the Inner Unit of the deep transversus abdominis, postural multifidi muscles of the spine, the respiratory diaphragm, and the pelvic floor, kinetically linking the torso with the lower extremities [45].

Tests then proceed through balancing seated ability, called Balance Point exercise in the Pilates language, to exert ground force reaction engagement up into the ischial tuberosities, thereby eliciting the spinal vestibular reflexes [46]. This exercise may be adapted for those with spinal fixation modifying the exercise by balancing with the hands to the side upon the mat and breathing for five repetitions.

One characteristic of classic Pilates exercises is the promotion of spinal articulation, a term called spinal rolling, essentially functional lumbo-pelvic rhythm [47].

In general, these exercises are contraindicated for those with spinal fixation. Precaution is also warranted in that end range and prolonged spinal rotation is generally not advised for those with spinal asymmetry. Sagittal rolling exercises are also not advised for the general populace with spinal asymmetry until spinal articulation and control are achieved. Yet braced lateral rolling, holding the knees with the hands in deep hip flexion on the floor helps those at all levels of ability with synovial membrane activation, common in exercise for osteoarthritis, giving meaning to the motto, "Motion is Lotion."

For those without spinal fixation, both lateral rolling exercises along with the squat to stand rolling spinal flexion in the sagittal plane are of tremendous value in educating the youth to consistently coordinate deep internal spinal and pelvic stabilizers, coordinating lumbo-pelvic rhythm, navigating from a squat to a full standing position with elevated arms.

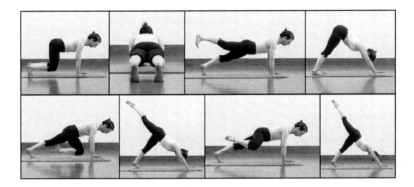

Figure 3. SSPOT-2 exercises.

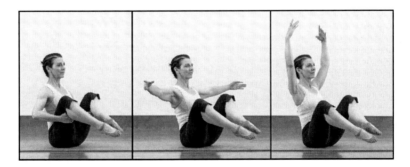

Figure 4. SSPOT-2 exercises.

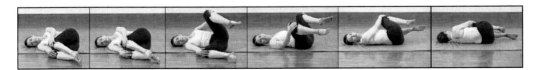

Figure 5. SSPOT-2 exercises.

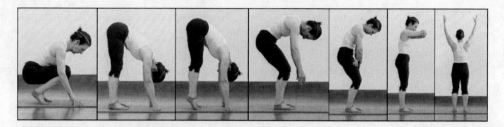

Figure 6. SSPOT-2 exercises.

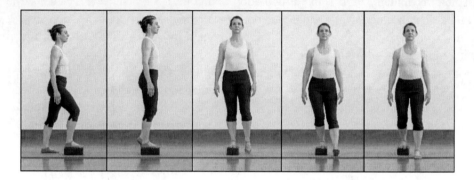

Figure 7. SSPOT-2 exercises.

The last part of the SSPOT-2 focuses upon the step-down from a yoga block or tall book. This functional action displays lower extremity compensations, such as a hip hike or Trendelenberg gait with increased internal hip rotation potentially causing hip, knee ankle, and foot injuries through repetitive compensatory motion [48]. Improvements in functional re-education and muscle balance are accomplished by using core control with lower extremity stance that is beneficial for both operative and non-operative youth. This test offers the perfect segue into the special section on operative youth.

Special Needs for Youth with Spinal Fixation

It is the responsibility of qualified movement educators to collaborate with the youth's medical team under the special circumstances of working with operative youth. Generally, an exercise program beyond the initial physical therapy recommendations should not begin before a three-month post-operative anniversary.

Although fixation surgically repairs structural spinal elements to form a stable bond, the body's functional tendencies may remain. The youth may misconceive that core strength or postural attention is no longer necessary. Many youth have spent considerable time in a rigid brace prior to surgery, potentially weakening core musculature and discouraging weight-bearing activities. For these reasons, it is recommended to focus upon reacquisition of the engagement and strengthening of deep abdominal and spinal musculature in static positions with little or no spinal motion in a neutral position. Adding breathing and isometric sitting challenges greatly aid this group.

Progressing youth into the positions of resisted isometric quadruped and kneeling exercises give additional stabilizing challenge without compromising structures. Operative youth may respond more favorably within the first post-operative year to standing, quadruped, and sitting exercise positions. However, as mentioned previously, the Plank Series of progressions and the Step-Down are the most appropriate components of the SSPOT-2 for operative youth.

Rib Shift Control

It is of utmost importance to acquire rib shift control post-operatively, yet is an important skill for everyone.

The fixation of surgery is strong yet soft tissue dis-use and pre-programmed neurological functional habits are still present. The half body from the waist up is very heavy. Rib Shift Control is a Body Skill for operative clients to learn to stand up inside the fixation by elongating and keeps the ribcage inside a stacked frame of the vertical pelvis.

Long-Sit Challenge

The Long-Sit Challenge benefits the line of the legs. It progresses the Long Sit test position of the SSPOT-2 while using balls and bands to oppose the twisting of the legs.

For operative youth, the addition of a wedge placed underneath the gluteus maximus on the traditional concave torso side allows fascial lengthening to improve functional sitting. A strong stretchy band is placed around the thighs, while a rubber band surrounds the great toes, and a ball is placed between the knees. A wedge can also be placed underneath the lighter side for operative clients between the ischial tuberosity and the coccyx to improve postural muscle activation. The youth performs a breathing exercise while holding a weighted ball overhead while also attempting to line up the second toe with the mid-patella and mid-hip joint.

Another important necessity for post-operative youth features single leg standing, a component of the Step-Down test. Strength in single standing allows correction in trunk to leg alignment and foot to core stability. It is recommended to start with the stronger standing side first.

Wobble Board Activities

A simple prop to magnify this effect of single leg stance is the use of a Wobble Board. Centering the talus, the keystone of the leg to foot connection aids in adopting a new normal of weight shift and control.

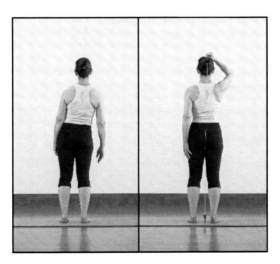

Figure 8. Wobble Board activities.

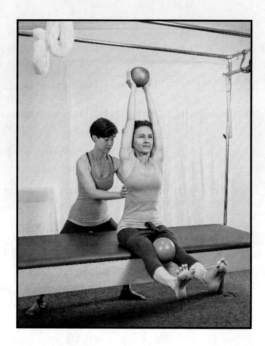

Figure 9. Wobble Board activities.

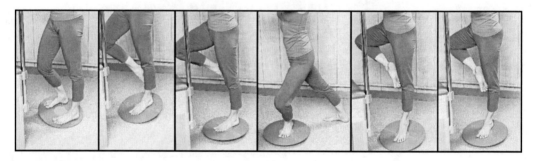

Figure 10. Wobble Board activities.

To sum, the Scoliosis Specific Physical Orthopedic Test™, comprised of the SSPOT-1 and SSPOT-2, provides a gateway through which a youth begins a journey of self-exploration, self-efficacy, and empowerment.

An astute and trained movement educator is a jewel in the individual scoliosis patient's care team, giving the time and personal relationship that is often not practical within the confines of medical settings. The promise of the use of the Pilates Method for AIS appears bright. Evidence supports the convergence of movement education with therapy and science. The general public now has access to an invaluable tool for youth to develop an active and satisfying life through this intelligent movement form.

REFERENCES

[1] Kane, William J. (1977). "Scoliosis Prevalence: A Call for a Statement of Terms." *Journal of Clinical Orthopedics and Research*, July/August, 43–46.

[2] *Scientific Spine Tanner Scale.* (2011). July 17, Accessed March 23, 2018. http://scientificspine.com/spine-scores/tanner-scale.html.
[3] Brighton, Kenneth L. (2007). *Coming of Age: The Education and Development of Young Adolescents.* Westerville, OH: National Middle School Association.
[4] Association of Middle Level Education (AMLE). (2014). "*Developmental Characteristics of Young Adolescents.*," Accessed March 21, 2018. https://www.amle.org/BrowsebyTopic/WhatsNew/WNDet/TabId/270/ArtMID/888/ArticleID/455/Developmental-Characteristics-of-Young-Adolescents.aspx.
[5] Phrompaet, Sureeporn., Atit, Paungmali., Ubon, Pirunsan. & Patraporn, Sitilertpisan. 2011. "Effects of Pilates Training on Lumbo-pelvic Stability and Flexibility." *Asian Journal of Sports Medicine*, 2(1), 16–22. Accessed March 25, 2018. doi: 10.5812/asjsm.34822.
[6] Bian, Zhijie., Hongmin, Sun., Chengbao, Lu., Li, Yao., Shengyong, Chen. & Xiaoli, Li. 2013. "Effect of Pilates Training on Alpha Rhythm." *Computational and Mathematical Methods in Medicine.* Accessed March 25, 2018. doi:10.1155/2013/295986.
[7] Rouhiainen, Leena. (2010). The Evolvement of the Pilates Method and its Relation to the Somatic Field. *Nordic Journal of Dance*, Vol 2, 57–69. Accessed March 1, 2018. http://www.nordicjournalofdance.com/TheEvolvement.pdf.
[8] Kim, Hak-Sun. (2014). "Evidence-based of Non-operative Treatment in Adolescent Idiopathic Scoliosis." *Asian Spine Journal*, 8, no. 5, 695–702. Accessed March 25, 2018. doi: 10.4184/asj.2014.8.5.695.
[9] Wells, Cherie., Gregory, S. Kolt., Paul, W. M. Marshall., Bridget, Hill. & Andrea, Bialocerkowski. (2014). "The Effectiveness of Pilates Exercise in People with Chronic Low Back Pain: A Systematic Review." *PLOS One*, 9, no. 7. Accessed March 25, 2018. doi: 10.1371/journal.pone.0100402.
[10] Keays, Kim S., Susan, R. Harris., Joseph, M. Lucyshun. & Donna, L. MacIntyre. (2008). "Effects of Pilates Exercises on Shoulder Range of Motion, Pain, Mood, and Upper Extremity Function in Women Living with Breast Cancer: A Pilot Study." *Physical Therapy*, 88, 494–510.
[11] Queiroz, Bergson C., Mariana, F. Cagliari., Cesar, F. Amorim. & Isabel, C. Sacco C. (2010). "Muscle Activation during Four Pilates Core Stability Exercises in Quadruped Position." *Archives of Physical Medicine and Rehabilitation*, 91, no. 1, 86–92. Accessed March 5, 2018. 10.1016/j.apmr.2009.09.016.
[12] Negrini, Stefano. Angelo Gabriele Aulisa., Lorenzo, Aulisa., Jean-Claude, deMoray., Jacel, Durmala., Theodore, B Grivas., Patrick, Knott., Tomasz, Kotwicki., Toru, Marumaya., Silvia, Minozzi., Joseph, P O'Brien., Dimitris, Papadopoulos., Manuel, Rigo., Charles, H Rivard., Michele, Romano., James, H Wynn., Monica, Villagrasa., Hans-Rudolph, Weiss. & Fabio, Zaina. (2012). "2011 SOSORT Guidelines: Orthopaedic and Rehabilitation Treatment of Idiopathic Scoliosis during Growth." *Scoliosis*, 7(3), 1–35. Accessed March 20, 2018. doi:10.1186/1748-7161-7-3.
[13] Bialek, Marianna. & Andzej, M'hango. (2008). "FITS Concept: Functional Individual Therapy of Scoliosis." *Studies in Health Technology and Informatics, 135,*

250–261. Accessed March 1, 2018. https://www.researchgate.net/publication/5451855_FITS_concept_Functional_Individual_Therapy_of_Scoliosis.
[14] "What is Life Style Medicine?" (2015). January 1. *American College of Life Style Medicine.* Accessed January 26, 2017. http://www.lifestylemedicine.org/What-is-Lif.
[15] Levine, David B. (2013, May 28). "*History of Scoliosis Surgery at HSS.*" Retrieved February 25, 2017, from Hospital for Special Surgery: https://www.hss.edu/playbook/history-of-scoliosis-surgery-at-hss/#.WK-XzoWcGMo.
[16] Reamy, Brian V. & Joseph, B. Slakey. (2001). Adolescent Idiopathic Scoliosis: Review and Current Concepts. *American Family Physician*, 64(1, July 1), 111–116. Accessed January 20, 2017/ http://www.aafp.org/afp/2001/0701/p111.html.
[17] Blom, Marie-Jose. (2012). "Pilates and Fascia: The Art of 'Working In.'" In *Fascia: The Tensional Network of the Human Body: The Science and Clinical Applications in Manual and Movement Therapy*, edited by R. Schleip, T. W. Findley, L. Chaitow, and P. Huijing, 449–456. Edinburgh, UK: Churchill Livingstone.
[18] Klippinger, Karen. (2017, July 30). Interview with Dr. Karen Klippinger, Professor of Anatomy by author. Alameda, CA, USA.
[19] Weiss, Hans-Rudolf. & Marc, Moramoarco. (2013). "Risks and Long Term Complications of Adolesecent Idiopathic Scoliosis Surgery versus Non-surgical and Natural History Outcomes." *Hard Tissue*, 2, no. 3 (April 30), 1–12. Accessed August 29, 2017. http://www.oapublishinglondon.com/article/498.
[20] Miller, Elise B. (2003). *Yoga for Scoliosis*. Oakland, CA: Shanti Productions.
[21] Lenke, Lawrence G., Randal, R. Betz., Jurgen, Harms., Andrew, Merola., Thomas, Haher., Thomas, Lowe., Peter, Newton., Keith, H. Bridwell. & Kathe, Blankl. (2001). "Adolescent Idiopathic Scoliosis: A New Classification to Determine Extent of Spinal Arthrodesis." *Journal of Bone and Joint Surgery*, 83, no. 8, 1169–1181.
[22] van Loon, Piet J. M. (2012). "Scoliosis Idiopathic? The Etiologic Factors in Scoliosis Will Affect Preventive and Conservative Therapeutic Strategies." In *Recent Advances in Scoliosis*, edited by Theodoros B. Grivas, 211–234. London, U.K: Intechopen. Accessed March 30, 2017. doi:10.5772/38199.
[23] Grivas, Theodoros B., Geoffrey Burwell, R., Kechagias, Vasileoios., Christina, Mazioti., Apostolous, Fountas., Dimitra, Kolovou. & Evagelos, Christodoulou. (2016). "Idiopathic and Normal Lateral Lumbar Curves: Muscle Effects Interpreted by 12th Rib Length Asymmetry with Pathomechanic Implications for Lumbar Idiopathic Scoliosis." *Scoliosis and Spinal Disorders*, 11, Supp 2(35), 39–91. Accessed December 27, 2017. doi:10.1186/s13013-016-0093-8.
[24] Stokes, Ian A. (1989). "Rib Cage Asymmetry in Idiopathic Scoliosis." *Journal of Orthopedic Research*, 7, no. 4, 599–606. Accessed December 26, 2017. doi:10.1002/jor.1100070419.
[25] Lin, Jiu-jeng., Wei-Hsiu, Chen., Po-Quang, Chen. & Jau-Yih, Tsauo. (2010). "Alteration in Shoulder Kinematics and Associated Muscle Activity in People with Idiopathic Scoliosis." *Spine*, 35, no. 11, 1151–1157.
[26] Catanzariti, Jean-Francois., Marc-Alexandre, Guyot., Olivier, Agnani., Samantha, Damaille., Elisabeth, Kolanowski. & Cécile, Donze. (2014). "Eye-hand Laterality

and Right Thoracic Idiopathic Scoliosis. *European Spine Journal*, 23, no. 6, 1232–1236. Accessed March 5, 2018. doi:10.1007/s00586-014-3269-z.

[27] Lambert, Francois M., David, Malvinaud., Joan, Glaunes., Catherine, Bergot., Hans, Straka. & Pierre-Paul, Vidal. (2009). "Vestibular Asymmetry as the Cause of Idiopathic Scoliosis: A Possible Answer from Xenopus." *Journal of Neuroscience*, 29, no. 40, 12477–12483. Accessed March 10, 2018. doi:10.1523/JNEUROSCI.2583-09.

[28] Bialek, Marianna., Patrycja, Pawlak. & Kotwicki, Tomasz. (2009). "Foot Loading Asymmetry in Patients with Scoliosis." *Scoliosis*, 4, Supp 0, 19, 1. doi:10.1186/1748-7161-4-S1-O19.

[29] Sperandio, Evandro. Anderson Sales Alexandre., Lui, C. Yi., Patricia, Rios Poletto., Alberrto, Gotfryd., Milana, Vidotto. & Victor, Dourado. (2014). "Impact of Scoliosis Severity on Functional Capacity in Patients with Adolescent Idiopathic Scoliosis." *The Spine Journal.*, Accessed March 30, 2018. doi:10.1016/j.spinee.2014.01.041.

[30] Kimmerle, Marliese. (2010). "Lateral Bias, Functional Asymmetry, Dance Training, and Dance Injuries." *Journal of Dance Medicine and Science*, 14, no. 2. Retrieved September 26, 2017. http://research_gate.net/44635340_Lateral_bias_functional_asymmetry_dance_training_and_dance.

[31] PwangBo, Pil-Neo. (2016). "Psychological and Physical Effects of Schroth and Pilates Exercise on Female High School Students with Idiopathic Scoliosis." *Journal of Korean Physical Therapy*, 28(6), 364–368. Accessed March 1, 2018. doi:10.1857/jkpt. 2016.28.6.364.

[32] Richardson, Carolyn A. & Julie, A. Hides. (2004). "The Rationale for a Motor Control Programme for the Treatment of Spinal Muscle Dysfunction. In *Grieve's Modern Manual Therapy: The Vertebral Column*, 3rd ed., edited by Jeffrey D. Boyling and Gwendolen A. Jull, 443–450. Edinburgh, U.K.: Churchill Livingstone.

[33] Pilates, Joseph Hubertus. (1945). "The Basic Fundamentals of a Natural Physical Education." In *Return to Life*, 25–30. Miami, Florida: Pilates Method Alliance, Inc.

[34] Anderson, Brent D. & Aaron, Spector. (2000). "Introduction to Pilates-based Rehabilitation." *Orthopedic Physical Therapy Clinics of North America*, 9, no. 3, 395–411. Accessed March 4, 2018. https://www.pilates.com/resources/librarydocs/Intro-pilates-rehab.pdf.

[35] Khosla, Shaun., Stephen, Tredwell., Robert, B. Day., Shinn, S. L. & Orvalle, W. K. Jr. (1980). "An Ultra-structural Study of Multifidus Muscle in Progressive Idiopathic Scoliosis." Changes Resulting from a Sarcolemmal Defect at the Myotendinous Junction." *Journal of Neurological Science*, 46, no 1 (April), 13–31. Accessed March 10, 2018. https://www.ncbi.nlm.nih.gov/pubmed/7373342.

[36] Burwell, R. Geoffrey., Emma, M. Clark., Peter, H. Dangerfield. & Alan Moulton, Alan. (2016). "Adolescent Idiopathic Scoliosis (AIS): A Multi-factorial Case Concept for Pathogenesis and Embryonic Origin." *Scoliosis and Spinal Disorders*, 11, no. 8, 1–9. Accessed March 10, 2018. doi:10.1186/s13013-016-0063.

[37] White, Alison. & Lew, Hardy. (1998). "An In-depth Analysis of the Uses of Imagery by High-level Slalom Canoeists and Artistic Gymnasts." *The Sport Psychologist*, 12, 387–403. Accessed March 2, 2018. doi: 10.1123/tsp.12.4.387.

[38] Muscolino, Joseph E. & Cipriani, Simona. (2004). "Pilates and the 'Powerhouse.'" *Journal of Body Work and Movement Therapy*, *8*, 15–24. Accessed March 6, 2018. https://www.learnmuscles.com/wp-content/uploads/2016/06/2004_Pilates_and_the_powerhourse_II_FADE.pdf.

[39] Kotwicki, Tomasz., Stefano, Negrini., Theodoro, B. Grivas., Manual, Rigo., Toru, Maruyama., Jacek, Durmala. & Fabio, Zaina. (2009). Members of the International Society on Scoliosis Orthopedic and Rehabilitation Treatment (SORSORT). "Methodology of Evaluation of Morphology of the Spine and the Trunk in Idiopathic and Other Spinal Deformities—6th SOSORT Consensus Paper." *Scoliosis*, *4*, no. 1, 1–16. Accessed March 17, 2018. doi: 10.1186/1748-7161-4-26.

[40] Chowanska, Joanna. Tomasz Kotwicki., Krzystof, Rosadzinski. & Ziebigniew, Sliwinski. (2012). "School Screening for Scoliosis: Can Surface Topography Replace Examination with Scoliometer?" *Scoliosis*, *7*, no. 9. Accessed February 20, 2018. doi:10.1186/1748-7161-7-9. *Journal* (Winter), 59–83.

[41] Schliep, Robert. & Divo, Gitta Muller. (2012). "Training Principles for Fascial Connective Tissues: Scientific Foundation and Suggested Practical Applications. *Journal of Bodywork and Movement Therapies*, *17*, no. 1, 1–13. Accessed February 20, 2018. doi:10.1016/j.jbmt.2012.06.007.

[42] Myers, Thomas W. (2001). *Anatomy Trains: Myofascial Meridians for Manual and Movement Therapists.* Edinburgh: Churchill Livingstone.

[43] Koch, Karl D., Renee, Buchanan., John, D. Birch., Richard, Browne., Ann, Morton. & Robert, Gatchel. (2001). "Adolescents Undergoing Surgery for Idiopathic Scoliosis." *Spine*, *26*, no. 19, 2119–2124. Accessed March 25, 2018. doi:10.1097/00007632-200110010-00015.

[44] Hach, Silvia. & Simone, Schutz-Bosbach. (2014). "In (or Outside of) Your Neck of the Woods: Laterality in Spatial Body Representation." *Frontiers in Psychology*, *1*, (February). Accessed January 30, 2018. doi:10.3389/fpsyg.2014.00123.

[45] Huson, Anthony. (1997). "Kinematic Models and the Human Pelvis." In *Movement, Stability, and Low Back Pain*, edited by Andry Vleeming, Vert Mooney, Chris J. Snijders, Thomas A. Dorman, and Rob Stoeckart, 123–131. Edinburgh: Churchill Livingstone.

[46] Bronstein, Adolfo M. (2018). "Vestibular Reflexes and Positional Maneuvers." *Journal of Neurology, Neurosurgery and Psychiatry*, *74*, no. 3. Accessed March 25, 2018. doi:10.1136/jnnp.74.3.289.

[47] Tafazzol, Alireza., Navid, Arjmand., Aboulfazle, Shirazi-Ali. & Pournianpour, Mohamed. (2013). "Lumbopelvic Rhythm during Forward and Backward Sagittal Trunk Rotations; Combined *In Vivo* Measurement with Inertial Tracking Device and Biomechanical Modeling." *Clinical Biomechanics.*, January, Accessed March 23, 2018. 10.1016/j.clinbiomech.2013.10.021.

[48] Pope, Ross. (2003). "The common compensatory pattern." *American Academy of Osteopathy Journal.* (Winter), pp. 59-83.

[49] Curtis, Alexa C. (2015). "Defining Adolescence, "*Journal of Adolescent and Family Health*, Vol. 7, Iss. 2, Article 2, pp. 25.

[50] Liederbach, Marijeanne. (2008). "Dance Medicine: Strategies for the Prevention and Care of Injuries to Dancers" In: Epidemiology of Dance Injuries: Biopsychosocial Considerations in the Management of Dancer Health. *Orthopaedic Section Independent Study Courses*, 1- 24, January. Accessed April 9, 2018. DOI:10.17832/isc.2008.18.3.1.

Chapter 12

ADOLESCENT IDIOPATHIC SCOLIOSIS: CONSERVATIVE TREATMENTS

Andre J. Kaelin[1,*] and Federico Canavese[2]
[1]Clinique des Grangettes, Geneva, Switzerland
[2]CHU Estaing, Service de Chirurgie Infantile

ABSTRACT

Adolescent Idiopathic Scoliosis (AIS) represents the most frequent tridimensional spinal deformity. Progression of curves is linked mainly to the rapid growth around puberty. The natural history can lead to large spinal and thoracic deformities, which could impose surgical treatments. In that specific adolescent period it is possible with very accurate treatments to alt curves progression. In this chapter we describe the different types of braces used worldwide their indications, technical applications, results and failures.

INTRODUCTION

The strategy for the treatment of idiopathic scoliosis depends essentially upon the size and pattern of the deformity, and its potential for progression due to the remaining growth. During the past decade, several studies have confirmed that the natural history of adolescent idiopathic scoliosis can be positively affected by non-operative treatment, particularly bracing [1-6]. The primary objective of non-operative treatment is to successfully arrest progressive curves or to correct curves that cause or may likely cause disability. Orthotic device selection is based on the effectiveness of acute curves correction, on the type and level of curve and the anticipated tolerance of the patient. Avoidance of unnecessary surgery, cosmetic improvement, and an increase of vital capacity as well as pain control, are also of major importance [7-14].

In 1985, the Scoliosis Research Society (SRS) initiated a controlled clinical trial study to investigate the effectiveness of bracing as treatment for scoliosis. Patients of the same age, curve pattern and curve severity were divided into two groups, one treated with bracing and one untreated. Results published in 1993 demonstrated that brace treatment is effective compared to natural history [2]. In another study [3], the records and radiographs of more than 1000 scoliotic patients treated by bracing were reviewed and compared with unbraced patients [15]. This retrospective study confirmed that bracing is an effective treatment to slow or arrest the progression of most spinal curvatures in skeletally immature patients compared with those untreated by this method. Furthermore, a meta-analysis of 20 studies showed that bracing 23 hours per day was significantly more successful than any other non-operative treatment [4, 6]. Nevertheless, there are some patients for whom brace treatment is not effective [16].

Other forms of non-surgical treatment, such as chiropractic or osteopathic manipulation, acupuncture, exercise or other manual treatments, or diet and nutrition, have not yet been proven effective in controlling spinal deformities.

Global scoliosis screening programs targeted on pre-pubertal children are still debated in the literature [42, 43]. The debate addresses mainly the cost/benefit and not the effectiveness of mass screening programs. In order to detect early enough low grade curves and to follow their possible progression, clinical back asymmetry assessments is mandatory. Thus, screening is already part of AIS conservative treatment.

WHEN TO BEGIN TREATMENT

Observation is appropriate treatment for small curves, curves that are at low risk of progression, and those with a natural history that is favorable at the completion of growth. Indications for brace treatment are a growing child presenting with a curve of 25° to 40° or with curves less than 25° that have shown documented progression of 5° to 10° in six months (progression of more than 1° per month). Curves of 20° to 25° in those with pronounced skeletal immaturity (Risser 0, Tanner 1 or 2) should also be treated immediately. Braces should generally be worn full time with treatment lasting from two to four years, until the end of bone growth [17, 18].

By contrast, contraindications for bracing are a child who has completed growth, or a growing child with a curve of over 45°, or under 25° without documented progression [2, 3, 6, 19]. True thoracic lordosis is also a contraindication for orthotic treatment due to the effect of orthoses on the thoracic spine. A child with a non-supportive home situation or who refuses to wear a brace should not be considered for brace treatment. Prevalence for AIS in girl is seven times higher than in boys but girls response to brace treatment is more favorable due to more spine flexibility, shorter growth pubertal spur and shorter length of treatment, compliance to brace treatment is also higher in girls and in boys [2,3,19,20]. Body habitus has been found to be a predictive factor of poor outcome in the orthotic treatment of adolescent idiopathic scoliosis. Overweight adolescent patients will have greater curve progression and be less successful with bracing. In addition, the ability of a brace to transmit corrective forces to the spine through the ribs and soft tissue may be compromised in these patients and this factor should be taken into account when making treatment decisions [20].

A prospective, multicenter study conducted by Nachemson et al. in several countries showed that the success rate of bracing was significantly higher compared to observation and surface electrical stimulation [2]. A meta-analysis of 20 studies further supported this finding and showed that the weighted mean proportion of success was low for lateral electrical surface stimulation and for observation, and progressively higher for bracing at 8, 16, or 23 hours per day. The study concluded that bracing 23 hours per day was significantly more successful than any other treatment [4]. Furthermore, a recently published systematic review concluded that bracing adolescent idiopathic scoliosis is effective in the long term [21]. However, it remains controversial as to whether or not a bracing program can decrease the frequency of surgery [22, 23]. A recently published systematic review used the number of surgically treated patients as an indicator of failure of bracing and reported a broad spectrum ranging from 1% to 43% [24, 25].

DURING TREATMENT

Brace construction must follow some rules in order to provide the best possible correction. The pelvis is first levelled so there is no side effect created by a pre-existing leg length discrepancy. The brace must fit the iliac crests, so the correction areas build-in will have the best sagittal and horizontal correction effects. When patients are first fitted with a brace, a x-ray is performed, the correction must at least be 50% for the initial Cobb angle. There is an initial adjustment period of usually one to two weeks. Initially, the patient is prescribed to wear the brace for a specific number of hours per day and the orthosis is left slightly loose to allow the patient to gradually adjust to it. The brace is increasingly tightened daily until the appropriate level of snugness is reached. If any areas of tenderness or skin irritation develop, the brace is adjusted for optimal fit. Repeated roentgenograms should be performed approximately every four to six months with the brace removed to follow the progression of the curve. The brace should be removed for a minimum of 12-24 hours before roentgenograms are taken so that the spine can go back to its deformed position and imaging can accurately detect curve deterioration.

This is not, however, a clinical practice accepted by all surgeons. Another option is to assess patients at follow-up with roentgenograms taken in the brace to monitor the effectiveness of the orthosis in controlling the deformity. This will allow for brace adjustments which are often necessary as patients grow. Roentgenograms out of the brace would be only required in the evidence of curve progression despite compliant bracing or at completion of brace treatment to assess the true size of the deformity and make definitive decisions in terms of the need for surgery.

A progression of 6 or more degrees during brace treatment is considered as a bad result, need for surgical stabilization are considered failure of brace treatment.

HOURS PER DAY

Studies conducted on the number of hours per day of brace wearing show that the more hours per day the brace is worn, the better the result. The brace is usually prescribed for full-time wear with time out for bathing, swimming, physical education and sport. The child should be encouraged to be active in sporting activities while continuing to wear the brace if possible. Contact sports are not allowed with the brace to protect other participants. These activities generally represent an average of two to four hours a day to ensure brace-wearing of 21 to 23 hours daily.

Use of the brace part-time or only at night has been advocated by some physicians and is widely used in some institutions. However, there is a paucity of long-term follow-up data to prove the effectiveness of this wearing regimen in adolescents, and all series on effective orthotic treatment were with full-time wear. Some small series with a short follow-up after bracing suggest that part-time wear can be effective. However, these reports do not compare their results to natural history or full-time bracing.

Wiley et al. analyzed the results of bracing according to the wearing regimen. Patients were divided into non-compliant (less than 12 hours per day), part-time (between 12 and 18 hours per day), and full-time brace wearing (between 18 and 23 hours per day). The initial curves were similar in the three groups. Patients who wore the brace less than 12 hours per day were associated with an average curve progression from 41.3° to 56.3°, and those who wore the brace part-time progressed from 37.6° to 41.2°. Significant curve improvement was noted in the full-time patient group and curves measured 35.7° at final follow-up compared to 39.3° at brace fitting. In addition, the surgical rate also depended on brace compliance with 73% in non-compliant patients compared to 9% in the fully compliant group [26].

Green [27] reported that 16 hours per day of bracing was effective in slowing curve progression. He studied a heterogeneous group of patients with curves between 23° and 49° and found that only 9% curves progressed 5° or more. However, both Boston and Milwaukee braces were used for treatment and follow-up was limited. Similarly, Emans et al. [28] found part-time brace wear to be as effective as full-time wear for smaller curves. Allington and Bowen [29] reported no difference in the efficacy of full-time versus part-time wear using the Wilmington brace for curves of 30° – 40°, but observed that 58% of patients progressed more than 5° degrees in the brace. Peltonen et al. [30] also noted that the results of 12 hours per day of bracing were similar to the results of 23 hours per day.

WHEN TO STOP TREATMENT

Brace weaning begins when the patient reaches skeletal maturity, determined as the finding of a Risser sign of 3 in girls and 4 in boys, i.e., more than 12 months post- menarche and lack of growth in height for 6 months. Over a period of two to three months, the time of brace wear is decreased progressively and a roentgenogram is then performed of the patient without the brace. If the spine remains stable, brace weaning continues over another two to three months with a further progressive decrease in brace wear. After the second phase of weaning, another roentgenogram without the brace is performed to verify the stability of the spine. If stability is maintained, the weaning program continues until the patient is completely independent of the brace. On the other hand, if the brace is weaned off and there is deterioration of the residual curve, this may constitute an indication for surgical correction of the scoliosis. If the patient is skeletally mature, there is no evidence to support that continuing bracing regime provides any treatment benefit.

COMPLICATIONS OF BRACE TREATMENT

Brace treatment have some disadvantages. Treatment with a brace can be rather bothersome [31, 32] Patients, usually young adolescents aged between 10 and 16 years, have to wear the brace for 18 to 23 hours a day during several years, the brace is often visible, and can be uncomfortable to wear [33, 34]. Moreover, noncompliance with brace wear is often an issue and varies from refusal to wear the orthosis, to premature discontinuation of the use of the brace, to less than full-time use of the brace. Lack of compliance is related to several factors, including the unacceptable appearance of the brace to the body image-conscious teenager, and the discomfort from chin and throat contact (especially Milwaukee brace) or from the pelvic or axillary portion of the brace (especially TLSO braces). A recent study showed that scoliosis patients are willing to undergo brace treatment only if it provides sizeable reduction of the risk of surgery [34]. While some studies report little variation in compliance between Milwaukee brace when compared to TLSO braces, other show significant less compliance with the Milwaukee brace when compared to TLSO's [3, 35].

Other problems encountered due to brace treatment include skin irritation, a temporary decrease in vital capacity, and mild chest wall and inferior rib deformation. Skin irritation is a common problem and more frequent in warm climates and during the summer months due to the increase in heat and sweat. To reduce the likelihood or occurrence of skin irritation, frequent changing of the cotton undergarment is recommended, but discontinuation of brace treatment due to skin irritation is uncommon. The vital capacity may be temporarily reduced in patients treated with thoraco-lumbo-sacral orthosis and mild chest wall and inferior rib deformation can appear during treatment.

Chest wall and rib deformation commonly occurs if bracing is performed at ages where the chest is very plastic and easily deformed with drooping of the ribs on the convexity of the scoliosis, where corrective forces are applied. When brace use is discontinued, the mild rib cage deformity usually disappears. However, if full-time bracing starts at very young age at continues for a numbers of years, chest wall and rib deformation may become permanent and may not reverse [7-14].

BRACE TYPES

Cervico-Thoraco-Lumbo-Sacral Orthosis (Milwaukee Brace)

The Milwaukee brace is an historical bracing system, also named cervico-thoraco-lumbo-sacral orthosis (CTLSO), is a full torso brace extending from the pelvis to the base of the skull. It was originally designed by Blount and Schmidt in 1946 for postoperative care when surgery required long periods of immobilization and it has subsequently been used for thoracic and double curves. Milwaukee braces are often custom-made from a mould of the patient's torso. One anterior and two posterior bars are attached to a pelvic girdle made of leather or plastic, as well as a neck ring. The ring has an anterior throat mould and two posterior occipital pads, which fit behind the patient's head. Lateral pads are strapped to the bars and adjustment of these straps holds the spine in alignment.

Curve patterns that should be treated in a Milwaukee brace are thoracic curves that have an apex at or above T8, double thoracic, and other double curves when the apex of the thoracic component is above T8, i.e., double thoracic and lumbar, or double thoracic and thoracolumbar patterns.

Success Rate

Curves between 20° and 29° with a Risser sign between 0 and 1 progressed 28% less than untreated curves of similar magnitude (40% versus 68%, respectively). Treated curves of similar magnitude, but a Risser sign of 2 or more, progressed 10% less than untreated curves (10% versus 23%, respectively). Similarly, curves between 30° and 39° with a Risser sign between 0 and 1 progressed 14% less than untreated curves of similar magnitude (43% versus 57%, respectively). Treated curves of similar magnitude, but a Risser sign of 2 or more, progressed 21% less than untreated curves (22% versus 43%, respectively) [3, 15].

Boston Brace (TLSO)

Hall and Miller jointly created the Boston brace in 1972 [33] and Watson, Hall and Stanish first reported on its efficacy on 1977 [35]. The brace opens at the back and corrects curvatures by pushing the spine with small pads placed against the ribs, which are also used for partial rotational correction. These pads are usually placed in the back corners of the brace so that the body is thrust forward against the front of the brace, which acts to hold the body upright. Areas of relief are provided opposite the sites of corrective force to allow the patient to pull the spine away by active muscular effort [28]. The brace also has a 15° lumbar lordosis built into it. The brace runs from just above the seat of a chair (when a person is seated) to around shoulder blade height and is not particularly useful in correcting very high curves [5, 25, 26, 28, 35]. In the early 1990's, the original brace design was modified to add 15° lumbar lordosis into the pelvic module to better derotate the spine [33].

Success Rate

The brace has been shown to be particularly effective for curves ranging from 20° to 59° between T8 and L2. At the beginning of treatment, brace correction is about 50%, decreasing to 15% by the time of brace discontinuance. With Boston brace treatment, approximately half of the curves (49%) remain unchanged, 39% are stabilized with a final correction of 5° to 15°, 4% are stabilized with a correction superior to 15°, 4% lose between 5° to 15°, and 3% progress more than 15°. A study by Emans et al. reported that 11% of patients underwent surgery during the period of bracing [28].

Lyon Brace

The Lyon brace was designed by Stagnara in 1947 and is also known as the Stagnara brace, this brace system is the first, which had prospective studies and consistent documented efficacy. It is composed of a pelvic section with axillary, thoracic and lumbar plates connected in units by two vertical aluminum rods, one anterior and one posterior. The pelvic section is composed of two lateral valves, one for each hemipelvis. The valves are connected by metal pieces to the vertical aluminum rods. Forces are applied at the two neutral vertebrae and a counterforce is applied at the apex of the curve. It is usually prescribed for progressive scoliosis with lumbar or low thoracolumbar curves between 30° to 50° [36, 37].

Success Rate

The overall efficacy of the Lyon brace is 95%. However, it drops to 87% for thoracic curves and to 80% in patients with Risser sign 0.

Chêneau Brace

Jacques Chêneau designed the original Chêneau brace in 1979. The brace is commonly used for the treatment of scoliosis and thoracic hypokyphosis in many European countries, Israel and Russia. However, it is not commonly prescribed in North America and the United Kingdom. The Chêneau brace utilizes large, sweeping pads to push the body against its curve and into blown out spaces and is usually coupled with the Schroth physical therapy method. The Schroth theory holds that the deformity can be corrected through retraining muscles and nerves to learn what a straight spine feels like, and by breathing deeply into areas crushed by the curvature to help gain flexibility and to expand [38, 39]. The brace helps patients to perform their exercises throughout the day. It is asymmetrical and used for patients of all degrees of severity and maturity, and often worn 20 to 23 hours daily. The brace principally contracts to allow for lateral and longitudinal rotation and movement [40].

Night-Time Braces

Despite the development of low-profile TLSO, such as the Boston brace, full compliance with a brace program that demands 18 to 23 hours of daily wear through skeletal maturity is difficult for adolescents. Night-time bracing systems were developed to improve patient compliance by reducing the total time in the brace and eliminating the social anxiety created by daytime wear.

Night-time braces are more effective in patients with isolated, flexible Thoraco-lumbar and lumbar curves. They are also recommended to patients noncompliant with a full-time wear program, patients in whom other types of orthotic management had failed, and patients nearing skeletal maturity who may not require full-time wear [17, 33, 45].

There have been previous studies comparing a nighttime orthosis to more traditional methods [17, 46-49]. Katz and Durrani retrospectively recommended the use of the Boston brace in curves between 36 to 45 degrees because it prevented curve progression of 6 degrees or more in 57% of patients, as compared with only 17% success in using the Charleston Orthosis. The Boston orthosis also controlled curves of 25 to 35 degrees more effectively than did the Charleston orthosis, preventing progression in 71% of patients versus 53% in using Charleston Orthosis [17]. Howard et al. also found that the TLSO was superior at preventing curve progression when compared with the Charleston brace [50]. Gepstein et al., however, found no statistical difference in the surgery rate of 13.5% using the TLSO and 11% using the

Charleston Brace [51]. Similarly, Janicki et al. found the Providence nighttime orthosis more effective in avoiding surgery and preventing curve progression than a TLSO in a comparable population of patients with AIS having initial curves of 25 to 40 degrees [52].

Charleston Brace

The Charleston bending brace was designed with the idea that compliance would increase if the brace was worn only at night. Hooper and Reed collaborated in 1978 on the early development of this new side-bending brace for nocturnal wear. The orthosis is asymmetrical and fights against the body's curve by overcorrecting the deformity. It grips the hips much like the Boston brace and rises to approximately the same height, but pushes the patient's body to the side. It is used in single, thoracolumbar curves in patients 12 to14 years of age (before structural maturity) who have flexible curves in the range of 25° to 35° [47, 48, 50].

Success Rate
Patients with a curve over 25° and a Risser sign between 0 and 2 showed a rate of surgery between 12% and 17% [47, 48, 50]. In a 2002 study, it has been shown to be equally effective as the Boston brace [50].

Providence Brace

The Providence brace was developed by D'Amato, Griggs and McCoy in the mid-1990s. The brace works by the application of controlled, direct, lateral and rotational forces on the trunk to move the spine toward the midline or beyond the midline. It does not bend the spine as with the Charleston bending brace. The goal is to use the centerline as a reference and bring the apexes of the scoliotic curve to that line or beyond through the application of lateral forces. This involves the use of three-point-pressure systems and void areas that are located opposite these pressures. Compared with natural history and the prospective study data of Nachemson et al. [2], the Providence brace is effective in preventing curve progression of deformities less than 35° and low apex curves of over 35°. It is more successful in curves with apex curves at or below T9 compared to curves with apex cephalad to T8 [52-54].

Success Rate
Recent studies showed that the Providence night brace generally achieves an average of about 90% for brace correction of the primary curve and during follow-up, progression of the curve of more than 5° degrees should be expected in about 25% of cases. The night brace may be recommended for the treatment of adolescent idiopathic scoliosis with curves less than 35° in lumbar and thoracolumbar cases [52-54].

Soft Brace

SpineCor Brace

The SpineCor brace was developed by Coillard and Rivard in the mid-1990s. The brace has a pelvic unit made of plastic, from which strong elastic bands wrap around the body, pulling against curves, rotations, and imbalances. It is most successful when patients have relatively small and simple curvatures and are structurally young and compliant. The SpineCor bracing method is an adjustable, flexible, and non-invasive technique providing correction that continues as a child moves and grows. The brace is usually worn 20 hours a day and the patient can remove it for no more than two hours a day.

Success Rate

A 2003 study reported that after two years, the SpineCor brace is able to correct scoliotic curves by 5° degrees in 55% of patients. The remaining 45% were stabilized (38%) or worsened by more than 5° (7%). Recent studies demonstrated a trend different from the findings of the SpineCor developing team and reported a lower success rate than rigid spinal orthosis [54-57]. According to Wong et al. [55], in patients with curves between 20° and 30° before skeletal maturity, a rigid brace showed better results than the elastic one at 45 months follow-up: 31.8% in the SpineCor group had 5 or more degrees of curve progression versus 4.7% in rigid brace.

OTHER CONSERVATIVE TREATMENTS

Opinions differ in the international literature on the efficacy of conservative approaches to scoliosis treatment. Alternative forms of non-surgical treatment, such as chiropractic or osteopathic manipulation, acupuncture, exercise or other manual treatments, or diet and nutrition, have not yet been proven to be effective in controlling spinal deformities.

Although a subject of debate, most experts agree that physiotherapy alone will not affect the progression of a structural scoliosis. However, there is agreement that a selective physical therapy program in conjunction with brace treatment is beneficial. The triad of out-patient physiotherapy, intensive in-patient rehabilitation, and bracing has proven effective in conservative scoliosis treatment in central Europe [38, 39].

Acupuncture involves penetration of the skin by thin, solid, metallic needles that are stimulated either manually or electrically and it is commonly used for pain control throughout the world, although the putative mechanisms are still unclear. To date, only one study has been published and the effects of acupuncture in the treatment of patients with scoliosis require further investigation [58].

Electrotherapy was hailed as a promising therapy, but failed to alter the natural history of idiopathic scoliosis. With electrotherapy, the lateral muscles on the convexity of the curve are stimulated electrically. It has been shown that no benefit was observed in approximately half of the patients treated by night- time electrotherapy and that the difference in progression between bracing programs and electrical stimulation was significantly different [59].

OUR PREFERRED TECHNIQUE FOR BRACE TREATMENT IN AIS

Screening programs allows early detection, and to individualize adolescents with curves progression. Brace indications are: curve documented progression over 20° (Figure 1: X-Ray at diagnosis. Figure 2: X-ray at brace indication), curves diagnosed between 25° and 45°, gross trunk imbalance in patients still in active growth. The apex of structural curves must be D6 or caudal, in apex D5 and above braces have no real effect. The candidate for bracing and his family must understand the purpose of the treatment its length, goal and limits.

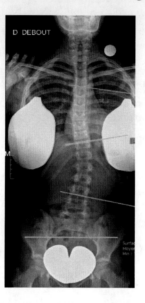

Figure 1. X-ray at diagnosis, immature girl, at 12 years 4 months old. Right thoracic curve 17°, left lumbar 21°, leg length discrepancy of 1 cm. Due to the lack-of documented progression the patient was set in a surveillance program.

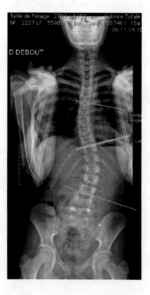

Figure 2. X-ray at 12 years and 8 months, documented progression to 25° in the right thoracic curve and 33° in the left lumbar one. Indication for brace treatment and a lift under the left foot.

Adolescent Idiopathic Scoliosis: Conservative Treatments 165

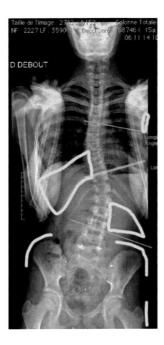

Figure 3. X-ray with the design of correction's pads for the orthopedic technician.

On a full spine X-Ray in standing position (classic or EOS), we assess the pelvic position, and we draw the area where we plan to apply pressure forces for correction. The forces are applied in pair in order to perform also derotation forces. (Figure 3: Brace planning on x-ray).

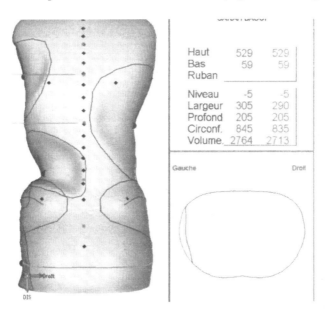

Figure 4. Vorum screen capture, the software has the patient measurement and size taken with a laser gun, it propose an initial correction, which is adjusted on the screen. The program computes 3D corrections keeping always the same volume for the thorax and the abdomen.

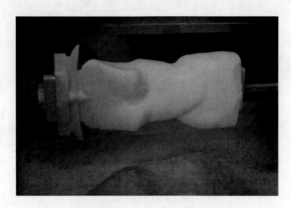

Figure 5. The data are sent to a milling machine, which trims a polyurethane mold. The polypropylene heated foil is applied on the mold, and then cut at the patient's size, the pads are fixed inside the brace.

Our choice of brace's construct is based on the Boston system, with anterior opening, and pressure area and expansion windows after Cheneau principles.

In the orthotic workshop, the patient is scanned by a laser measurement system and the data are collected in the software: VORUM™. We define the final shape of the brace on a screen with a 3-D model [41], alterations to increase the curve correction, are made in constant trunk volume, the program manages also voids opposite to correction area. (Figure 4: Vorum screen capture brace design)

Digital data are sent to a milling unit, where a polyurethane block is shaped to a positive mold. (Figure 5: polyurethane mold after milling)

A 2½ mm polypropylene sheet, is soften by heat, it is applied on the mold, and then cut to the patient longitudinal size. Foam pads increase correction effect. (Figure 6: Adjusted brace with Velcro straps and pads for increased correction)

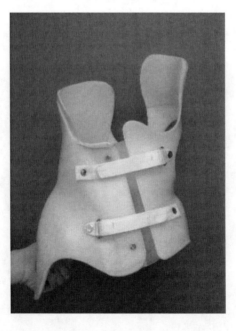

Figure 6. Brace at the end of process with trim shaped, velcro straps and pad inside to increase the correction effect especially in rotation correction.

Insertion of metallic landmarks allows seeing the correction's pads zones. After proper fitting on the patient, an initial X-Ray demonstrate a correction of at least 50% of the original curve, if not pads are modified in position and thickness and if necessary, a new brace is built-up. 50% correction of initial Cobb angle is the best indicator for a successful treatment. (Figure 7: Immediate correction at first in brace)

Once the best correction achieved, patient wear his orthosis progressively from 2h periods daily to a program of 20h/24h in around 2 weeks. Physical therapy exercises keep flexibility and good muscle tonus.

After 6 to 8 weeks a clinical assessment check the skin, the patient morphology and the compliance, during the length of the treatment clinical and X-Rays out of brace for 24h are organized at least every six months, usually the brace is changed if growth exceed 8cm or 8kg.

Weaning begins at Risser 3 in girls and Risser 4 in boys, after first menstruation and when growth stops; the three conditions must be fulfilled.

Weaning is performed in a period of 6 months.

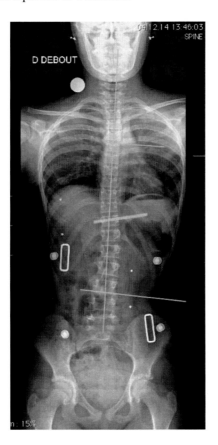

Figure 7. X-ray done just after the first brace fitting with immediate correction. The index of brace's treatment success is the correction index (Cobb pre brace -Cobb in-brace/Cobb pre-brace*100); the correction must be at least 50%. For this case, the thoracic curve decreases from 25° to 12° = a correction index of 52%, the lumbar curve decreases from 33° to 14° = 58%. The metallic dots are x-ray visible landmarks for the corrective pads. Allowing easy correction if needed. Rotational correction is also obtained. Note the bone immaturity, the Risser sign does not appear.

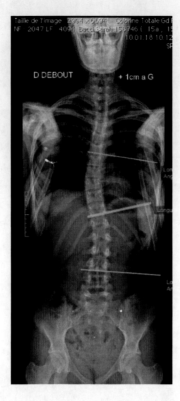

Figure 8. X-ray at 16 years 7 months old, 2 years after the end of brace's treatment, at bone maturity. The curves are stabilized at an angle below the initial angle, the thoracic curve decreased from 25§ to 20° and the lumbar for 33° to 16°.

We perform clinical and X-RAYS 1 years and 2 years after brace's stop. (Figure 8: X-Ray at two years follow-up after brace stop)

Table 1. Results of the prospective study on 43 patients, the initial correction index is 60.8%, the final correction at 2 years follow-up is 2°, improvement of the apex rotation and of the overall balance

Number of Patients in Study	43
Mean Cobb Angle at Bracing	28.3°
Initial Angle in Brace	11.1°
Correction Index (%)	60.8%
Correction in°	17.2
AP Balance Out of Brace	1.48 cm
AP Balance in Brace	0.77 cm
Rotation (NASH-MOE) Pre-Brace	Index : 1.56
Rotation (NASH-MOE) in-Brace	Index : 1.05
Mean Time in Brace	22 Months
Growth in Brace	9 cm
Weight Gain in Brace	11 kg
Mean Cobb° at 2 Y F-U	26°
Surgery (Failure)	2/43 (4.6%)

From 2009 to 2011 a prospective study included 43 patients treated with this brace concept. 37 girls and 6 boys, mean age at bracing: 12 years and 6 months. 20 were single curves and 23 multiple curves. The best correction's percentage is in thoraco-lumbar area (81%), then in lumbar area (62%) and thoracic area (61%). This series has two cases (4.3%) of failure leading to surgery, one because of an imbalanced thoraco-lumbar of 37° with important imbalance, the other for progression due to lack of compliance. The results at 2 years follow-up after brace's stop are collected in the Table 1 and demonstrate a mean long-term follow-up curves correction of 2° from 28° to 26°.

CONCLUSION

Brace treatment is the only method that has been proven to alter the natural history of idiopathic scoliosis. However, different orthosis and many bracing regimens exist. Observation is appropriate for small curves, whereas bracing is generally indicated for progressive curves or for curves over 25° in a skeletally immature child. Braces are generally prescribed for more than 20 hours a day and the results of brace treatment correlates to treatment compliance. Problems encountered with bracing are limited [44].

REFERENCES

[1] Fernandez-Filiberti, R; Flynn, J; Ramirez, N; Trautmann, M; Alegria, M. Effectiveness of TLSO bracing in the conservative treatment of idiopathic scoliosis. *J Pediatr Orthop*, 1995, 15, 176-81.

[2] Nachemson, A; Peterson, L. and members of the Brace Study Group of the Scoliosis Research Society. Effectiveness of treatment with a brace in girls who have adolescent idiopathic scoliosis. *J Bone Joint Surg Am*, 1995, 77, 815-22.

[3] Lonstein, JE; Winter, RB. The Milwaukee brace for the treatment of adolescent idiopathic scoliosis: A review of 1020 patients. *J Bone Joint Surg Am*, 1994, 76, 1207-21.

[4] Rowe, DE; Bernstein, SM; Riddick, MF; Adler, F; Emans, JB; Gardner-Bonneau E. A meta-analysis of the efficacy of non-operative treatments for idiopathic scoliosis. *J Bone Joint Surg Am*, 1997, 79, 664-74.

[5] Olafsson, Y; Saraste, H; Soderlund, V; Hoffsten, M. Boston brace in the treatment of idiopathic scoliosis *J Pediatr Orthop*, 1995, 15, 524-7.

[6] Asher, MA; Burton, DC. Adolescent idiopathic scoliosis: natural history and long term treatment effects. *Scoliosis*, 2006, 1, 2.

[7] Noonan, KJ; Dolan, LA; Jacobson, WC; Weinstein, SL. Long-term psychosocial characteristics of patients treated for idiopathic scoliosis. *J Pediatr Orthop*, 1997, 17, 712-7.

[8] Götze, C; Liljenqvist, UR; Slomka, A; Götze, HG; Steinbeck, J. Quality of life and back pain: Outcome 16.7 years after Harrington instrumentation. *Spine*, 2002, 27, 1456-64.

[9] Betz, RR; Bunnell, WP; Lamrecht-Mulier, E; *et al.* Scoliosis and pregnancy. *J Bone Joint Surg Am,* 1987, 69, 90-96.

[10] Danielsson, AJ; Nachemson, AL. Childbearing, curve progression, and sexual function in women 22 years after treatment for adolescent idiopathic scoliosis. A case-control study. *Spine,* 2001, 26, 1449-56.

[11] Barrios, C; Pérez-Encinas, C; Maruenda, JI; Laguía, M. Significant ventilatory functional restriction in adolescents with mild or moderate scoliosis during maximal exercise tolerance test. *Spine,* 2005, 30, 1610-5.

[12] Chong, K; Letts, R; Cumming, G. Influence of spinal curvature on exercise capacity. *J Ped Orthop,* 1981, 1, 251-4.

[13] Jackson, RP; Simmons, EH; Stripinis, D. Incidence and severity of back pain in adult idiopathic scoliosis. *Spine,* 1983, 8, 749-56.

[14] Pehrsson, K; Danielsson, A; Nachemson, A. Pulmonary function in patients with adolescent idiopathic scoliosis: A 25 year follow-up after surgery or start of brace treatment. *Thorax,* 2001, 56, 388-93.

[15] Lonstein JE; Carlson JM. The prediction of Curve progression in untreated idiopathic scoliosis during growth. *J Bone Joint Surg Am* 1984, 66, 1061-71.

[16] Noonan, KJ; Weinstein, SL; Jacobson, WC; Dolan, LA. Use of the Milwaukee brace for progressive idiopathic scoliosis. *J Bone Joint Surg Am,* 1996, 78, 557-67.

[17] Katz, DE; Richards, BS; Browne, RH; Herring, JA. A comparison between the Boston brace and the Charleston bending brace in adolescent idiopathic scoliosis. *Spine,* 1997, 22, 1302-12.

[18] Landauer, F; Wimmer, C; Behensky, H. Estimating the final outcome of brace treatment for idiopathic thoracic scoliosis at 6 months follow-up. *Pediatric Rehabilitation,* 2003, 6, 201-7.

[19] Carr, WA; Moe, JH; Winter, RB; Lonstein, JE. Treatment of idiopathic scoliosis in the Milwaukee brace. *J Bone Joint Surg Am,* 1980, 62, 599-612.

[20] O'Neill, PJ; Karol, LA; Shindle, MK; Elerson, EE; BrintzenhofeSzoc, KM; Katz, DE; et al. Decreased orthotic effectiveness in overweight patients with adolescent idiopathic scoliosis. *J Bone Joint Surg Am,* 2005, 87, 1069-74.

[21] Maruyama, T. Bracing adolescent idiopathic scoliosis: a systematic review of the literature of effective conservative treatment looking for end results 5 years after weaning. *Disabil Rehabil,* 2008, 30, 786-91.

[22] Weiss, HR; Weiss, G; Schaar, HJ. Incidence of surgery in conservatively treated patients with scoliosis. *Pediatr Rehabil,* 2003, 6, 111-8.

[23] Rigo, M; Reiter, CH; Weiss, HR. Effect of conservative management on the prevalence of surgery in patients with adolescent idiopathic scoliosis. *Pediatr Rehabil,* 2003, 6, 209-14.

[24] Dolan, LA; Weinstein, SL. Surgical rates after observation and bracing for adolescent idiopathic scoliosis: an evidence-based review. *Spine,* 2007, 32, S91-S100.

[25] *Lange, JE; Steen, H; Brox, JN.* Long-term results after Boston brace treatment in adolescent idiopathic scoliosis. *Scoliosis,* 2009, 4, 17.

[26] Wiley, JW; Thomson, JD; Mitchell, TM; Smith, BG; Banta, JV. Effectiveness of the Boston brace in treatment of large curves in adolescent idiopathic scoliosis. *Spine*, 2000, 25, 2326-32.

[27] Green, NE. Part-time bracing of adolescent idiopathic scoliosis. *J Bone Joint Surg Am*, 1986, 68, 738–43.

[28] Emans, JB; Kaelin, A; Bancel, P; Hall, JE; Miller, ME. The Boston Bracing system for idiopathic scoliosis: follow-up results in 295 patients. *Spine*, 1986, 11, 792–801.

[29] Allington, NJ; Bowen, JR. Adolescent idiopathic scoliosis: treatment with the Wilmington brace. *J Bone Joint Surg Am*, 1996, 78, 1056–62.

[30] Peltonen, J; Poussa, M; Ylikoski, M. Three year results of bracing in scoliosis. *Acta Orthop Scand*, 1988, 59, 487–90.

[31] Matsunaga, S; Hayashi, K; Naruo, T; Nozoe, S; Komiya, S. Psychologic management of brace therapy for patients with idiopathic scoliosis. *Spine*, 2005, 30, 547–50.

[32] Tones, M; Moss, N; Polly, DW. Jr. A review of quality of life and psychosocial issues in scoliosis. *Spine*, 2006, 31, 3027–38.

[33] Fayssoux, RS; Cho, RH; Herman, MJ. A history of bracing for Idiopathic Scoliosis in North America. *Clin Orthop Relat Res*, 2010, 468, 654-64.

[34] Bunge, EM; de Bekker-Grob, EW; van Biezen, FC; Essink-Bot, ML; de Koning, HJ. Patients' Preferences for Scoliosis Brace Treatment: A Discrete Choice Experiment. *Spine*, 2010, 35, 57-63.

[35] Watts, HG; Hall, JE; Stanish, W. The Boston brace system for the treatment of low thoracic and lumbar scoliosis by the use of a girdle without superstructure. *Clin Orthop*, 1977, 126, 87–92.

[36] Stagnara P; de Mauroy JC. *Résultats à long terme du traitement orthopédique lyonnais. in Actualités en rééducation fonctionnelle et réadaptation.* [Long-term results of Lyonnais orthopedic treatment. in News in Functional Rehabilitation and Rehabilitation.] Ed. Masson; Paris; 1977, 2° série 33-36.

[37] Stagnara, P; Desbrosses, J. Scolioses essentielles pendant l'enfance et l'adolescence: résultats des traitements orthopédiques et chirurgicaux. [J. Essential scoliosis during childhood and adolescence: results of orthopedic and surgical treatments.] *Rev Chir Orthop*, 1960, 46, 562-575.

[38] Weiss, HR. Conservative treatment of idiopathic scoliosis with physical therapy and orthoses. *Orthopade*, 2003, 32, 146-56.

[39] Weiss, HR. Rehabilitation of adolescent patients with scoliosis--what do we know? A review of the literature. *Pediatr Rehabil*, 2003, 6, 183-94.

[40] Chêneau, J. *Orthese de scoliose; 1ère Edition.* [Scoliosis orthosis; 1st Edition.] Chêneau, J., Saint Orensm, 1990.

[41] Cobetto, N; Aubin, CE; Le May, S; Desbiens-Blais, F; Labelle, H; Parent, S. Braces Optimized With Computer-Assisted Design and Simulations Are Lighter, More Comfortable, and More Efficient Than Plaster-Cast Braces for the Treatment of Adolescent Idiopathic Scoliosis. *Spine Deform.*, 2014 Jul, 2(4), 276-284. doi: 10.1016/j.jspd.2014.03.005.

[42] Screening for the Early Detection for Idiopathic Scoliosis in Adolescents. *SRS/POSNA/AAOS /AAP Position Statement*. https,//www.srs.org/about-srs/quality-and-safety/position-statements/screening-for-the-early-detection-for-idiopathic-scoliosis-in-adolescents.

[43] Labelle, H; Stephens, B Richards, De Kleuver, M; Grivas, TB; Luk, KDK; Hee, Kit Wong; Thometz, J; Beauséjour, M; Turgeon, I; Fong, DYT. Screening for adolescent idiopathic scoliosis: an information statement by the scoliosis research society international task force. *Scoliosis.*, 2013, 8, 17.

[44] Mehlman, CT. *Idiopathic Scoliosis Treatment & Management*; https://emedicine.medscape.com/article/1265794-treatment.

[45] Rigo, M. Intra-observer reliability of a new classification correlating with brace treatment. *Pediatric Rehabilitation,* 2004, 7, 63.

[46] Trivedi, JM; Thomson, JD. Results of Charleston bracing in skeletally immature patients with idiopathic scoliosis. *J Pediatr Orthop*, 2001, 21, 277-80.

[47] Price, CT; Scott, DS; Reed, FEJ; Riddick, MF. Nighttime bracing for adolescent idiopathic scoliosis with the Charleston bending brace. Preliminary report. *Spine*, 1990, 15, 1294-9.

[48] Price, CT; Scott, DS; Reed, FEJ; Sproul, JT; Riddick, MF. Nighttime bracing for adolescent idiopathic scoliosis with the Charleston Bending Brace: long-term follow-up. *J Pediatr Orthop*, 1997, 17, 703-7.

[49] Yrjönen, T; Ylikoski, M; Schlenzka, D; Kinnunen, R; Poussa, M. Effectiveness of the Providence nighttime bracing in adolescent idiopathic scoliosis: a comparative study of 36 female patients. *Eur Spine J*, 2006, 15, 1139-43.

[50] Howard, A; Wright, JG; Hedden, D. A comparative study of TLSO, Charleston, and Milwaukee braces for idiopathic scoliosis. *Spine*, 1998, 23, 2404-2411.

[51] Gepstein, R; Leitner, Y; Zohar, E; Angel, I; Shabat, S; Pekarsky, I; et al. Effectiveness of the Charleston bending brace in the treatment of single-curve idiopathic scoliosis. *J Pediatr Orthop*, 2002, 22, 84-74.

[52] Janicki, J; Poe-Kochert, C; Armstrong, DG; Thompson, GH. A comparison of the thoracolumbosacral orthoses and providence orthosis in the treatment of adolescent idiopathic scoliosis: results using the new SRS inclusion and assessment criteria for bracing studies. *J Pediatr Orthop*, 2007, 27, 369-74.

[53] Federico, DJ; Renshaw, TS. Results of treatment of idiopathic scoliosis with the Charleston Bending Brace. *Spine*, 1990, 15, 886-7.

[54] D'Amato, CR; Griggs, S; McCoy, B. Nighttime Bracing With the Providence Brace in Adolescent Girls with Idiopathic Scoliosis. *Spine*, 2001, 26, 2006-12.

[55] Wong, MS; Cheng, JC; Lam, TP; Ng, BK; Sin, SW; Lee-Shum, SL; et al. The effect of rigid versus flexible spinal orthosis on the clinical efficacy and acceptance of the patients with adolescent idiopathic scoliosis. *Spine*, 2008, 33, 1360-5.

[56] Coillard, C; Vachon, V; Circo, AB; Beauséjour, M; Rivard, CH. Effectiveness of the SpineCor brace based on the new standardized criteria proposed by the scoliosis research society for adolescent idiopathic scoliosis. *J Pediatr Orthop*, 2007, 27, 375–9.

[57] Coillard, C; Leroux, MA; Zabjek, KF; Rivard, CH. SpineCor – a non-rigid brace for the treatment of idiopathic scoliosis: post-treatment results. *Eur Spine J*, 2003, 12, 141–8.

[58] Weiss, HR; Bohr, S; Jahnke, A; Pleines, S. Acupucture in the treatment of scoliosis - a single blind controlled pilot study. *Scoliosis*, 2008, 3.

[59] Cassella, MC; Hall, JE. Current treatment approaches in the nonoperative and operative management of adolescent idiopathic scoliosis. *Phys Ther*, 1991, 71, 897-909.

Chapter 13

FUSIONLESS TECHNIQUES FOR JUVENILE AND ADOLESCENT IDIOPATHIC SCOLIOSIS

Kedar Padhye, MD and Ron El-Hawary[†], MD
*Division of Orthopedic Surgery, IWK Health Centre,
Halifax, Nova Scotia, Canada*

ABSTRACT

Scoliosis is a complex, three-dimensional deformity of the spine resulting from both known and unknown causes. It is estimated that in children who are 5 years old, there is up to 12.5 cm of vertical growth of the spine remaining. Furthermore, the lungs do not fully develop until the age of 8; the alveolar maturation process continues from birth, resulting in an increase in the number of alveoli, alveolar ducts, and terminal saccules. After the age of lung maturity, surgical management of scoliosis has been focused on correcting the curvature and obtaining a solid fusion of the growing spine, thereby halting further progression of the deformity. In recent times, there has been growing interest in fusionless techniques like vertebral body tethering (VBT), vertebral body stapling (VBS), and Apifix-Posterior Dynamic Deformity Correction for the treatment of juvenile and adolescent idiopathic scoliosis. This chapter aims to discuss in detail the indications, surgical techniques, early outcomes, and the complications associated with these procedures.

Keywords: fusionless, anterior vertebral body tethering, stapling, spine, idiopathic scoliosis

INTRODUCTION

Scoliosis is a complex, three-dimensional deformity of the spine resulting from both known and unknown causes. The current standard of care for skeletally immature patients with idiopathic scoliosis and moderate curves (25°– 40°) is thoracolumbosacral orthosis [1]. The

---

[*] Corresponding Author Email: Kedar.Padhye@iwk.nshealth.ca.
[†] Corresponding Author Email: Ron.El-hawary@iwk.nshealth.ca.

BrAIST study demonstrated the effectiveness of bracing to prevent progression to 50° [2]. However, several reports question the success rate of bracing [3–5], and some patients experience lower body image and emotional stress, which may be greater than those caused by the deformity itself [4, 5]. These issues can lead to an increase in the incidence of non-compliance in this population [6–8]. Those patients who fail bracing and whose curves reach 50° are often offered a fusion. Fusion remains a viable option but limits spine mobility and may lead to adjacent segment disease [9, 10].

In recent times, there has been growing interest in fusionless techniques such as vertebral body tethering (VBT), vertebral body stapling (VBS), and ApiFix- Posterior Dynamic Deformity Correction for the treatment of juvenile and adolescent idiopathic scoliosis [11–14]. The goal of these fusionless techniques has been to prevent deformity progression as well as maintain mobility of the spine. This chapter aims to discuss in detail the indications, surgical techniques, early outcomes, and the complications associated with these procedures.

NORMAL GROWTH

Development of the spine and thoracic cage is a complex series of events during growth of the child. The slightest error or modification can lead to anomalies or deformity that has an impact on the spine, thoracic cavity and lung development influencing the circle of growth [15–19].

Only comprehensive knowledge of normal growth parameters allows us to have a better understanding of abnormalities resulting in a spinal deformity [20, 21]. As a spinal deformity progresses, the spinal growth is affected along with the size and shape of the thoracic. In a "domino effect," this distortion of the thorax eventually interferes with lung development and cardiac function, leading to the development of potentially lethal thoracic insufficiency syndrome and cor-pulmonale [17]. Severe spinal deformities and early spinal fusion can have a negative impact on the cardiovascular and respiratory systems. The pattern and timing varies according to the degree and evolution of the deformity [15, 18, 20–28].

Normal growth of the spine comprises of a series of acceleration and deceleration phases divided into three periods of the child's growth. The first period ranges from birth to five years, is characterized by a gain in sitting height of 27 cm, with 12 cm of growth occurring during the first year of life. The second period between ages five to ten years is a quiescent phase, where the sitting height increases by 2.5 cm/year. The third period corresponds to puberty and is characterized by a gain in sitting height of approximately 12 cm [20–22]. At the initiation of puberty, the average growth in the sitting height is approximately 12.5 cm for boys and 11.5 cm for girls. Two-thirds of this growth occurs during the "peak height velocity" or "acceleration phase." The average growth in sitting height during the "deceleration phase" is approximately 4 cm for boys and 3.5 cm for girls [16, 19–22].

The height of the spine accounts for 60% of the total sitting height, and the head and pelvis account for the remaining 40%. The T1-S1 segment accounts for approximately 50% of the sitting height; two-thirds of this segment is from thoracic spine and one-third from the lumbar spine. The T1-S1 segment grows approximately 10 cm during the first five years of life (2 cm/year), approximately 5 cm between ages five and 10 (1 cm/year), and approximately 10 cm between age 10 and skeletal maturity (1.8 cm/year). T1-T12 is the posterior pillar of the thoracic cage and is an important segment. It measures, on an average, approximately 12 cm at birth, 18 cm at five years of age, and 27 cm at skeletal maturity. The thoracic spine constitutes 30% of the sitting height, and each thoracic vertebra and its disc account for 2.5% of the sitting height. In normal children, the longitudinal growth of the thoracic spine is approximately 1.3 cm/year between birth and five years, 0.7 cm/year between the ages of five and 10 years, and 1.1 cm/year during puberty. A precocious arthrodesis of the T1-T12 segment affects thoracic growth and lung development. The L1-L5 length is, on an average, approximately 7.5 cm at birth and 16 cm at skeletal maturity. The lumbar spine constitutes approximately 18% of the sitting height, and a single lumbar vertebra and its disc account for 3.5% of the sitting height [29].

An early fusion of the spine can have negative repercussions on thoracic growth and lung development. Karol et al. [27] showed that a thoracic spine height of 18-22 cm or more is necessary to avoid severe respiratory insufficiency. They showed that children undergoing an early spinal fusion have a reduced thoracic depth and a shorter T1-T12 segment compared to normal subjects [27]. The capacity may decrease by 50% of the predicted volume if more than 60% of the thoracic spine, or 8 thoracic vertebrae, are fused before 8 years of age [17, 30–36]. Gollogly et al. [36], showed that lung parenchyma volume is a function of age. The lung parenchyma volume is approximately 400 cc at birth, 900 cc at 5 years of age, 1500 cc at 10 years of age, and is approximately 4500 cc for boys and 3500 for girls at skeletal maturity. Therefore, early-onset scoliosis adversely affects thoracic growth at the critical period of maximum "respiratory growth," inducing irreversible changes in the thoraco-pulmonary structure [16, 19–22, 24, 25, 29, 30, 34–38].

A young patient's remaining growth is usually assessed by four maturity indices [39–42]:

1) The Risser sign (a skeletal marker of the pelvis)
2) Hand and wrist skeletal maturity
3) Peak height velocity (PHV),
4) Menarchal status in females (a physiologic marker).

The Risser sign is a radiographic measurement based on the ossification of the iliac apophysis, which is divided into four quadrants, beginning on the lateral aspect of the iliac apophysis and progressing medially. A modified Risser grading system has been created in which a new group, Risser 0 with closed triradiate cartilage, and Risser 1 were found to be the best predictors of the beginning of rapid curve progression [43].

Sanders et al. [42] came up with a simplified classification based on the epiphyses of the phalanx, metacarpal, and distal radius. They concluded that this method reliably predicts maturity and probability of progression to surgery.

Peak height velocity (PHV) is a measurement of the maximal skeletal growth that occurs during the adolescent growth spurt [41, 44, 45]. Calculated from changes in a patient's height measurements over time, PHV is reported to be about 8.0 cm/yr. for girls and 9.5 cm/yr. for boys [40, 43]. The reported average age at PHV in North American girl's is approximately 11.5 years. Closure of the triradiate cartilage, a radiographic index of maturity, occurs after PHV and before Risser grade 1 and menarche. Although PHV requires analysis of serial height measurements collected over time, it is the earliest and best index available to demonstrate that growth is slowing and the risk for curve progression is diminishing. In boys, use of PHV is a superior predictor compared to the Risser sign and chronologic age, and closure of the triradiate cartilage approximates the time of PHV. The Tanner index of maturity, which is based on an assessment of breast and genital development, is another clinical index that has been used to determine a child's remaining growth and thus can indirectly predict the risk for curve progression [40].

Fusionless procedures not only rely on the operative technique and the implants used but also on the spines growth potential. Finding this narrow window of opportunity is crucial when fusionless techniques are used. Understanding the normal growth of the spine is essential to calculate the growth potential and thereby helps as a guide to choosing the appropriate fusionless technique.

VERTEBRAL BODY STAPLING (VBS)

Stapling across physes of the long bones has been accepted for many years as a predictable method of treating limb malalignment in young children [46, 47]. Animal studies using a rat tail model confirm the ability to modulate vertebral growth plates with skeletal fixation devices [48]. In 1951, Nachlas and Borden performed vertebral interbody stapling across the physeal endplates and discs in a dog scoliosis model [49]. Correction was seen in many dogs, and in some, the curve progression was arrested. Some staples failed because they spanned two interspaces instead of just one. Results for humans with congenital scoliosis were presented as early as 1954 [50], but the results were disappointing with limited correction, staple loosening or breakage. However, recent studies have shown encouraging results when the curve magnitude is between 20 to 35 degrees in cases of idiopathic scoliosis [51].

Our current indications for VBS are (1) age <13 years in girls and <15 years in boys; (2) Risser 0 to 2 with 1 year of growth remaining by wrist radiograph; (3) thoracic or lumbar coronal curve <35° with minimal rotation and flexible to <20°; and (4) thoracic kyphosis <40°.

Contraindications include (1) Congenital scoliosis (2) Curves above T4 or below L4 (3) True thoracic kyphosis greater than 40 degrees.

Authors Preferred Surgical Technique

We prefer the double lumen endo-catheter tube following intubation for general anesthesia. After intubation, arterial line for blood pressure monitoring, urinary catheter and electrodes for intraoperative neuromonitoring (IONM) are placed. The patient is placed in a lateral decubitus position on a flat top of a radiolucent table with all bony prominences well-padded with the convex side of the curve facing upwards. The axillary role is placed under the patient. Fluoroscopy is used to landmark the planned instrumented vertebrae in the lateral projection. We prefer two mid-axillary anterior portals (12mm) and three posterior working portals (15mm) through the intercostal spaces. First superior-anterior portal is used to visualize the chest cavity. At this stage, the right lung is deflated to better visualize the vertebral column. Two to three discs can be stapled through one portal. A 30-degree scope is inserted in the supero-anterior portal to visualize the extent of the exposure. Inter-vertebral disc spaces are identified. Parietal pleura is not excised and segmental vessels are preserved where possible. If a segmental vessel comes in the way of the staples, it can be retracted by making a small incision in the parietal pleura or cauterized. A radio-opaque trial inserter is used to obtain the appropriate dimension of the staple and to create pilot holes. Vertical force can be used on the spine to visualize the possible correction before insertion of the staple. One of three posterior portals can be used to obtain a 'pipeline' view in order to thoracoscopically simulate a lateral view while fluoroscopy is used to judge anteroposterior trajectory. The smallest staple that spans the disc and growth plate is used. Shape memory Nitinol alloy (Medtronic, Memphis, TN) based staples that have been cooled over a basin of ice are placed over the pilot holes. Before inserting the stapes radiographic confirmation is done. Two single staples or one double staple can be used at each disc space spanning the ends of the curve. If there is significant hypo-kyphosis at the apex (<10 degrees) staples can be positioned anterior to the body of the vertebra or a third staple could be added. If the patient has two structural curves, both curves should be stapled. We prefer to obtain maximum correction on the operating table which is obtained by the corrective positioning of the patient on the table and by applying adequate pressure to the spinal segment before insertion of the staple. If the staple is not in the desired position, it can be pulled with a clamp and re-positioned. Final confirmatory anterior-posterior and lateral fluoroscopic images are taken and a thorough irrigation with saline is performed. Appropriate size chest tube is inserted through the lowest of the posterior portals through a subcutaneous tunnel, one interspace cranial to the incision. Following the closure of the wound, the chest-tube is set at 20 cm of H2O suction. (Figures 1-6).

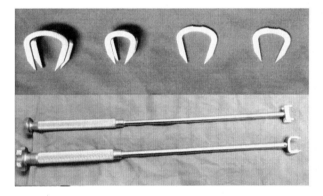

Figure 1. Single and double prong staples along with its trial inserter and final inserter.

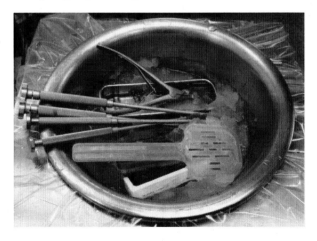

Figure 2. Shape memory alloy (Nitinol alloy) based staples kept in iced saline which allows it to expand.

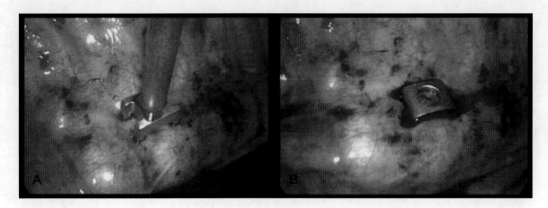

Figure 3A and 3B. Thoracoscopic view while insertion of the trial followed by insertion of the double staple across the disc space.

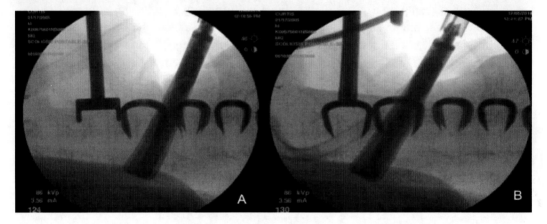

Figure 4A and 4B. Fluoroscopic confirmation of placement of trial and the final implant across the disc space.

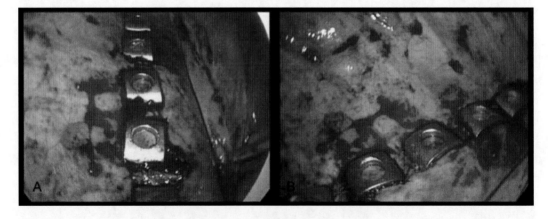

Figure 5A and 5B. Final implant position through the posterior and anterior thoracoscopic portals.

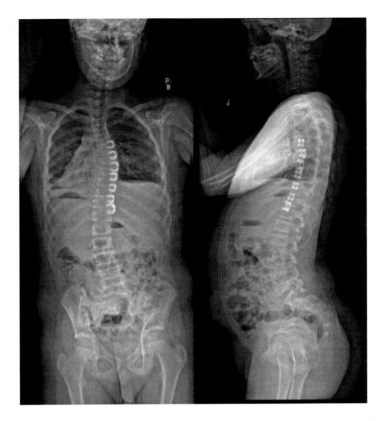

Figure 6. Postoperative x-rays of an 11-year-old boy with right main thoracic curve treated with VBS.

Postoperative Care

The chest tube is usually removed on the second postoperative day. All patients receive opioid analgesia combined with anti-inflammatory drugs. Chest physiotherapy in the form of incentive spirometry is encouraged. A chest x-ray is done for three postoperative days to rule out atelectasis, pneumothorax or hemothorax. Activities, as tolerated, are started after chest tube comes out.

Review of Literature

Vertebral Body Stapling has been used in humans in congenital scoliosis as early as 1954 [50], but the results were disappointing. Correction of the scoliosis was limited because the children had little growth remaining and the curves were severe, with considerable rotational deformity. Some staples broke or became loose, possibly because of motion through the intervertebral discs. However, recent studies have shown encouraging results when the curve magnitude is between 20 to 45 degrees [12, 13, 52, 53].

Since the advent of Nitinol alloy-based stapes, results have been promising. These staples are unique in that the prongs are straight when cooled but clamp down into the bone in a "C" shape when the staple returns to body temperature, thus providing secure fixation. This Nitinol staple has been tested in a goat scoliosis model by Braun et al. [54], and has been shown to be safe and have utility for arresting iatrogenic curves of <70° in the goat. Laituri et al. [53], reported curve improvement in 7 children (aged 8–11yrs) with idiopathic scoliosis with a mean curve magnitude 34 degrees (range 25° to 41°) correcting to a mean curve magnitude of 23 degrees (range 16 to 30). Although Laituri et al. [53], did not report on lumbar curves, Betz et al. [13], found that 87% of all lumbar curves in children with idiopathic scoliosis measuring 25° to 45° and 79% of thoracic curves with a curve measuring 25° to 35° had a successful outcome at least 2 years after being treated with VBS. They studied 28 patients with a minimum of 2-year follow-up and found an 86% success rate of thoracic curves of less than 35° and a 100% success rate in lumbar curves. Cuddihy et al. [55], suggested that the thoracic curves bending more than 50% of preoperative measurement correction had a success rate of 71.4% in comparison to 25% success in the curves with less than 50% flexibility. Curve flexibility did not have any effect on results in the lumbar group. A factor that might contribute to the greater success rate of VBS for lumbar curves in the previous literature is the more rapid growth of this region of the spine than that of the thoracic region. Another factor is the relative flexibility of the lumbar spine, which provides more operative correction than that of the thoracic spine, where the ribs may constrain correction [52].

In a recent study by Bumpass et al. [12], control rate for thoracic curves <35 degrees was 79%, nearly identical to Betz et al. [13], who reported 78% control. For thoracolumbar curves <35 degrees, they achieved a 70% control rate, less than the 87% as reported by Betz et al. Their series also highlights an interesting case of over-correction that first required staple removal and later spinal fusion. They removed staples when the spine was nearly neutral, but the patient continued to develop a significant reversed curvature. They suggested that the patient possibly had a hemiepiphysiodesis of the stapled levels as significant physeal damage has been reported in the literature in a bovine study by Shillington et al. [56]. They postulated that growth modulation from VBS may actually be due to the staples causing closure of the vertebral physes, rather than a true Hueter–Volkmann effect created by staple compression.

In a recent study by Cahill et al. [51] reported a success rate of 74% in thoracic curves (71% for the subgroup that reached maturity) with preoperative Cobb angles less than 35 degrees and 82% in lumbar curves (89% for the subgroup that reached maturity) with preoperative Cobb angles less than 45 degrees. Their study reports a mean postoperative follow-up of 3.4 years for 24 patients who reached skeletal maturity. The authors indicate that results of the study are important because the patients included in this study were all at high risk of progression. Their patients were either Risser 0 or 1 at time of VBS with a thoracic curve magnitude between 25 and 35 and/or a lumbar curve magnitude between 25 and 45. They did not report any adverse "flattening" (decrease in lordosis) of the lumbar spine when VBS is performed in the lumbar spine but kyphosis is imparted to the thoracic spine which they considered beneficial effect in a hypokyphotic deformity. Presently, due to the lack of long-term reports on VBS in the literature, it is unknown if there will be degenerative changes in the disc or if there are negative effects on the mobility of the spine on a long-term.

Complications

The risk of pulmonary complications with the thoracoscopic approach for scoliosis surgery is reported at 21% and includes atelectasis, pneumothorax, hemothorax, chylothorax and pleural effusion [57]. Complications associated specifically with VBS include broken staples, staple dislodgement, curve overcorrection, congenital diaphragmatic hernia rupture, contralateral pleural effusion, and superior mesenteric artery syndrome [12, 53, 58, 59].

VERTEBRAL BODY TETHERING (VBT)

The concept of vertebral body tethering (VBT) is to prevent vertebral growth on the convex side while allowing growth on the concave side. This dynamic epiphysiodesis of the convex side aims to equilibrate the height of both concave and convex sides of the vertebra without fusion [60]. Anterior VBT has been extensively studied in animal models. Newton et al. [61, 62], have demonstrated the ability of a unilateral tether to induce deformity in a bovine model with radiographical evidence of disc wedging and rotation while retaining spine flexibility. Braun et al. [63] have demonstrated similar results in a goat model.

Although promising, specific medical devices have only been recently developed for this technique.

Authors-Current Indications for VBT

1) Risser 0 to 2.
2) Age >10 years.
3) Single thoracic curve (T5-T12), single lumbar curve (T12, L1-L3/4).
4) Cobb angle 40-65 degrees
5) Flexibility > 50%
6) Kyphosis < 40 degrees.
7) Double curve.

Contraindications

1) Age < 10 years.
2) Risser 3 and above.

Authors Preferred Surgical Technique

Following general anesthesia, a double lumen endo-catheter intubation is performed. After intubation, the arterial line for blood pressure monitoring, urinary catheter, and electrodes for intraoperative neuromonitoring (IONM) are placed. The patient is placed in a lateral decubitus position on a flat top of a radiolucent table with all bony prominences well-padded with the convex side of the curve facing upwards. The axillary role is placed under the patient. Fluoroscopy is used to landmark the planned instrumented vertebrae in the lateral projection. We prefer two mid-axillary anterior portals (12mm) and three posterior working portals (15mm) through the intercostal spaces. First supero-anterior portal is used to visualize the chest cavity. At this point, the right lung is deflated to better visualize the vertebral column. A 30-degree scope is inserted in the supero-anterior portal to visualize the extent of the exposure. The pleura is dissected off the vertebral bodies at all levels from the upper end to the lower end vertebrae (Figure 7A). This is done in a sequential fashion along the length of the curve. Segmental vessels at each level are cauterized or de-functioned with a harmonic blade (Figure 7B). Rib heads can be prominent at T5-7 and sometimes need resection prior to insertion of staples and screws. A three-prong staple is placed in the anterior aspect of the vertebral body adjacent to the rib head. Sequentially at all levels, screws of appropriate size are inserted (Figures 8A and 8B). At each level starting cranially, we prefer to use the scope in the posterior portals to obtain a 'pipeline' view in order to judge anterior/posterior trajectory. Utmost care is be taken at this level in order to prevent posterior trajectory of the screws into the spinal canal. Fluoroscopy is used at every level on AP/lateral projection to confirm screw placement. At each level, once the screw is inserted a tether is placed in the tulip of each screw sequentially and set-screw is used to secure the tether (Figure 9). We prefer to tension the tether at each level sequentially as we insert screws. Tether tensioning can also be performed all at once after insertion of screws in the planned levels. Correction of the curve occurs through both tensioning of the tether and translation of the spine. Residual tether is trimmed leaving at least 2 cm at both ends to accommodate potential tether re-adjustment (Figure 10). At each apical level, a long handle blade can be used to incise the anterior longitudinal ligament and perform annulotomy in case of a stiff curve. Care must be taken not to disrupt the end plates in order to avoid unwanted fusion. We prefer to use intra-operative neurological monitoring throughout the procedure. At the end of the procedure, a final copy of the fluoroscopy images are saved and a thorough irrigation with saline is performed. Appropriate size chest tube is inserted through the lowest of the posterior portals through a subcutaneous tunnel, one interspace cranial to the incision. Following the closure of the wound, the chest-tube is set at 20 cm of H_2O suction.

Postoperative Care

The chest tube is usually removed on the second postoperative day. All patients receive opioid analgesia combined with anti-inflammatory drugs. Chest physiotherapy in the form of incentive spirometry is encouraged. A chest x-ray is done for three postoperative days to rule out atelectasis, pneumothorax or hemothorax. Activities, as tolerated, are started after chest tube comes out.

Fusionless Techniques for Juvenile and Adolescent Idiopathic Scoliosis 185

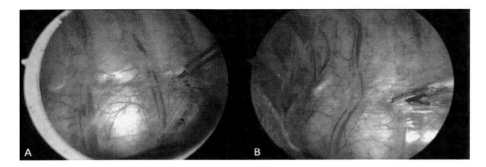

Figure 7. A- Pleura is dissected off the vertebral body with the help of hook cautery. B- Segmental artery is de-functioned with the help of harmonic.

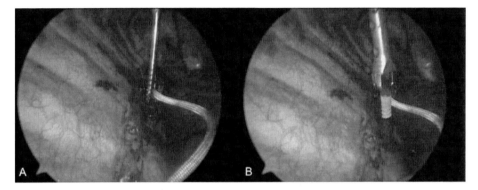

Figure 8. A- Insertion of 3 prong staple followed by tapping. B- "Pipeline" view through one of the posterior portals showing insertion of screw.

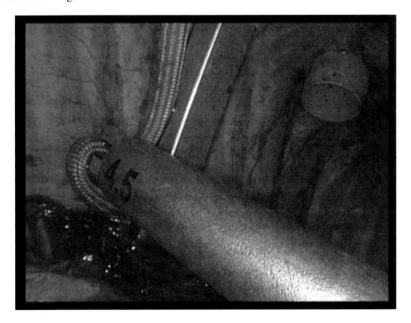

Figure 9. Tensioning of the tether is performed at each level prior to insertion of the screw at the following levels.

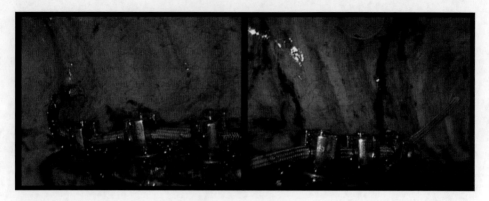

Figure 10. 2cm long tether is left at both end in case readjustment or further tensioning is needed.

Review of Literature

Newton et al. [64], demonstrated that, in an immature porcine model, a flexible polyethylene tether attached via pedicle screws along the anterolateral aspect of the spine could alter the spinal morphology and induce a scoliotic deformity. This alteration was achieved while concurrently maintaining disc health and maximizing axial growth in a series of 12 mini pigs whose growth rates were similar to that of an adolescent growth spurt. Braun et al. [65], noted tethering to be superior to staples in deformity correction in their caprine model. The authors of these experimental studies also reported on the health of the discs in the tethered segments and found no evidence of irreversible growth cartilage or disc injury [62, 64, 66, 67]. Decreased disc thickness, increased proteoglycan synthesis, and a change in collagen distribution between the 280 concave and convex sides were reported; however, there was no change in water and glycosaminoglycan content within the tethered discs. The clinical implications and reversibility of these changes remain unknown.

Crawford and Lenke [68] reported a skeletally immature patient who underwent anterior VBT and demonstrated progressive correction of his curvature over a 5-year time span. Similarly, Samdani et al. [69] reported their first series of 11 skeletally immature patients with 2-year follow-up and found continued progressive correction of the tethered thoracic curve, the nonstructural lumbar curve, and the rib prominence. Patients had a mean age of 12.3 ± 1.6 years and mean Risser grade of 0.6 ± 1.1 with an average preoperative curve magnitude of $44.2° \pm 9.0°$ which corrected to $20.3° \pm 11°$ on the first erect X-ray, with continued improvement at 2 years to a mean $13.5° \pm 11.6°$. The authors noted a 70% correction of the curves with VBT over a 2-year follow-up. Most recently, Samdani et al. [70] presented on 25 patients treated with VBT who have now reached skeletal maturity. These patients mean age was 12.5 ± 1.4 years with a mean Risser of 0.5 ± 1.0. The average preoperative Cobb was $40.9° \pm 7.1°$ which corrected to $20.1° \pm 8.4°$ on the first erect X-ray with progressive improvement to skeletal maturity to a mean $14.0° \pm 11.1°$, noting a 66.1% correction over time. There were two patients who required subsequent surgery for overcorrection of their curves that required loosening of the tether. The authors did not report on any patient requiring a conversion to fusion surgery. In a recent report by Boudissa et al. [71], 6 patients of mean age of 11.2 ± 1.2 (9–12) years with a mean follow-up was 21.6 months (18–24) correcting main thoracic curve magnitude from $45° \pm 10°$ (35–60) to $38° \pm 7°$ (30–50), and the mean lumbar curve magnitude of $33° \pm 5°$ (30–40) to 25° ± 9° (15–40). They reported that all patients were well-balanced in the frontal plan and the sagittal plan on full spine X-rays and there were no complications.

The disadvantage of this technique is that currently there are few specific devices developed for it. Also, there is a possibility of overcorrection, which has been difficult to predict as there are no long-term studies in the literature to date. Other complications reported are atelectasis, tether loosening, and subsequent readjustment. Although initial results have been encouraging, long-term benefits are yet to be reported.

APIFIX: POSTERIOR DYNAMIC DEFORMITY CORRECTION

In progressive scoliosis, a good correction of the deformity can be achieved with current surgical techniques, but the postoperative spinal motion is significantly diminished due to the fusion of the spine [72]. To overcome these negative consequences of extensive fusion procedures, recent research has been aimed at developing techniques that allow scoliosis correction with posterior instrumentation without fusion [11, 73]. A new less-invasive and the potentially fusionless scoliosis correction system is a posterior concave periapical distraction device (ApiFix Ltd, Misgav, Israel), which spans a minimum of 3 to 4 motion segments (Figure 12).

Device Details

The device has an overall length range of 65–105 mm and is expanded in increments of 1.3 mm, for a total extension of 20–30 mm, depending on length (Figure 11). The device has a ratchet mechanism that allows unidirectional elongation of an expandable rod. The ratchet mechanism consists of a toothed area and locking tooth. Both are made of Titanium alloy. The locking tooth rotates around a 2 mm pin and interacts with the toothed area to allow only unidirectional movement. The locking tooth is pressed via a flat spring to prevent backward slippage. The spring part is made from Nitinol (NiTi). The entire device is made from Titanium alloy with ADLC coating (amorphous diamond-like ceramic). This ceramic coating minimizes friction and wear. The ceramic coating has also the ability to inhibit bacterial growth that may reduce the incidence of post-operative deep wound infection. The expandable rod with polyaxial rings at its extremities is attached by 2 pedicle screws around the apex of the main spinal curvature. As stated before the rod can expand by either 20 mm or 30 mm depending on the pre-distraction rod length. Rod expansion is incremental and gradual, making the deformity correction safer than "all at once" acute rod distraction in the standard type surgery. Spanning the correction process over several weeks to months allows the soft tissues to accommodate any incremental correction. The long, incremental process reduces the load on the screws and allows the body to slowly rebuild itself in the correct position/shape. The implant has a control pin that can abort the ratchet mechanism and put the device in a free neutral mode or a locked position creating a stiff fusion like a rod.

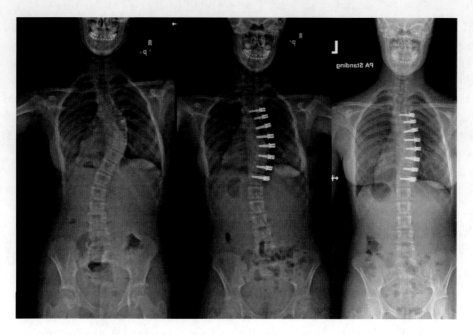

Figure 11. 12-year-old female with juvenile idiopathic scoliosis (JIS). Progressive improvement of the curve at 1 year follow up.

The device is a unilateral construct that connects 2 periapical pedicle screws through polyaxial mobile ball-and-socket joints with a rod. The device is inserted on the concave side of the curve. The rod includes a ratchet that can elongate when the patient performs exercises after surgery, especially with side bending toward the convexity. By side bending, the ratchet allows elongation of the rod and thereby corrects the scoliotic curve. The ratchet does not allow for shortening when the patient stands upright again and thus it preserves the correction. The device can be used as itself in shorter curves or with extenders spanning longer curves (option of two cranial screws and two caudal screws). Extenders are freely mobile in the coronal plane and has semi-constrained angular mobility in the sagittal plane.

Authors-Current Indications

1) Age 11 to 18 years.
2) Risser level 0 to 5.
3) Single thoracic/single lumbar or single thoracolumbar major curve.
4) Cobb angle 35 to 60 degrees.
5) Flexible to ≤ 35 degrees

Contraindications

1) Double major/triple major curve.
2) Cobb angle > 60 degrees
3) Stiff curve

Authors Preferred Surgical Technique

After adequate general anesthesia and endotracheal intubation patient is carefully positioned prone on the spine top of the Radiolucent table. All bony prominences are well padded. Halo femoral traction is preferred as it aids with correction. The posterior spine is prepared and drapped. Fluoroscopy is utilized to landmark the pedicles on the concave side of the curve. Appropriate sized midline skin incision is taken (in case of a large curve, two small skin incisions can be used exposing the end vertebrae using a minimally invasive surgical technique). Subcutaneous tissue is dissected in line with the skin. Fascia is incised in the midline and subperiosteal dissection is performed to expose the tips of the transverse processes of the desired vertebrae. For intervening segment, a paramedian approach through the thoracolumbar fascia, approximately one cm lateral to the spinous processes is performed. Muscle splitting is done and deep retractors are placed. Pedicle screws are inserted at the desired vertebral level. In cases of small curves, ApiFix device can be used in isolation; while in cases of longer curves, device extenders can be used on either end of the device. Once the device is placed and secured to the screws, it is placed in rachet position and distracted to obtain maximum correction. Once the adequate correction is obtained the device is placed in locked position. Final confirmatory anterior-posterior and lateral fluoroscopic images are taken and a thorough irrigation with saline is performed (Figure 12-13)

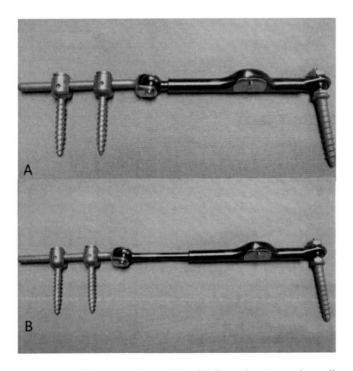

Figure 12. ApiFix device made of titanium alloy with ADLC coating (amorphous diamond-like ceramic). The spring part is made from Nitinol (NiTi). 13A- **Device in its "fully loaded" position.** 13B- Device with full excursion. The device can be used by itself in shorter curves or with extenders spanning longer curves. Extenders are freely mobile in the coronal plane with some angular mobility in the sagittal plane.

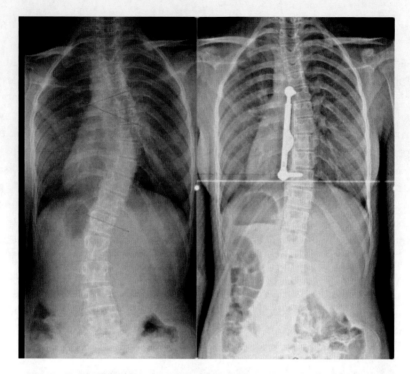

Figure 13. Preoperative (left) and Postoperative (right) x-rays of a 15-year-old girl with right thoracic curve measuring 44 degrees, Risser 3 corrected to 19 degrees with the help of ApiFix device. Radiographs courtesy of Professor Y. Floman.

Postoperative Management

Two to three weeks after the surgery the patients are directed to perform five basic Schroth exercises that enable gradual elongation of the ratchet mechanism leading to a reduction of the spinal curve. These exercises consist of a hand hanging from a bar or door, lateral bending maneuvers while standing or sitting and side stretching while lying on the side over a firm roll. The patient is instructed to perform the exercises for 30 minutes on a daily basis. Exercises are continued for 3–6 months after surgery.

Review of Literature

Since ApiFix is a new device, not much has yet been published in the literature. Floman et al. [11] demonstrated the effectiveness of the periapical distraction device by reducing the Cobb angle from 43-53 degrees to 22-33 degrees in a small case series with a follow-up ranging from 6 months to 2 years. The authors stated that the new device is a less rigid construct than traditional rigid pedicle screw-rod instrumentation and as a result, preserves a more physiologic spinal ROM after treatment with this device. No screw loosening or breakage was encountered in their series. They report biomechanical test on the run-out load of 5,000,000 cycles showed the ApiFix to be 3-fold stronger than standard fusion constructs (unpublished data). According to the authors, three factors may contribute to ApiFix's success: polyaxial connections that prevent mechanical failure, gradual curve correction by spinal motion and spinal growth modulation.

A recent biomechanical study reports the periapical distraction device in free mode roughly halved spinal range of motion of flexion-extension (FE) (human 40.0% and porcine 55.9%), while lateral bending (LB) was only slightly affected (human 18.2% and porcine 17.9%) and axial rotation (AR) was unaffected. In comparison, the rigid pedicle screw-rod instrumentation resulted in a far larger decrease in ROM of FE (human 80.9% and porcine 94.0%), LB (human 75.0% and porcine 92.2%), and AR (human 71.3% and porcine 86.9%). The study also reported that the periapical distraction device did not significantly affect adjacent segment motion.

In contrast, after rigid pedicle screw-rod instrumentation, the range of motion of AR decreased by 18.1% in the cranial adjacent segment of the human spines and increased by 23.9% in the caudal adjacent segment of the porcine spines.

Early results from the device are promising and the hope in the future is to have minimum implants in the spine without compromising the range of motion [11, 73].

CONCLUSION

In the past few years, there has been a paradigm shift from traditional fusion surgeries towards motion preserving fusionless surgeries in moderate idiopathic scoliosis. Modern technology and newer implant design and manufacture has given a rebirth to the classic idea of growth modulation.

REFERENCES

[1] Richards BS, Bernstein RM, D'amato CR, Thompson GH. Standardization of Criteria for Adolescent Idiopathic Scoliosis Brace Studies: Srs Committee on Bracing and Nonoperative Management. *Spine* (Phila Pa 1976) [Internet]. 2005 Sep 1 [cited 2018 Mar 26];30(18):2068–75. Available from: https://insights.ovid.com/crossref?an=00007632-200509150-00013.

[2] Weinstein SL, Dolan LA, Wright JG, Dobbs MB. Effects of Bracing in Adolescents with Idiopathic Scoliosis. *N Engl J Med* [Internet]. 2013;369(16):1512–21. Available from: http://dx.doi.org/10.1056/nejmoa1307337.

[3] Dolan LA, Weinstein SL. Surgical Rates After Observation and Bracing for Adolescent Idiopathic Scoliosis. *Spine* (Phila Pa 1976) [Internet]. 2007 Sep;32(Supplement):S91--S100. Available from: https://doi.org/10.1097%2Fbrs.0b013e318134ead9.

[4] Fällström K, Cochran T, Nachemson A. Long-term effects on personality development in patients with adolescent idiopathic scoliosis. Influence of type of treatment. *Spine* (Phila Pa 1976) [Internet]. 1986 Sep [cited 2018 Feb 24];11(7):756–8. Available from: http://www.ncbi.nlm.nih.gov/pubmed/3787349.

[5] Misterska E, Glowacki M, Latuszewska J. Female Patients' and Parents' Assessment of Deformity- and Brace-Related Stress in the Conservative Treatment of Adolescent Idiopathic Scoliosis. *Spine* (Phila Pa 1976) [Internet]. 2012;37(14):1218–23. Available

from: http://content.wkhealth.com/linkback/openurl?sid=WKPTLP:landingpage&an=00007632-201206150-00006.

[6] Hasler CC, Wietlisbach S, Büchler P. Objective compliance of adolescent girls with idiopathic scoliosis in a dynamic (SpineCor) brace. *J Child Orthop* [Internet]. 2010 Jun;4(3):211–8. Available from: https://doi.org/10.1007%2Fs11832-010-0249-7.

[7] DiRaimondo CV, Green NE. Brace-Wear Compliance in Patients with Adolescent Idiopathic Scoliosis. *J Pediatr Orthop* [Internet]. 1988 Mar;8(2):143–6. Available from: https://doi.org/10.1097%2F01241398-198803000-00004.

[8] Helfenstein A, Lankes M, Öhlert K, Varoga D, Hahne HJ, Ulrich HW, et al. The Objective Determination of Compliance in Treatment of Adolescent Idiopathic Scoliosis With Spinal Orthoses. *Spine* (Phila Pa 1976) [Internet]. 2006 Feb;31(3):339–44. Available from: https://doi.org/10.1097%2F01.brs.0000197412.70050.0d.

[9] Danielsson AJ, Nachemson AL. Back Pain and Function 22 Years After Brace Treatment for Adolescent Idiopathic Scoliosis: A Case-Control Study{\textemdash}Part I. *Spine* (Phila Pa 1976) [Internet]. 2003 Sep;28(18):2078–85. Available from: https://doi.org/10.1097%2F01.brs.0000084268.77805.6f.

[10] Green DW, Lawhorne TW, Widmann RF, Kepler CK, Ahern C, Mintz DN, et al. Long-Term Magnetic Resonance Imaging Follow-up Demonstrates Minimal Transitional Level Lumbar Disc Degeneration After Posterior Spine Fusion for Adolescent Idiopathic Scoliosis. *Spine* (Phila Pa 1976) [Internet]. 2011;36(23):1948–54. Available from: http://dx.doi.org/10.1097/brs.0b013e3181ff1ea9.

[11] Floman Y, Burnei G, Gavriliu S, Anekstein Y, Straticiuc S, Tunyogi-Csapo M, et al. Surgical management of moderate adolescent idiopathic scoliosis with ApiFix®: a short peri- apical fixation followed by post-operative curve reduction with exercises. *Scoliosis* [Internet]. 2015;10(1):4. Available from: http://scoliosisjournal.biomedcentral.com/articles/10.1186/s13013-015-0028-9.

[12] Bumpass DB, Fuhrhop SK, Schootman M, Smith JC, Luhmann SJ. Vertebral Body Stapling for Moderate Juvenile and Early Adolescent Idiopathic Scoliosis. *Spine* (Phila Pa 1976) [Internet]. 2015;40(24):E1305–14. Available from: http://content.wkhealth.com/linkback/openurl?sid=WKPTLP:landingpage&an=00007632-201512150-00014.

[13] Betz RR, Ranade A, Samdani AF, Chafetz R, D'Andrea LP, Gaughan JP, et al. Vertebral body stapling: a fusionless treatment option for a growing child with moderate idiopathic scoliosis. *Spine* (Phila Pa 1976). 2010;35(2):169–76.

[14] Samdani AF, Ames RJ, Kimball JS, Pahys JM, Grewal H, Pelletier GJ, et al. Anterior Vertebral Body Tethering for Idiopathic Scoliosis. *Spine* (Phila Pa 1976) [Internet]. 2014 Sep [cited 2017 Oct 14];39(20):1688–93. Available from: http://content.wkhealth.com/linkback/openurl?sid=WKPTLP:landingpage&an=00007632-201409150-00014.

[15] Canavese F, Dimeglio A, Volpatti D, Stebel M, Daures J-P, Canavese B, et al. Dorsal Arthrodesis of Thoracic Spine and Effects on Thorax Growth in Prepubertal New Zealand White Rabbits. *Spine* (Phila Pa 1976) [Internet]. 2007 Jul;32(16):E443--E450. Available from: https://doi.org/10.1097%2Fbrs.0b013e3180bc2340.

[16] Dimeglio A. Growth of the Spine Before Age 5 Years. *J Pediatr Orthop B* [Internet]. 1992;1(2):102–7. Available from: https://doi.org/10.1097%2F01202412-199201020-00003.

[17] Akbarnia BA, Campbell RM, Dimeglio A, Flynn JM, Redding GJ, Sponseller PD, et al. Fusionless procedures for the management of early-onset spine deformities in 2011: what

do we know? *J Child Orthop* [Internet]. 2011 Jun;5(3):159–72. Available from: https://doi.org/10.1007%2Fs11832-011-0342-6.

[18] Goldberg CJ, Gillic I, Connaughton O, Moore DP, Fogarty EE, Canny GJ, et al. Respiratory Function and Cosmesis at Maturity in Infantile-onset Scoliosis. *Spine* (Phila Pa 1976) [Internet]. 2003 Oct;28(20):2397–406. Available from: https://doi.org/10.1097%2F01.brs.0000085367.24266.ca.

[19] Dimeglio A, Canavese F. Progression or not progression? How to deal with adolescent idiopathic scoliosis during puberty. Vol. 7, *Journal of Children's Orthopaedics*. 2013. p. 43–9.

[20] Dimeglio A. *Growth in Pediatric Orthopaedics*. 2001;549–55.

[21] Dimeglio A, Canavese F. The growing spine: How spinal deformities influence normal spine and thoracic cage growth. *Eur Spine J*. 2012;21(1):64–70.

[22] DiMeglio A, Dimeglio A, Canavese F, Charles YP, Charles P. Growth and adolescent idiopathic scoliosis: when and how much? *J Pediatr Orthop* [Internet]. 2011;31(1):S28-36. Available from: http://www.ncbi.nlm.nih.gov/pubmed/21173616.

[23] Charles YP, Diméglio A, Marcoul M, Bourgin JF, Marcoul A, Bozonnat MC. Influence of Idiopathic Scoliosis on Three-Dimensional Thoracic Growth. *Spine* (Phila Pa 1976) [Internet]. 2008 May;33(11):1209–18. Available from: https://doi.org/10.1097%2Fbrs.0b013e3181715272.

[24] Canavese F, Dimeglio A, Stebel M, Galeotti M, Canavese B, Cavalli F. Thoracic cage plasticity in prepubertal New Zealand white rabbits submitted to T1{\textendash}T12 dorsal arthrodesis: computed tomography evaluation, echocardiographic assessment and cardio-pulmonary measurements. *Eur Spine J* [Internet]. 2013 Jan;22(5):1101–12. Available from: https://doi.org/10.1007%2Fs00586-012-2644-x.

[25] Canavese F, Dimeglio A, D$\prime$Amato C, Volpatti D, Granier M, Stebel M, et al. Dorsal arthrodesis in prepubertal New Zealand white rabbitsfollowed to skeletal maturity: Effect on thoracic dimensions, spine growth and neural elements. *Indian J Orthop* [Internet]. 2010;44(1):14. Available from: https://doi.org/10.4103%2F0019-5413.57280.

[26] Swank SM, Winter RB, Moe JH. Scoliosis and Cor Pulmonale. *Spine* (Phila Pa 1976) [Internet]. 1982 Jul;7(4):343–54. Available from: https://doi.org/10.1097%2F00007632-198207000-00004.

[27] Karol LA, Johnston C, Mladenov K, Schochet P, Walters P, Browne RH. Pulmonary Function Following Early Thoracic Fusion in Non-Neuromuscular Scoliosis. *J Bone Jt Surg* [Internet]. 2008 Jun;90(6):1272–81. Available from: https://doi.org/10.2106%2Fjbjs.g.00184.

[28] Emans JB, Ciarlo M, Callahan M, Zurakowski D. Prediction of Thoracic Dimensions and Spine Length Based on Individual Pelvic Dimensions in Children and Adolescents. *Spine* (Phila Pa 1976) [Internet]. 2005 Dec; 30(24):2824–9. Available from: https://doi.org/10.1097%2F01.brs.0000190865.47673.6a.

[29] Canavese F. Normal and abnormal spine and thoracic cage development. *World J Orthop* [Internet]. 2013;4(4):167. Available from: http://www.wjgnet.com/2218-5836/full/v4/i4/167.htm.

[30] Mehta HP, Snyder BD, Callender NN, Bellardine CL, Jackson AC. The reciprocal relationship between thoracic and spinal deformity and its effect on pulmonary function in a rabbit model: A pilot study. *Spine* (Phila Pa 1976). 2006;31(23):2654–64.

[31] Campbell RM, Hell-Vocke AK. Growth of the thoracic spine in congenital scoliosis after expansion thoracoplasty. *J Bone Jt Surg - Ser A*. 2003;85(3):409–20.

[32] Campbell RM, Smith MD, Mayes TC, Mangos JA, Willey-Courand DB, Kose N, et al. The effect of opening wedge thoracostomy on thoracic insufficiency syndrome associated with fused ribs and congenital scoliosis. *J Bone Jt Surg - Ser A*. 2004;86(8):1659–74.

[33] Dubousset J, Wicart P, Pomero V, Barois A, Estournet B. [Thoracic scoliosis: exothoracic and endothoracic deformations and the spinal penetration index]. *Rev Chir Orthop Reparatrice Appar Mot*. 2002;88(0035–1040 (Print)):9–18.

[34] Berend N, Rynell AC, Ward HE. Structure of a human pulmonary acinus. *Thorax*. 1991;46(2):117–21.

[35] Pehrsson K, Larsson S, Oden A, Nachemson A. Long-term follow-up of patients with untreated scoliosis: A study of mortality, causes of death, and symptoms. *Spine* (Phila Pa 1976). 1992;17(9):1091–6.

[36] Gollogly S, Smith JT, White SK, Firth S, White K. The Volume of Lung Parenchyma as a Function of Age: A Review of 1050 Normal {CT} Scans of the Chest With Three-Dimensional Volumetric Reconstruction of the Pulmonary System. *Spine* (Phila Pa 1976) [Internet]. 2004 Sep;29(18):2061–6. Available from: https://doi.org/10.1097%2F01.brs.0000140779.22741.33.

[37] DeGroodt EG, Van Pelt W, Borsboom GJJM, Quanjer Ph. H, Van Zomeren BC. Growth of lung and thorax dimensions during the pubertal growth spurt. *Eur Respir J*. 1988;1(2):102–8.

[38] Charles YP, Diméglio A, Marcoul M, Bourgin JF, Marcoul A, Bozonnat MC. Influence of idiopathic scoliosis on three-dimensional thoracic growth. *Spine* (Phila Pa 1976). 2008;33(11):1209–18.

[39] Risser JC. The Classic: The Iliac Apophysis: An Invaluable Sign in the Management of Scoliosis. *Clin Orthop Relat Res* [Internet]. 2010 Mar 18 [cited 2018 Mar 10];468(3):646–53. Available from: http://www.ncbi.nlm.nih.gov/pubmed/19763720.

[40] Tanner JM, Whitehouse RH, Takaishi M. Standards from birth to maturity for height, weight, height velocity, and weight velocity: British children, 1965. I. *Arch Dis Child* [Internet]. 1966 Oct 1 [cited 2018 Mar 10];41(219):454–71. Available from: http://www.ncbi.nlm.nih.gov/pubmed/5957718.

[41] Sanders JO, Little DG, Richards BS. Prediction of the Crankshaft Phenomenon by Peak Height Velocity. *Spine* (Phila Pa 1976) [Internet]. 1997 Jun 1 [cited 2018 Mar 10];22(12):1352–6. Available from: https://insights.ovid.com/crossref?an=00007632-199706150-00013.

[42] Sanders JO, Khoury JG, Kishan S, Browne RH, Mooney JF, Arnold KD, et al. Predicting Scoliosis Progression from Skeletal Maturity: A Simplified Classification During Adolescence. *J Bone Jt Surgery-american Vol* [Internet]. 2008 Mar 1 [cited 2018 Mar 10];90(3):540–53. Available from: https://insights.ovid.com/crossref?an=00004623-200803000-00011.

[43] Nault M, Parent S, Phan P, Roy-Beaudry M, Labelle H, Rivard M. A Modified Risser Grading System Predicts the Curve Acceleration Phase of Female Adolescent Idiopathic Scoliosis. *J. Bone & Joint Surgery* [Internet]. 2010 May 1 [cited 2018 Mar 10];92(5):1073–81. Available from: https://insights.ovid.com/crossref?an=00004623-201005000-00002.

[44] Little DG, Song KM, Katz D, Herring JA. Relationship of Peak Height Velocity to Other Maturity Indicators in Idiopathic Scoliosis in Girls*. *J Bone Jt Surgery-american Vol* [Internet]. 2000 May 1 [cited 2018 Mar 10];82(5):685–93. Available from: https://insights.ovid.com/crossref?an=00004623-200005000-00009.

[45] Song KM, Little DG. Peak height velocity as a maturity indicator for males with idiopathic scoliosis. *J Pediatr Orthop* [Internet]. [cited 2018 Mar 10];20(3):286–8. Available from: http://www.ncbi.nlm.nih.gov/pubmed/10823591.

[46] Zuege RC, Kempken TG, Blount WP. Epiphyseal stapling for angular deformity at the knee. *J Bone Jt Surg* [Internet]. 1979 Apr;61(3):320–9. Available from: https://doi.org/10.2106%2F00004623-197961030-00001.

[47] Stevens PM, Maguire M, Dales MD, Robins AJ. Physeal Stapling for Idiopathic Genu Valgum. *J Pediatr Orthop* [Internet]. 1999 Sep;19(5):645. Available from: https://doi.org/10.1097%2F01241398-199909000-00018.

[48] Mente PL, Aronsson DD, Stokes IAF, Iatridis JC. Mechanical modulation of growth for the correction of vertebral wedge deformities. *J Orthop Res* [Internet]. 1999 Jul;17(4):518–24. Available from: https://doi.org/10.1002%2Fjor.1100170409.

[49] Nachlas IW, Borden JN. the Cure of Experimental Scoliosis By Directed Growth Control. *J Bone Jt Surg* [Internet]. 1951 Jan;33(1):24–34. Available from: http://insights.ovid.com/crossref?an=00004623-195133010-00002.

[50] Smith AD, Von Lackum WH, Wylie R. An Operation for Stapling Vertebral Bodies in Congenital Scoliosis. *J Bone Jt Surg* [Internet]. 1954 Apr;36(2):342–8. Available from: http://insights.ovid.com/crossref?an=00004623-195436020-00011.

[51] Cahill PJ, Auriemma M, Dakwar E, Gaughan JP, Samdani AF, Pahys JM, et al. Factors Predictive of Outcomes in Vertebral Body Stapling for Idiopathic Scoliosis. *Spine Deform* [Internet]. 2018 [cited 2018 Mar 26];6(1):28–37. Available from: https://ac-els-cdn-com.ezproxy.library.dal.ca/S2212134X17301120/1-s2.0-S2212134X17301120-main.pdf?_tid=601b4be0-314c-11e8-a7cb-00000aab0f26&acdnat=1522106662_c0d 163157ccf852e2a63b937ec3a4227.

[52] Theologis AA, Cahill P, Auriemma M, Betz R, Diab M. Vertebral body stapling in children younger than 10 years with idiopathic scoliosis with curve magnitude of 30 degrees to 39 degrees. *Spine* (Phila Pa 1976) [Internet]. 2013;38(25):E1583-8. Available from: http://www.ncbi.nlm.nih.gov/pubmed/23963018%5Cnhttp://graphics.tx.ovid.com /ovftpdfs/FPDDNCGCFEMBNH00/fs047/ovft/live/gv031/00007632/00007632-201312010-00013.pdf.

[53] Laituri CA, Schwend RM, III GWH. Thoracoscopic Vertebral Body Stapling for Treatment of Scoliosis in Young Children. *J Laparoendosc Adv Surg Tech* [Internet]. 2012;22(8):830–3. Available from: http://online.liebertpub.com/doi/abs/10.1089/lap.2011.0289.

[54] Braun JT, Ogilvie JW, Akyuz E, Brodke DS, Bachus KN. Fusionless Scoliosis Correction Using a Shape Memory Alloy Staple in the Anterior Thoracic Spine of the Immature Goat. *Spine* (Phila Pa 1976) [Internet]. 2004 Sep;29(18):1980–9. Available from: https://doi.org/10.1097%2F01.brs.0000138278.41431.72.

[55] Cuddihy L, Danielsson AJ, Cahill PJ, Samdani AF, Grewal H, Richmond JM, et al. Vertebral Body Stapling versus Bracing for Patients with High-Risk Moderate Idiopathic Scoliosis. *Biomed Res Int*. 2015;2015.

[56] Shillington MP, Labrom RD, Askin GN, Adam CJ. A biomechanical investigation of vertebral staples for fusionless scoliosis correction. *Clin Biomech.* 2011;26(5):445–51.

[57] Padhye K, Soroceanu A, Russell D, El-Hawary R. *Thoracoscopic Anterior Instrumentation and Fusion as a Treatment for Adolescent Idiopathic Scoliosis: A Systematic Review of the Literature.* Accept Spine Deform. 2018.

[58] Trobisch PD, Samdani A, Cahill P, Betz RR. Vertebral body stapling as an alternative in the treatment of idiopathic scoliosis. *Oper Orthop Traumatol.* 2011;23(3):227–31.

[59] Theologis AA, Cahill P, Auriemma M, Betz R, Diab M. Vertebral Body Stapling in Children Younger Than 10 Years With Idiopathic Scoliosis With Curve Magnitude of 30° to 39°. *Spine* (Phila Pa 1976) [Internet]. 2013;38(25):E1583–8. Available from: http://dx.doi.org/10.1097/brs.0b013e3182a8280d.

[60] Courvoisier A, Eid A, Bourgeois E, Griffet J. Growth tethering devices for idiopathic scoliosis. *Expert Rev Med Devices* [Internet]. 2015;12(4):449–56. Available from: http://dx.doi.org/10.1586/17434440.2015.1052745.

[61] Newton PO, Fricka KB, Lee SS, Farnsworth CL, Cox TG, Mahar AT. Asymmetrical Flexible Tethering of Spine Growth in an Immature Bovine Model. *Spine* (Phila Pa 1976) [Internet]. 2002 Apr;27(7):689–93. Available from: https://doi.org/10.1097%2F00007632-200204010-00004.

[62] Newton PO, Farnsworth CL, Faro FD, Mahar AT, Odell TR, Mohamad F, et al. Spinal growth modulation with an anterolateral flexible tether in an immature bovine model: disc health and motion preservation. *Spine* (Phila Pa 1976). 2008;33(7):724–33.

[63] Braun JT, Ogilvie JW, Akyuz E, Brodke DS, Bachus KN. Creation of an Experimental Idiopathic-Type Scoliosis in an Immature Goat Model Using a Flexible Posterior Asymmetric Tether. *Spine* (Phila Pa 1976) [Internet]. 2006 Jun;31(13):1410–4. Available from: https://doi.org/10.1097%2F01.brs.0000219869.01599.6b.

[64] Newton PO, Farnsworth CL, Upasani V V, Chambers RC, Varley E, Tsutsui S. Effects of Intraoperative Tensioning of an Anterolateral Spinal Tether on Spinal Growth Modulation in a Porcine Model. *Spine* (Phila Pa 1976) [Internet]. 2011 Jan;36(2):109–17. Available from: https://doi.org/10.1097%2Fbrs.0b013e3181cc8fce.

[65] Braun JT, Hoffman M, Akyuz E, Ogilvie JW, Brodke DS, Bachus KN. Mechanical Modulation of Vertebral Growth in the Fusionless Treatment of Progressive Scoliosis in an Experimental Model. *Spine* (Phila Pa 1976) [Internet]. 2006 May;31(12):1314–20. Available from: https://doi.org/10.1097%2F01.brs.0000218662.78165.b1.

[66] Hunt KJ, Braun JT, Christensen BA. The effect of two clinically relevant fusionless scoliosis implant strategies on the health of the intervertebral disc: analysis in an immature goat model. *Spine* (Phila Pa 1976). 2010 Feb;35(4):371–7.

[67] Upasani VV., Farnsworth CL, Chambers RC, Bastrom TP, Williams GM, Sah RL, et al. Intervertebral disc health preservation after six months of spinal growth modulation. *J Bone Joint Surg Am.* 2011 Aug;93(15):1408–16.

[68] Crawford CH, Lenke LG. Growth Modulation by Means of Anterior Tethering Resulting in Progressive Correction of Juvenile Idiopathic Scoliosis. *J Bone Jt Surgery-American Vol* [Internet]. 2010;92(1):202–9. Available from: http://dx.doi.org/10.2106/jbjs.h.01728.

[69] Samdani AF, Ames RJ, Kimball JS, Pahys JM, Grewal H, Pelletier GJ, et al. Anterior vertebral body tethering for idiopathic scoliosis: two-year results. *Spine* (Phila Pa 1976). 2014 Sep;39(20):1688–93.

[70] Samdani AF, Ames RJ, Kimball JS, Pahys JM, Grewal H, Pelletier GJ, et al. Anterior vertebral body tethering for immature adolescent idiopathic scoliosis: one-year results on the first 32 patients. *Eur Spine J Off Publ Eur Spine Soc Eur Spinal Deform Soc Eur Sect Cerv Spine Res Soc.* 2015 Jul;24(7):1533–9.

[71] Boudissa et al. - *Early outcomes of spinal growth tethering for idiopathic scoliosis with a novel device a prospective study with 2 year.pdf.*

[72] Danielsson AJ, Romberg K, Nachemson AL. Spinal Range of Motion, Muscle Endurance, and Back Pain and Function at Least 20 Years After Fusion or Brace Treatment for Adolescent Idiopathic Scoliosis. *Spine* (Phila Pa 1976) [Internet]. 2006 Feb;31(3):275–83. Available from: https://doi.org/10.1097%2F01.brs.0000197652.52890.71.

[73] Holewijn RM, de Kleuver M, van der Veen AJ, Emanuel KS, Bisschop A, Stadhouder A, et al. A Novel Spinal Implant for Fusionless Scoliosis Correction: A Biomechanical Analysis of the Motion Preserving Properties of a Posterior Periapical Concave Distraction Device. *Glob Spine J.* 2017.

In: Scoliosis: Diagnosis, Classification and Management Options   ISBN: 978-1-53614-464-2
Editors: F. Canavese, A. Andreacchio and H. Xu   © 2018 Nova Science Publishers, Inc.

Chapter 14

INSTRUMENTED POSTERIOR FUSION IN AIS: INDICATIONS, PREOPERATIVE PLANNING AND OUTCOME

Xiaodong Qin and Zezhang Zhu[*]

Spine Surgery Department, Drum Tower Hospital of Nanjing University Medical School, Nanjing, China

ABSTRACT

Adolescent idiopathic scoliosis is a three-dimensional deformity of the growing spine, affecting 2%–3% of adolescents. Surgery is the alternative treatment for severe idiopathic scoliosis, which is rapidly progressive. Instrumented posterior fusion has become the standard for the surgical treatment of nearly all types of curves over the past decade. Understanding operation indications, careful planning preoperatively and effectively evaluating outcomes are essential in corrective surgery of idiopathic scoliosis.

Keywords: adolescent idiopathic scoliosis, posterior spinal instrumented fusion, indication, preoperative planning, outcome

INTRODUCTION

Adolescent idiopathic scoliosis (AIS) is a complex three-dimensional deformity that constitutes the most common type of spinal deformity in puberty [1]. The treatment strategy of AIS depends mainly on the curve magnitude and curve. Observation is the appropriate treatment for small curves less than 25°. Brace is the appropriate treatment for a growing child presenting with a curve of 25°–40° or a curve less than 25° with documented progression [2]. Surgical treatment is essentially used for patients whose curves are greater than 45° while still growing or greater than 50° when growth has stopped [3]. The posterior spinal instrumented

---

[*] Corresponding Author Email: zhuzezhang@126.com.

fusion (PSIF) is utilized most often in the surgical treatment for AIS [4-6]. Milestones of this technique can be traced back to the instrumentation devised by Harrington and Cotrel-Dubousset [7-8]. PSIF is implemented through a posterior midline vertical skin incision. Curve correction is performed using pedicle screws or hooks implanted in posterior elements of the spine and connected with rods and transverse devices to form stable structures. The realignment corrective techniques include rod rotation, translation, and direct vertebral derotation, among others. PSIF has several advantages, such as providing good three-dimensional deformity correction and reducing the operation time, the number of fused vertebral levels and the rib hump, among others [9]. The purpose of this chapter is to analyze the indications, preoperative planning and outcomes of surgical treatment using PSIF for AIS patients.

INDICATIONS

The main goals of surgical treatment for AIS are to halt the progression of deformity to achieve three-dimensional correction of spinal alignment and to maintain the correction at long-term follow-up. However, spinal fusion surgery does not restore the normal spine and might have several adverse effects on patients, such as limitations in sports and physical activities. Hence, whether a surgical instrumented fusion is indicated for AIS remains controversial, especially for curves ranging from 40° to 50°. In general, PSIF can be performed when long-term outcomes would be better with a fused spine than with the untreated natural history of AIS. However, the understanding of these two situations over the long-term follow-up is lacking, leaving the indications for the surgical treatment of these patients open to debate.

Curvature Magnitude

The curve magnitude of scoliosis measured as the Cobb angle is the primary determinant of the risk for curve progression. When the Cobb angle is greater than 50°, there is a significant risk for progression; the risk with curves between 40° and 50° might be dependent on the growth potential, and with curves less than 40° the risk of progression appears to be low [10]. Therefore, surgical treatment is indicated for patients whose curves are greater than 45° while still growing or greater than 50° when growth has stopped [3].

Growth Potential

The growth potential reflected by skeletal maturity should be taken into consideration when making the decision whether to operate, especially for curves between 40° and 50°. Patients with skeletal immaturity have a high risk of curve progression (Figure 1) and ultimately require surgical intervention [11]. We reviewed a cohort of 54 patients with a Cobb angle between 40° and 50° at the first visit, who refused surgery and insisted on receiving brace treatment in Nanjing Spine Center [12]. These patients were followed up for a mean period of 3.7 years (range 1.2-5.4 years). On the whole, the curve progressed in 35 patients, remained stable in 12 patients and improved in the other 7 patients. All the patients with curve progression finally received surgery. The mean grade of the initial Risser sign in patients with curve progression was significantly lower than that in patients with stable or improved curves (0.3 ± 0.8 vs. 1.2 ± 1.4, p=0.02) (Table 1). Therefore, the effectiveness of conservative treatment significantly decreased when applied to patients with an immature skeleton with a curve magnitude between 40° and 50°. The majority of these patients will inevitably undergo surgical intervention.

Accurate skeletal maturity assessment is important for the prediction of curve progression and clinical management of scoliosis. In addition to the Risser sign and menarche, there are several other methods to evaluate skeletal maturity. Sanders et al. [13] proposed that the Tanner-Whitehouse-3 (TW3) radius, ulna, and small bones of the hand (RUS) score system were highly correlated with curve progression in AIS. He further simplified the RUS score into a digital skeletal age (DSA) score system and confirmed that the DSA score was also correlated with the curve acceleration phase [13]. However, the DSA score system is still time-consuming and requires the use of an atlas with a substantial learning curve. Our Joint Scoliosis Research Center attempted to further simplify the current skeletal maturity staging system by focusing on the morphology of a minimum number of essential hand ossification centers that we hoped would reliably predict the skeletal maturity information from the whole hand in a quicker and easier manner. We developed a new thumb classification based on the epiphyses of the distal and proximal phalanges together with the adductor sesamoid bone, which we call the "thumb ossification composite index (TOCI)" (Figure 2) [14]. We found that 70.1% of the AIS patients attained their peak height velocity (PHV) at TOCI stage 5, which had the comparable accuracy of predicting PHV with previous score systems. Therefore, this new proposed TOCI could provide a simplified staging system for assessment of the skeletal maturity of subjects with AIS. Additionally, we performed a genetic study and identified several genetic determinants of PHV in AIS [15]. Polymorphisms of rs4794665 in C17orf67 and rs12459350 in DOT1L were associated with a combined predisposition to AIS susceptibility and higher pubertal PHV. Hence, genetic testing might be helpful in the clinical management of AIS in the future.

Other Variables

According to our clinical experience, there are several other unproven variables used in the decision to operate. Loss of physiologic sagittal alignment may be a factor in favor of surgery because a physiologic spinal profile is considered one of the important determinants of being free of back pain. Coronal balance and clinical appearance are also important factors in favor of surgery. For radiographic and clinical coronal imbalance patients with a curve magnitude between 40° and 50°, we recommend performing the corrective surgery at a young age (Figure 3). Additionally, the length of the curve is an important variable. The more vertebrae there are within the curvature, the more severe the clinical deformity.

Table 1. Comparison of clinical parameters between patients with and without curve progression

Groups	N	Initial age	Initial Risser	Initial weight	Initial Cobb angle
Curve progression	35	12.8±2.8	0.3±0.8	42.2± 9.7	43.4±3.3
Stable/improved curve	19	14.0±2.0	1.2±1.4	40.9 ± 11.2	43.3±3.1
P value		0.1	0.02	0.15	0.9

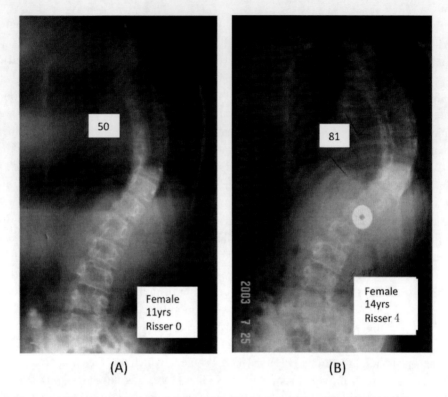

Figure 1. Female AIS patient, 11 years old, Risser 0, Cobb angle 50° at first visit (A). Three years later, Risser 4, curve progressed with a Cobb angle of 81°(B).

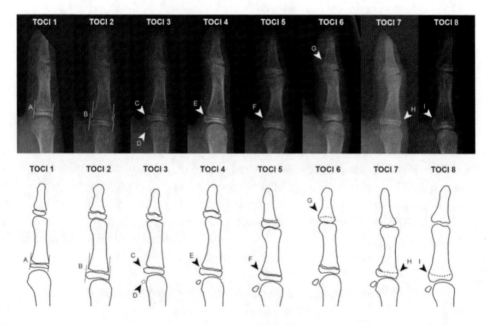

Figure 2. TOCI stages 1 through 8 and the corresponding ossification pattern and sequence of the adductor sesamoid, distal phalangeal epiphysis, and proximal phalangeal epiphysis.

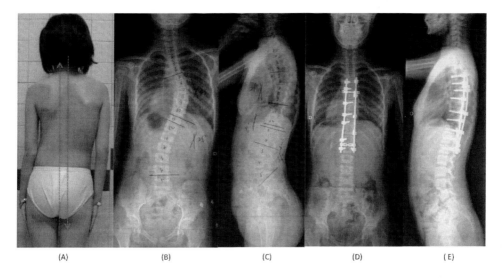

Figure 3. Preoperative appearance and PA, lateral radiographs of a 14-year-old girl demonstrate a 42° thoracic curve, coronal imbalance with trunk shift to the right (A,B,C). Two years of postoperative radiographs demonstrate a well-balanced spine (D,E).

PREOPERATIVE PLANNING

Clinical and Radiologic Evaluation

Preoperative planning requires a thorough clinical and radiologic evaluation. The history and physical examination is critical for the planning, including the family history of scoliosis, activity level and medical comorbidities, among others. Additionally, the preoperative lung function and heart Doppler ultrasound test are important to assess cardiopulmonary function for AIS patients. For severe scoliosis with poor lung function, we recommend the use of the BiPAP ventilator-method to improve lung function before surgery [16]. Clinical deformities such as shoulder balance, trunk shift and rib prominence will be useful for surgical planning. Radiographic measurements are obtained from long-cassette standing anteroposterior (AP) and lateral radiographs of the spine. A set of flexibility films should also be collected, including right and left side-bending (SB) films. Several radiographic parameters are measured to assess the deformity. The Cobb angle and flexibility of each spinal curve will determine whether a curve is structural and should be included in the fusion segment. The tilt of the lower instrumented vertebrae (LIV), apical vertebra translation to the central sacral vertical line (CSVL), as well as coronal balance by relating C7 to the CSVL are assessed. Vertebral rotation is measured using the Nash-Moe method [17]. The sagittal balance is assessed on the lateral radiographs considering the distance from the C7 plumb line (C7PL) to the first sacral vertebral body, and thoracic kyphosis and lumbar lordosis are evaluated. The shoulder balance can also be evaluated on AP films, including the measurement of the T1 tilt, clavicle angle and radiographic shoulder height (RSH) (Figure 4). Additionally, CT scans and MRI of the whole spine are of significant importance to evaluate the spine morphology and exclude potential neurological pathologies.

On the basis of radiographic measurement, the curves are classified using the method described by Lenke et al. [3]. A thorough understanding of the Lenke classification system is essential in preoperative planning. The type of curve implies the extent of fusion: structural curves require fusion, whereas nonstructural regions will not be fused. The selection of fusion levels according to the Lenke classification is discussed as follows.

Lenke Type 1

The Lenke type 1 curve is the main thoracic (MT) curve, which is the most common curve type of AIS. To determine the upper instrumented vertebrae (UIV), the shoulder balance should be assessed. For the right MT curve with the right shoulder elevated, selecting T4/T5 as UIV would be appropriate. Non-fusion of the proximal thoracic (PT) will allow left shoulder elevation to occur with MT correction, making the shoulders level postoperatively. For a MT curve with level shoulders, selecting T3/T4 as the UIV is often indicated. For a right MT curve with the left shoulder elevated, extension of fixation to T2 is usually necessary to prevent a postoperative shoulder imbalance.

Sparing spinal levels from surgical fusion is always one of the goals of preoperative planning, especially at the lumbar spine. Hence, selective fusion of the MT curve has become the mainstay of operative treatments for AIS patients with Lenke type 1A. Several studies have documented good outcomes when the last touching vertebra (LTV), defined as the last cephalad vertebra touched by the CSVL, was selected as the LIV [18]. We further classified LTV into substantially touched vertebra (STV) and non-substantially touched vertebra (nSTV), and we found that selecting STV as LIV could yield a promising outcome for a Lenke 1A curve with a low incidence of distal adding-on [19]. To understand the specific association between LIV selection and distal adding-on, please refer to the chapter "How to Control Shoulder Balance and Prevent Adding On in Patients with AIS Undergoing Surgery." For Lenke type 1B curves, LIV selection is based on the SV at the thoracolumbar junction, unless a thoracolumbar kyphosis is present. For Lenke type 1C curves, whether to perform a selective fusion largely remains controversial. The Cobb angle, apical vertebral rotation (AVR), and apical vertebral translation (AVT) of both the thoracic and lumbar curves must be measured. When the Cobb angle ratio of the MT to the thoracolumbar/lumbar (TL/L) curves and the respective ratio of AVR and AVT are >1.2, selective thoracic fusion can be performed with a low incidence of postoperative coronal decompensation [20].

Several techniques are used in correction surgery for thoracic curves such as rod derotation and translation. The majority of these techniques begin from the concave side, which bears potential neurovascular risks. The technique of vertebral coplanar alignment (VCA) was introduced by Vallespir et al. [21] with the intention of correcting the rotation and translation and simultaneously restoring the normal sagittal profile of thoracic scoliosis. We compared the surgical outcomes of the VCA technique against the traditional derotation maneuver with segmental pedicle screw instrumentation for Lenke type 1 AIS [22]. The VCA technique could achieve a correction and clinical outcome as good as the derotation technique. The advantage lies in its superior renormalization effect of thoracic kyphosis compared with the derotation technique from the concave side (Figure 5).

Lenke Type 2

The Lenke type 2 curve is double thoracic curve, including a major structural MT curve and a minor structural PT curve. The LIV selection is similar to that for treating the Lenke type 1 curve (Figure 6). Traditionally, fusion of the rigid PT curve is recommended for the Lenke Type 2A curve [3]. In our experience, in addition to the flexibility of the PT curve, both the shoulder balance and correction rate of MT curve should be taken into account [23]. For a flexible PT curve with a right-elevated shoulder, proximal fusion to T4 is sufficient. In contrast, for a rigid PT curve with left-elevated or leveled shoulder, UIV should be selected as T2. For a rigid PT curve with a right-elevated shoulder, traditionally the PT curve should be fused, while non-fusion of PT curve can also achieve a good outcome when the MT curve is not overcorrected. To understand the specific association between UIV selection and shoulder balance, please refer to the chapter "How to Control Shoulder Balance and Prevent Adding On in Patients with AIS Undergoing Surgery."

Lenke Type 3

The Lenke type 3 curve is a double major curve, including a major structural MT curve and a minor structural TL/L curve. The UIV selection is similar to that of the Lenke type 1 curve, ranging from T3 to T5, depending on the shoulder position. The LIV is usually selected as L3 or L4. Stopping the distal fusion at L3 can save more mobile lumbar spinal segments, but it may increase the risk of decompensation; in contrast, stopping the distal fusion at L4 may improve coronal correction while leading to a higher incidence of disc degeneration and low back pain [23-25]. Kim et al. [26] suggested fusing the curve to L3 with favorable radiographic outcomes when L3 crosses the mid-sacral line with a rotation less than grade II in bending films. Otherwise, the fusion must be extended to L4. We have evaluated several preoperative radiographic factors that are associated with the selection of either L3 or L4 as LIV in posteriorly treated AIS with a large lumbar curve. Eighty-four AIS patients with a lumbar curve greater than 60° were included with a minimum follow-up of 2 years after posterior instrumentation with lumbar curves included in the fusion. The patients were grouped according to the selection of LIV as either the L3 group (n=24) or the L4 group (n=60). At the last follow-up, no differences were found in the clinical and radiographic parameters between the two groups. Preoperatively, the L3 group had lower L3 translation on the AP view, L3 translation on the concave SB film, L3 rotation on the convex SB film, and more L3/4 disc opening on the convex SB film. Hence, in our experience, L3 selection criteria are as follows: L3 being stable vertebra on the SB film; L4 derotation and being horizontal on the SB film; L3/4 disc opening on the SB film (Figure 7).

For some severe rigid thoracic curves of AIS, the multi-level Ponte osteotomy technique is often used to achieve a good correction outcome. This osteotomy technique was proposed by Alberto Ponte for the treatment of Scheuermann's kyphosis [28]. A modified posterior resection is now used in corrective surgery for AIS. Ponte osteotomy is mainly used for sagittal profile correction, while coronal correction also can be achieved by asymmetric osteotomies (Figure 8).

Lenke Type 4

The Lenke type 4 curve is a triple major curve, including structural PT, MT and TL/L curves. Similar to Lenke type 2, the UIV is often selected as T2 or T3, depending on the shoulder position. The LIV selection is again similar to that of Lenke type 3, either L3 or L4, depending on the SB film (Figure 9).

Lenke Type 5

The Lenke type 5 curve is the major curve in the TL/L region, with nonstructural PT and MT regions. Traditionally, this curve pattern can be treated with anterior spinal instrumentation and fusion (ASIF) from the upper end vertebra (EV) to the lower EV. Currently, there is a trend towards PSIF for the treatment of TL/L curves. Selection of the fusion level in PSIF is usually identical to that in ASIF. We compared the long-term radiographic outcomes of the sagittal profile reconstruction of the Lenke type 5 curve treated with anterior or posterior approach selective TL/L fusion. One hundred two Lenke 5 AIS patients who underwent TL/L spine fusion with a minimum of 2 years of follow-up were retrospectively evaluated. Fifty-six patients underwent ASIF, and the other 46 patients were treated with PSIF. Preoperative radiographic parameters and demographic data showed no significant differences between the two groups. The fusion levels were shorter in the anterior group (5.3 ± 0.5 vs. 5.9 ± 0.8, $P<0.001$). In the coronal plane, there was no significant difference in the correction rate between the two groups. In the sagittal plane, however, lumbar lordosis decreased $3.5°$ in the anterior group and increased $1°$ in the posterior group immediately after surgery. At the last follow-up, lumbar lordosis increased $0.9°$ in the anterior group and $4.3°$ in the posterior group, revealing a significant difference between the two groups. Hence, posterior fusion surgery can offer better restoration of the sagittal alignment of Lenke type 5 AIS patients than anterior fusion surgery in the long-term follow-up (Figure 10-11).

Posterior minimally invasive scoliosis surgery (MISS) assisted by O-arm navigation can be used in corrective surgery for Lenke 5 curves. We investigated the outcome of posterior MISS for the correction of Lenke type 5C AIS [28]. A cohort of 45 patients was retrospectively reviewed, of whom 15 underwent posterior MISS with O-arm navigation and 30 underwent PSIF. A comparison of radiographic parameters revealed no obvious differences between the two groups at the final follow-up. However, the MISS patients had significantly less estimated blood loss (EBL) during surgery. The evaluation of pain and self-image using the SRS-22 showed significantly higher scores in the MISS group than the PSIF group. Hence, for mild to moderate curves less than $70°$ with reasonable flexibility, posterior MISS is a feasible and effective alternative with reduced morbidity (Figure 12). Furthermore, high accuracy in pedicle screw placement during MISS can be achieved through O-arm navigation (Figure 13).

Lenke Type 6

The Lenke type 6 curve consists of a major structural TL/L curve with a minor structural MT curve. The UIV is usually selected from T2 to T5, depending on the shoulder balance. The LIV is usually selected as L3 or L4. The L3 selection criteria have been described before (Figure 14).

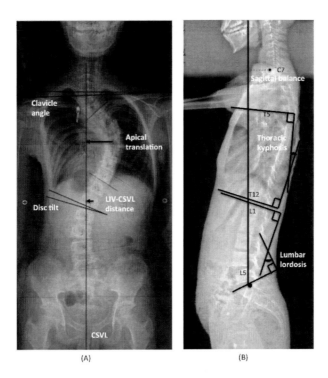

Figure 4. Definitions of radiographic parameters: CSVL, central sacral vertical line, the vertical line that bisects the proximal sacrum; clavicle angle, an angle between the horizontal line and the line through the upper endplate of the clavicles; apical translation, the distance in millimeters from the CSVL to the mid-point of the apical vertebra; LIV-CSVL, the distance in millimeters from the CSVL to the mid-point of the lowest instrumented vertebra; disc tilt, the tilt angle of the first disc below the LIV (A); sagittal balance, the distance from the C7 center to the sacral vertical axis; thoracic kyphosis, the angle between the upper endplate of T5 and the lower endplate of T12; lumbar lordosis, the angle between the upper endplate of L1 and the upper endplate of S1(B).

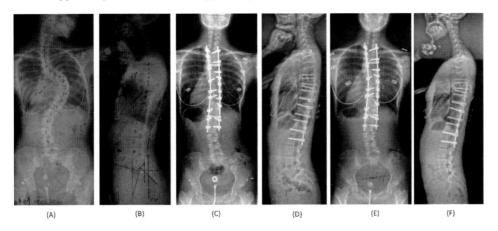

Figure 5. A 13-year-old girl with severe thoracic curve was operated on with the VCA technique. Coronal view shows a right thoracic curve of 82°, lateral view shows a thoracic kyphosis of 11° (A,B). Postoperative radiographs show the scoliosis corrected to 19° and the kyphosis increased to 23° (C,D). Two years of postoperative radiographs show good maintenance of the correction (E,F).

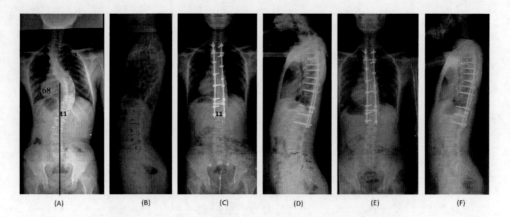

Figure 6. PA and lateral radiographs of a 16-year old boy with a Lenke type 2B curve, L1 was STV (A,B). Selection of L1 (STV) as LIV, postoperative radiographs show scoliosis corrected to 11° (C,D). Two years of postoperative radiographs show good maintenance of the correction (E,F).

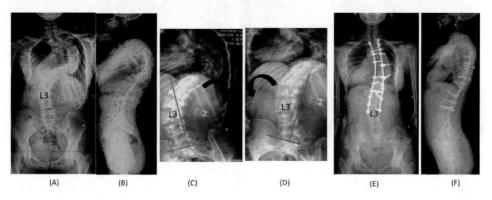

Figure 7. Preoperative PA and lateral radiographs of a 12-year-old girl with a Lenke type 3C curve (A,B). L3 was stable vertebra, L4 was horizontal, and L3/4 disc opening on SB film, hence, L3 could be selected as LIV (C,D). The lumbar curve was corrected to 14° with satisfactory results at four years of follow-up (E,F).

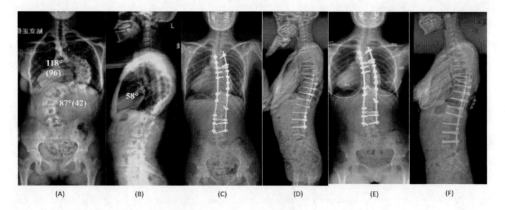

Figure 8. A 17-year-old girl with a Lenke type 3 C curve was operated on with multi-level Ponte osteotomy. Coronal view shows a 118° right thoracic scoliosis and 87° left lumbar scoliosis (A). Lateral view shows a thoracic kyphosis of 58° (B). Postoperative radiographs show the main thoracic curve corrected to 22° and the kyphosis decreased to 25° (C,D). Two years of postoperative radiographs show good maintenance of the correction (E,F).

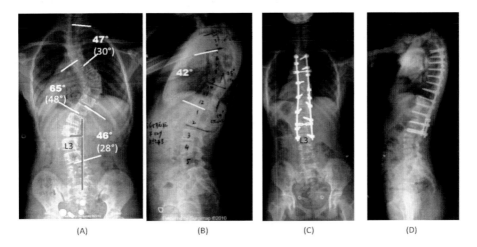

Figure 9. Preoperative standing posteroanterior and lateral radiographs of a 12-year-old girl with a Lenke type 4C curve (A,B). L3 was selected as LIV, 2 years of postoperative standing posteroanterior and lateral radiographs show satisfactory correction (C,D).

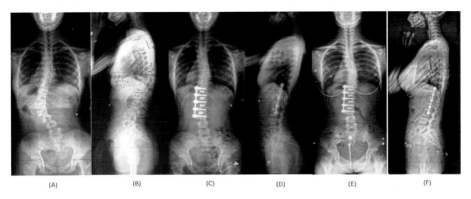

Figure 10. Preoperative PA and lateral radiographs of a 13-year-old girl with a Lenke type 5C curve, Cobb angle=54°, LL=44° (A,B). The patient underwent anterior spinal fusion from T11 to L3. Immediately after surgery, Cobb angle=8°, LL=40° (C,D). At the last follow-up at 5 years, Cobb angle=10°, LL=38° (E,F).

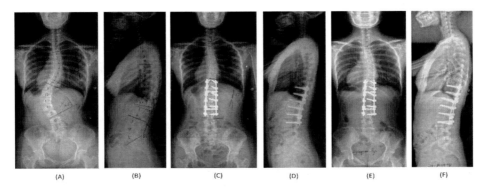

Figure 11. Preoperative PA and lateral radiographs of a 15-year-old girl with a Lenke type 5C curve, Cobb angle=60°, LL=44° (A,B). The patient underwent posterior spinal fusion from T10 to L3. Immediately after surgery, Cobb angle=12°, LL=48° (C,D). At the two-year follow up, Cobb angle=12°, LL=48° (E,F).

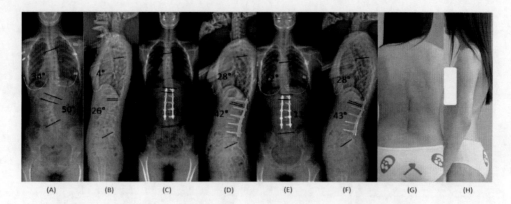

Figure 12. Preoperative PA and lateral radiographs of a 17-year-old girl with Lenke type 5C curve of 50° (A,B). The patient underwent posterior MISS from T12 to L4. Immediately after surgery, the correction rate of the main curve was 75% (C,D). At the last follow-up of 25 months, the correction rate of the main curve was 77.1% (E,F). The appearance of the patient 3 months after surgery (G,H).

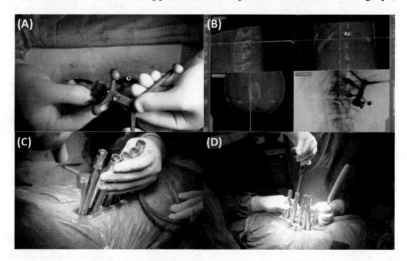

Figure 13. Two small (3–5 cm) midline skin incisions are used for the minimally invasive surgical technique (A). Intraoperative snapshot showing pedicle screw placement under navigational guidance (B). The rod is passed in a cephalocaudal manner with the assistance of screw extensions (C). Distraction and compression were performed with a special adjustable fulcrum, followed by final tightening (D).

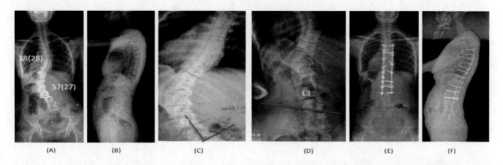

Figure 14. Preoperative PA and lateral radiographs of a 13-year-old girl with a Lenke type 6C curve (A,B). L3 was stable vertebrae and L4 was horizontal on SB film, hence, L3 could be selected as LIV (C,D). The lumbar curve was corrected to 8° with satisfactory results at two years of follow-up (E,F).

Outcome of Treatment

The postoperative outcome of AIS is associated with several different factors, ranging from clinical and radiographical measurements to health-related quality-of-life (HRQOL) assessments. Surgeons may be interested in one specific parameter, while patients may pay more attention to an entirely different set of outcomes. The "ideal" outcome should be measured by a combination of different variables. Hence, the accurate measurement of these variables is crucial in assessing and guiding treatment.

Radiographic Assessment

Outcome research in AIS started as an attempt to investigate the radiographic outcomes of surgical treatment with posterior instrumentation. Poor selection of fusion levels may cause radiographic decompensation such as progressive deformity, coronal imbalance and sagittal imbalance.

Coronal imbalance consists of shoulder imbalance, distal adding-on and trunk shift, among others. Shoulder imbalance is associated with inappropriate selection of UIV. Moreover, we found that overcorrection of the MT curve is also an important risk factor for postoperative shoulder imbalance [29]. The selection of fusion levels proximal to the appropriate LIV may lead to distal adding-on. Interestingly, the postoperative shoulder balance and postoperative distal adding-on were significantly associated with each other. Distal adding-on might progress during follow-up if the left shoulder is higher than the right side after surgery, while it might be stable or improved if the right shoulder is higher than the left one (Figure 15). An interesting phenomenon was observed: when distal adding-on progressed, the right shoulder might elevate. Hence, patients with higher left shoulders after surgery could rebalance the shoulders by progressive distal adding-on. In contrast, when distal adding-on improved, the left shoulder might elevate. Therefore, for some adding-on patients with higher right shoulders after surgery, the distal adding-on might remain stable or improve during follow-up.

Sagittal imbalance consists of proximal junctional kyphosis (PJK) and distal junctional kyphosis (DJK). The incidence of PJK has been reported to be 26% in AIS [30]. Several risk factors are associated with the onset of PJK, such as UIV close to the kyphosis apex, ligamentous damage during dissection and TK overcorrection, among others (Figure 16). An incidence of DJK of 14.6% was found in AIS with posterior spinal fusion [31]. Preoperative TL kyphosis is a risk factor for postoperative DJK, and extension of the fusion distal to the kyphotic segment should be recommended.

Functional Assessment

Radiographic measurements can only provide a static assessment of the spinal alignment, and they cannot represent functional movement of the spine. Although many studies have found improvements in spinal alignment after surgery, few studies have investigated postoperative changes in the capabilities of the spine for functional movement. The functional assessment can be measured by the range of motion (ROM) of the spine. Engsberg et al. compared pre- and post-operative global and regional spinal ROM with a camera system and probe markers attached to the skin [32]. The postoperative global spinal ROM significantly decreased during forward and lateral-bending movements. The ROM above and below the instrumented fusion region also decreased. This bending movement is a two-dimensional method of assessment, however, the scoliosis can still have three-dimensional rotations postoperatively that cannot be detected. Further investigations in this area are needed.

HRQOL Assessment

Patient satisfaction should be taken into account when assessing the outcome of surgery. The tools used to evaluate patient satisfaction are complicated because the outcome evaluation should include various factors such as daily living, personal perception, and overall well-being. The HRQOL questionnaire of the SRS-22 was designed to assess patient satisfaction for AIS. The questionnaire consists of 22 questions divided into 5 equally weighted domains as determined by factor analysis. The domains are function/activity, pain, self-perceived image, satisfaction with treatment, and mental health. Questions in each domain have 5 verbal response alternatives ranging from 1 to 5, with a value of 5 indicating the best outcome. The SRS-22 questionnaire is used to demonstrate the ability of operation to improve the outcome of AIS patients. In a multicenter study of 1510 patients, statistically significant improvements were observed in the pain domain score of the SRS-22 questionnaire at the 2-year postoperative follow-up [33].

In addition to the adaptation and validation in English-speaking countries, cross-cultural versions of the SRS-22 Questionnaire are available in Turkish, Chinese, and other languages [34-38]. The SRS-22 Questionnaire is currently widely used for the clinical evaluation of adolescents and young adults with scoliosis treated with surgery.

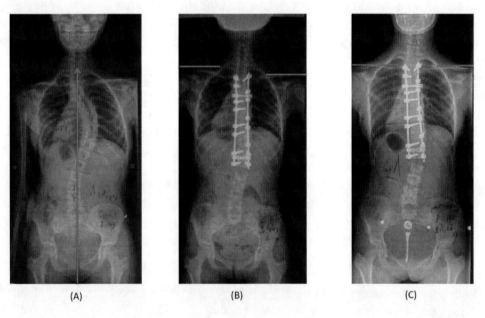

Figure 15. Preoperative radiograph of a 14-year-old boy with a Lenke 1A curve (A). Three-month postoperative radiograph shows adding-on with disc angulation of 6.1°. Left shoulder elevated with an RSH of 21.5 mm (B). Two-year postoperative radiograph shows adding-on progressed with disc angulation of 12.1°. Shoulders were level with an RSH of 5.5 mm (C).

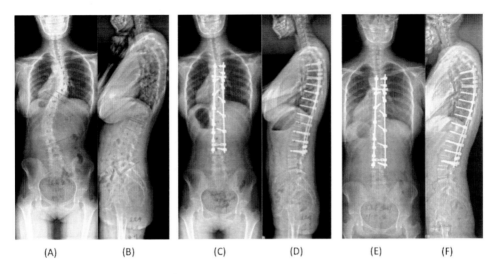

Figure 16. Preoperative PA and lateral radiographs of a 12-year-old girl with a Lenke type 6C curve (A,B). Postoperative radiographs show a good correction outcome in the coronal and sagittal planes with fusion from T4 to L3 (C,D). Two-year postoperative radiographs demonstrate proximal junctional kyphosis (E,F).

REFERENCES

[1] Weinstein SL, Dolan LA, Cheng JC, et al. Adolescent idiopathic scoliosis. *Lancet*, 2008, 371(9623):1527-1537. doi: 10.1016/S0140-6736(08)60658-3.

[2] Richards BS, Bernstein RM, D'amato CR, et al. Standardization of criteria for adolescent idiopathic scoliosis brace studies: SRS Committee on Bracing and Nonoperative Management. *Spine*, 2005, 30(18): 2068-2075. doi: 10.1097/01.brs.0000178819.90239.d0.

[3] Lenke LG, Edwards CC, Bridwell KH. The Lenke classification of adolescent idiopathic scoliosis: how it organizes curve patterns as a template to perform selective fusions of the spine. *Spine*, 2003, 28(20S): S199-S207. doi: 10.1097/01.BRS.0000092216.16155.33.

[4] Min K, Sdzuy C, Farshad M. Posterior correction of thoracic adolescent idiopathic scoliosis with pedicle screw instrumentation: results of 48 patients with minimal 10-year follow-up. *European Spine Journal*, 2013, 22(2):345-354. doi: https://0-doi-org.skyline.ucdenver.edu/10.1007/s00586-012-2533-3.

[5] Di SM, Lolli F, Bakaloudis G, et al. Apical vertebral derotation in the posterior treatment of adolescent idiopathic scoliosis: myth or reality?. *European Spine Journal*, 2013, 22(2):313-323. doi: https://0-doi-org.skyline.ucdenver.edu/10.1007/s00586-012-2372-2.

[6] Vora V, Crawford A, Babekhir N, et al. A pedicle screw construct gives an enhanced posterior correction of adolescent idiopathic scoliosis when compared with other constructs: myth or reality. *Spine*, 2007, 32(17):1869-74. doi: 10.1097/BRS.0b013e318108b912.

[7] Harrington PR. Treatment of scoliosis. Correction and internal fixation by spine instrumentation. *Journal of Bone & Joint Surgery American Volume*, 1962, 44(4):591-634.

[8] Cotrel Y, Dubousset J. A new technic for segmental spinal osteosynthesis using the posterior approach. *Rev Chir Orthop Reparatrice Appar Mot*, 1984, 70(6):489-494.

[9] Muschik MT, Kimmich H, Demmel T. Comparison of anterior and posterior double-rod instrumentation for thoracic idiopathic scoliosis: results of 141 patients. *European Spine Journal*, 2006, 15(7):1128-1138. doi: https://0-doi-org.skyline.ucdenver.edu/10.1007/s00586-005-0034-3.

[10] Weinstein SL, Ponseti IV. Curve progression in idiopathic scoliosis. *Journal of Bone & Joint Surgery American Volume*, 1983, 65(4):447-455.

[11] Asher MA, Burton DC. Adolescent idiopathic scoliosis: natural history and long term treatment effects. *Scoliosis*, 2006, 1(1):1-10. doi: https://0-doi-org.skyline.ucdenver.edu/10.1186/1748-7161-1-2.

[12] Zhu Z, Xu L, Jiang L, et al. Is Brace Treatment Appropriate for Adolescent Idiopathic Scoliosis Patients Refusing Surgery With Cobb Angle Between 40 and 50 Degrees. *Clinical spine surgery*, 2017, 30(2): 85-89. doi:10.1097/BSD.0b013e3182a1de29.

[13] Sanders JO, Browne RH, Mcconnell SJ, et al. Maturity assessment and curve progression in girls with idiopathic scoliosis. *Journal of Bone & Joint Surgery American Volume*, 2007, 89(1):64-73. doi: 10.2106/JBJS.F.00067.

[14] Hung AL, Chau W, Shi B, et al. Thumb Ossification Composite Index (TOCI) for Predicting Peripubertal Skeletal Maturity and Peak Height Velocity in Idiopathic Scoliosis. *Journal of Bone & Joint Surgery American Volume*, 2017, 99(17):1438-1446. doi: http://dx.doi.org/10.2106/JBJS.16.01078.

[15] Mao S, Xu L, Zhu Z, et al. Association between genetic determinants of peak height velocity during puberty and predisposition to adolescent idiopathic scoliosis. *Spine*, 2013, 38(12):1034-1039. doi: 10.1097/BRS.0b013e318287fcfd.

[16] Bao H, Yan P, Bao M, et al. Halo-gravity traction combined with assisted ventilation: an effective pre-operative management for severe adult scoliosis complicated with respiratory dysfunction. *European Spine Journal*, 2016, 25(8):2416-2422. doi: https://0-doi-org.skyline.ucdenver.edu/10.1007/s00586-016-4607-0.

[17] Nash CL, Moe JH. A study of vertebral rotation. *J Bone Joint Surg Am*, 1969, 51(2): 223-229.

[18] Murphy JS, Upasani VV, Yaszay B, et al. Predictors of Distal Adding-On in Thoracic Major Curves with AR Lumbar Modifiers. *Spine*, 2016, 42(4): E211–E218. doi:10.1097/BRS.0000000000001761.

[19] Qin X, Sun W, Xu L, et al. Selecting the Last "Substantially" Touching Vertebra as Lowest Instrumented Vertebra in Lenke Type 1A Curve: Radiographic Outcomes with a Minimum of 2-year Follow-Up. *Spine*, 2016, 41(12): E742-E750. doi: http://10.1097/BRS.0000000000001374.

[20] Lenke LG, Bridwell KH, Baldus C, et al. Preventing decompensation in King type II curves treated with Cotrel-Dubousset instrumentation. Strict guidelines for selective thoracic fusion. *Spine*, 1992, 17(8 Suppl):274-281.

[21] Vallespir GP, Flores JB, Trigueros IS, et al. Vertebral coplanar alignment: a standardized technique for three dimensional correction in scoliosis surgery: technical description and preliminary results in Lenke type 1 curves. *Spine*, 2008, 33(14):1588-1597. doi: 10.1097/BRS.0b013e3181788704.

[22] Qiu Y, Zhu F, Wang B, et al. Comparison of surgical outcomes of lenke type 1 idiopathic scoliosis: vertebral coplanar alignment versus derotation technique. *Journal of Spinal Disorders & Techniques*, 2011, 24(8):492-499. doi: 10.1097/BSD.0b013e3182060337.

[23] Jiang J, Qian BP, Qiu Y, et al. The mechanisms underlying the variety of preoperative directionalities of shoulder tilting in adolescent idiopathic scoliosis patients with double thoracic curve. *European Spine Journal*, 2018;27:305-311. doi: https://0-doi-org.skyline.ucdenver.edu/10.1007/s00586-017-5171-y.

[24] Danielsson AJ, Cederlund CG, Ekholm S, et al. The prevalence of disc aging and back pain after fusion extending into the lower lumbar spine: a matched MR study twenty-five years after surgery for adolescent idiopathic scoliosis. *Acta radiologica*, 2001, 42(2): 187-197.

[25] Wilk B, Karol LA, Johnston CE, et al. The effect of scoliosis fusion on spinal motion: a comparison of fused and nonfused patients with idiopathic scoliosis. *Spine*, 2006, 31(3): 309-314. doi: 10.1097/01.brs.0000197168.11815.ec.

[26] Sung-Soo K, Dong-Ju L, Jin-Hyok K, et al. Determination of the Distal Fusion Level in the Management of Thoracolumbar and Lumbar Adolescent Idiopathic Scoliosis Using Pedicle Screw Instrumentation. *Asian Spine Journal*, 2014, 8(6):804-812. https://doi.org/10.4184/asj.2014.8.6.804.

[27] Geck MJ, Macagno A, Ponte A, et al. The Ponte procedure: posterior only treatment of Scheuermann's kyphosis using segmental posterior shortening and pedicle screw instrumentation. *Journal of Spinal Disorders & Techniques*, 2007, 20(8):586-593. doi: 10.1097/BSD.0b013e31803d3b16.

[28] Zhu W, Sun W, Xu L, et al. Minimally invasive scoliosis surgery assisted by O-arm navigation for Lenke Type 5C adolescent idiopathic scoliosis: a comparison with standard open approach spinal instrumentation. *Journal of Neurosurgery Pediatrics*, 2017, 19(4):1-7. doi: https://thejns.org/doi/abs/10.3171/2016.11.PEDS16412.

[29] Jiang J, Qiu Y, Qian B, et al. Postoperative shoulder balances of Lenke 2 adolescent idiopathic scoliosis patients with preoperative right-elevated shoulder after selective thoracic fusion. *Chinese Journal of Bone & Joint Surgery*, 2015(1):21-26. doi:10.3969/j.issn.2095-9958.2015.01-005.

[30] Helgeson MD, Shah SP. Evaluation of proximal junctional kyphosis in adolescent idiopathic scoliosis following pedicle screw, hook, or hybrid instrumentation. *Spine*, 2010, 35(2):177-181. doi: 10.1097/BRS.0b013e3181c77f8c.

[31] Lowe TG, Lenke L, Betz R, et al. Distal junctional kyphosis of adolescent idiopathic thoracic curves following anterior or posterior instrumented fusion: incidence, risk factors, and prevention. *Spine*, 2006, 31(3):299-302. doi: 10.1097/01.brs.0000197221.23109.fc.

[32] Engsberg JR, Bridwell KH, Reitenbach AK, et al. Preoperative gait comparisons between adults undergoing long spinal deformity fusion surgery (thoracic to L4, L5, or sacrum) and controls. *Spine*, 2001, 26(18):2020-2028. doi: 10.1097/00007632-200109150-00016.

[33] Djurasovic M, Glassman SD, Sucato DJ, et al. Improvement in SRS22R Pain Scores after Surgery for Adolescent Idiopathic Scoliosis. *Spine*, 2016, 16(10):S343-344. doi: https://doi.org/10.1016/j.spinee.2016.07.443.

[34] Alanay A, Cil A, Berk H, et al. Reliability and validity of adapted Turkish Version of Scoliosis Research Society-22 (SRS-22) questionnaire. *Spine*, 2005, 30(21):2464-2468. http://10.1097/01.brs.0000184366.71761.84.

[35] Antonarakos PD, Katranitsa L, Angelis L, et al. Reliability and validity of the adapted Greek version of scoliosis research society–22 (SRS-22) questionnaire. *Scoliosis*, 2009, 4(1):14. https://doi.org/10.1186/1748-7161-4-14.

[36] Hashimoto H, Sase T, Arai Y, et al. Validation of a Japanese version of the Scoliosis Research Society-22 Patient Questionnaire among idiopathic scoliosis patients in Japan. *Spine*, 2007, 32(4):E141-E146. doi: 10.1097/01.brs.0000255220.47077.33.

[37] Glowacki M, Misterska E, Laurentowska M, et al. Polish adaptation of scoliosis research society-22 questionnaire. *Spine*, 2009, 34(10):1060-1065. doi: 10.1097/BRS.0b013e31819c1ec3.

[38] Qiu G, Qiu Y, Zhu Z, et al. Re-evaluation of reliability and validity of simplified Chinese version of SRS-22 patient questionnaire: a multicenter study of 333 cases. *Spine*, 2011, 36(8):545-550. doi: 10.1097/BRS.0b013e3181e0485e.

Chapter 15

ANTERIOR INSTRUMENTED FUSION IN ADOLESCENT IDIOPATHIC SCOLIOSIS: INDICATION, PREOPERATIVE PLANNING, AND OUTCOME

Michael Ruf and Jörg Drumm
Center for Spinal Surgery, Orthopedics, and Traumatology, Karlsbad, Germany

ABSTRACT

Adolescent idiopathic scoliosis is a complex three-dimensional deformity of the spine consisting of a lateral curvature, apical vertebral rotation, and an impairment of the sagittal profile. Surgical options include anterior and posterior approaches.

Anterior instrumented fusion is suitable in Lenke type 1 and 5 curves. It provides excellent results in coronal plane correction and is superior in restoration of the sagittal profile and apical derotation. Fusion is shorter compared to posterior correction, and complication rate is low. Pulmonary function is impaired postoperatively, but recovers within two years.

Keywords: adolescent idiopathic scoliosis, anterior approach, correction, derotation, thoracic kyphosis, pulmonary function

INTRODUCTION

Adolescent idiopathic scoliosis (AIS) is a complex three-dimensional deformity of the spine including a lateral curvature (frontal plane) combined with vertebral rotation (transverse plane) and impairment of the sagittal profile. Recent studies suggest that the sagittal profile during the growth period plays an important role in the development of AIS [1].

The idiopathic scoliosis usually occurs in otherwise healthy adolescents during the prepubertal growth spurt. The prevalence is between 0.5 and 5%. Girls are more frequent affected than boys (ratio about 7:1) [2].

AIS in a 10 to 12 year old patient is likely to progress. According to Nachemson et al., a curve of 30 to 60° has a probability to deteriorate of 90% [3].

The AIS is classified according to Lenke in six curve types (thoracic, double thoracic, double major, triple major, thoracolumbar/lumbar, and double major/prim. lumbar). Based on the type of the scoliosis, the degree and stiffness of the curve(s), the sagittal profile, and the age of the patient, different treatment options and different approaches are available [4].

Anterior correction of AIS was introduced by Alan Dwyer in the early seventies [5]. He used an anterior cable and screw instrumentation system to correct and stabilize scoliotic deformities. The technique showed good results in the frontal plane, however, due to the anterior compression, a tendency to kyphosis was inherent in this technique. This was favorable in the thoracic region, but disastrous in the lumbar spine [6]. In addition, the pseudarthrosis rate was high.

The anterior technique was further developed by Klaus Zielke [7]. He introduced a flexible solid threaded rod /screw system with the possibility for derotation with a special tool (derotator). In the following, the fusion rates improved; however, the problem of kyphosis in the lumbar spine remained.

Subsequent developments improved the results of anterior scoliosis surgery. The introduction of screw/rod systems with stiff rods (single and double rods) allowed for a new correction maneuver: correction was achieved by rotation of a prebent stiff rod. The problem of kyphosis in the lumbar spine was overcome by the use of structural grafts/cages in the disc space. By combination of these techniques (rod rotation, anterior support, and compression via the instrumentation) a complete correction of the deformity in all three planes was achieved with a high stability of the construct. Pseudarthrosis rate decreased [8–11].

INDICATION

Anterior correction in AIS should be considered in single thoracic and lumbar deformities with flexible compensatory curves. These are type 1 and type 5 curvatures according to Lenke's classification.

The indication for anterior correction and fusion depends on the degree of the scoliosis in the frontal plane, the amount of kyphosis/lordosis in the sagittal plane, the age of the patient, the expected further progression, and the cosmetic impairment (rib hump).

In the thoracic spine, the indication for surgery is starting with a Cobb angle of 40 to 50 degrees. The ideal patient for anterior instrumented fusion is the single thoracic curve (Lenke type 1 A-C) with hypokyphosis (T5-12 sagittal modifier – or N). Since the anterior correction includes a shortening of the anterior column of the spine and is therefore kyphogenic, it should not be applied in primarily hyperkyphotic cases (rare), or in very young children that tend to develop hyperkyphosis due to the anterior tether.

In the lumbar spine, indication for surgical correction is given with an angle of 35 to 40 degrees. Lenke type 5 curves are ideal for anterior instrumented fusion, since the length of fusion is shorter than in posterior correction and derotation is more effective.

PREOPERATIVE PLANNING

The aim of surgery is a three-dimensional correction with a well-balanced, straight spine and a fusion as short as possible. A physiological sagittal profile has to be restored. For a perfect cosmetic result the shoulder level should be horizontalized and the rib hump corrected.

Radiographs of the whole spine in ap. and lateral view as well as bending films are inevitable to assess the extent, localization and flexibility of the main curve as well as the compensatory curves. MRI of the whole spine is recommended to exclude intraspinal pathologies. In severe cases a low-dose CT and traction films should be considered.

The deformity is then classified according to Lenke [4].

In the thoracic spine (Lenke type 1) fusion is planned from end vertebra to end vertebra. For typical Lenke 1 curves the uppermost instrumented vertebra is T5 or T6, the lowest T11, T12, or L1. The approach is planned via a double thoracotomy, the upper one between 4th and 5th respectively between 5th and 6th rib with distal osteotomy of the rib, the lower one usually 4 rib spaces lower. Depending on the severity of the rib hump, the resection of the rib heads is projected. To regain thoracic kyphosis, a shortening of the anterior column is necessary by complete resection of the disc including the posterior annulus; in severe hypokyphosis the convex and anterior part of the endplates should be removed as well. Screws are inserted in the center of the vertebral body parallel to the endplates. Correction is achieved by cantilever technique, rotation of the prebent rod and final compression. To avoid a junctional thoracolumbar kyphosis, a structural graft or cage may be used at the lowest fused disc space Figure 1).

For lumbar curves (Lenke type 5) fusion is planned from end vertebra to end vertebra as well, typically T11 to L3. The approach is a thoraco-phreno-lumbotomy with sectioning of the diaphragm close to the costal insertion. After insertion of the screws correction is achieved by rotation of the prebent rod from scoliosis to lordosis. Structural spacers (i.e., cages) are inserted in the debrided disc spaces; compression is applied via the rod. Autologous bone or bone substitute are added for bony fusion.

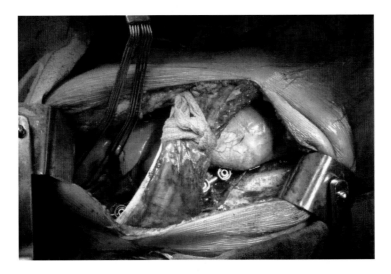

Figure 1. Surgical approach to the thoracic spine via a double thoracotomy.

Fixation can be performed with single or double rod instrumentation. Follow-up studies showed no significant difference in functional or radiographic outcome between both types of instrumentation [12].

OUTCOME

Clinical and Radiographic Results

Anterior instrumentation and fusion in AIS may deliver excellent results in short-term as well as long-term examinations.

In our own series of 50 patients with thoracic and lumbar scoliosis we evaluated clinical results with the SRS30 outcome score with a follow-up of 10 to 26 years (average 16 yrs.). We found an average score of 4.1 (pain 4.2/ function 4.2/ self-image 4.0/ mental health 3.9/ satisfaction 4.2); patients with thoracic scoliosis correction scored slightly better than patients with lumbar correction: 4.2 vs. 3.9 [13]. These results are similar to a control group of volunteers without scoliosis [14].

These favorable results are endorsed by several recent publications. Tis et al. [15] described a series of 85 patients with thoracic curves (Lenke 1) in a five year follow-up, Sudo et al. [16] a series of 25 patients with average 15 years follow-up, and Rushton and et al. [17] 18 patients with 2years follow-up. They found that anterior correction and fusion is a safe and reproducible procedure for thoracic AIS. Correction rate was between 51% and 64% in the coronal plane; complication rate was low. The SRS outcome score improved significantly.

Advantages of anterior versus posterior techniques are the true segmental derotation with excellent rib hump correction [18]. The rib hump showed better correction after anterior surgery than after a posterior correction procedures [17].

Maintenance of thoracic curve correction after anterior instrumentation and fusion provided a stable spontaneous correction of the secondary lumbar curve over time [19].

For thoracolumbar/lumbar curves (Lenke 5) excellent results are described in short- and long-term follow-up as well. Verma et al. found a SRS score of average 4.4 two years after surgery [20], Kelly et al. a score of 4.3 and Sudo et al. of 4.2, both at 17 years follow-up [21, 22]. The correction described in coronal plane was between 74% and 80%, with a powerful derotation of the apical vertebrae [20, 22, 23]. Complications like pseudoarthrosis and implant failures were rare [12, 23].

Sagittal Profile

Thoracic scoliosis is mostly associated with hypokyphosis or even lordosis in the sagittal plane. The three-dimensional degree of hypokyphosis is usually underestimated when plain lateral radiographs are used [24].

Anterior correction and fusion is able to correct this hypokyphosis and to restore a physiological sagittal profile. When comparing anterior and posterior approaches for correction of thoracic AIS, the results in frontal plane correction are similar; however, there is clear evidence that the anterior approach is superior in restoration of a normal thoracic kyphosis [17, 18, 25–27].

These results are of special interest, as a thoracic flat back seems to be a risk factor for lumbar degenerative disc disease after spinal fusion in a long-term follow-up [28].

On the other hand, in patients with preoperative hyperkyphosis a posterior approach should be considered. Furthermore, very young patients with a high growth potential are at risk to develop hyperkyphosis during further growth after anterior correction and fusion.

Fusion Length

In anterior scoliosis correction the fusion is usually performed from the upper end vertebra to the lower end vertebra. Current recommendations for posterior scoliosis correction whereas comprise more segments in thoracic as well as in thoracolumbar/lumbar curves. The difference in fusion length is between one and fore vertebrae [25, 27, 29–31].

In our opinion, it is of utmost importance to keep the fusion length in these young patients as short as possible. This is especially valid for mobility in the lumbar segments. It may be accepted that the stress in few residual mobile segments is higher, and that this will result in an increased rate of degenerative disc disease during lifetime.

Pulmonary Function

After anterior approach, due to the opening of the chest wall, the pulmonary function is more deteriorated than after posterior approach. However, it improves within the next months. After two years, pulmonary function is comparable to the preoperative values without significant differences between anterior and posterior approaches [32, 33].

This was also found for thoracolumbar/lumbar AIS patients who underwent a thoracophrenolaparotomy [34].

Correction Maneuver

Correction of thoracic deformity by an anterior approach is based on two mechanisms: First is the shortening of the anterior column of the spine, second the correction via the rigid rod. It has been shown that an aggressive anterior release with removal of the rib heads, complete resection of the annulus, disruption of the posterior longitudinal ligament and partial resection of the endplates of the adjacent vertebral bodies results in a considerable shortening of the anterior spine. This shortening is followed by a spontaneous correction of the scoliosis without application of any corrective force [35]. In this case series with anterior release and posterior instrumentation, the thoracic scoliosis corrected spontaneously from 80° to 50° after the anterior release, thoracic kyphosis improved from 11° to 32°. The reason for this effect is probably linked to the development of thoracic scoliosis: The imbalance of anterior and posterior spinal column length in favor of the anterior column may be a driving force in the development of thoracic AIS. The effect is a hypokyphotic and scoliotic spine. Anterior shortening reverses this imbalance; the spine straightens spontaneously, and kyphosis evolves. The second part of correction and the stabilization is then performed by the anterior instrumentation with a rigid rod by a cantilever procedure, rod rotation, and convex compression.

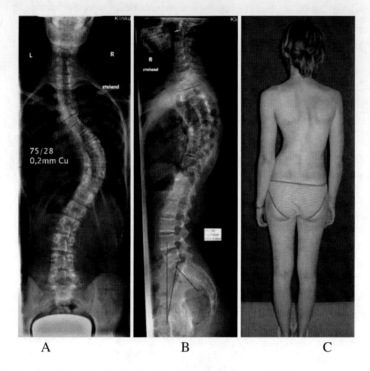

Figure 2A-C. 15 yrs. old girl with adolescent idiopathic thoracic scoliosis.

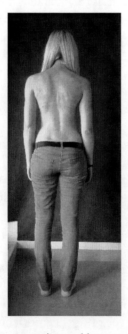

Figure 2D. Same girl 5 yrs. after anterior correction and instrumented fusion.

Anterior Instrumented Fusion in Adolescent Idiopathic Scoliosis

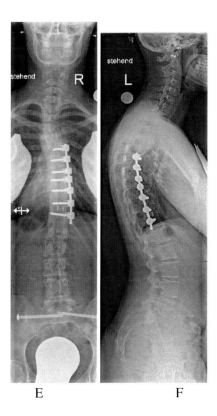

E F

Figure 2E and F. The radiographs 10 yrs. after surgery show the short instrumentation T6-T12 with solid fusion. In the meantime she had a car accident with a pelvic fracture but no problem with the thoracolumbar spine.

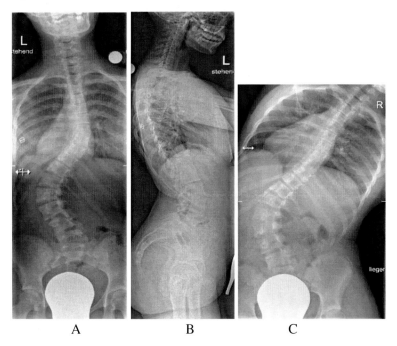

A B C

Figure 3A-E. (Continued).

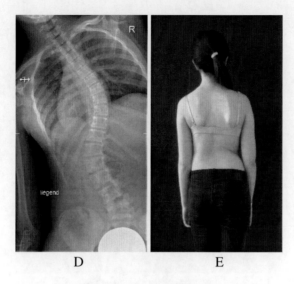

Figure 3A-E. A 15 yrs. old girl with a primary lumbar scoliosis (Lenke 3C).

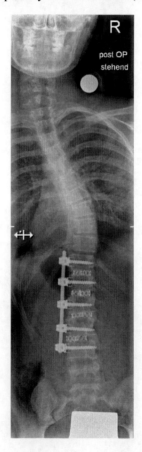

Figure 3F. Immediately postoperative following anterior correction and fusion.

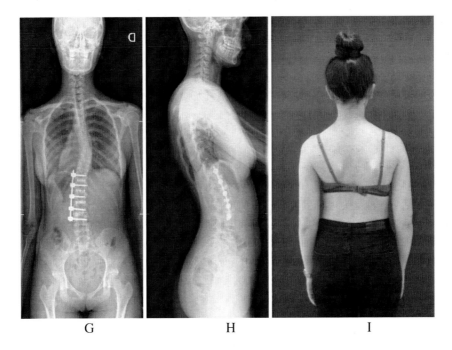

Figure 3G-I. Two yrs. later: well-balanced spine with a short instrumentation and fusion.

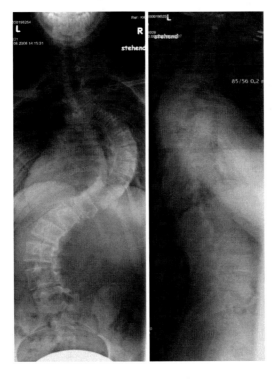

Figure 4A and B. Rigid scoliosis Lenke 4C in a 16-year-old girl.

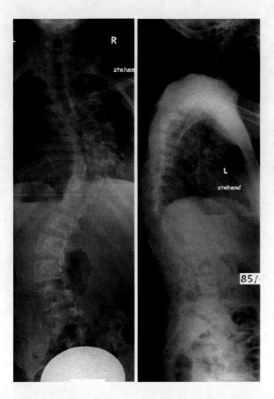

Figure 4C and D. One week after anterior release with shortening of the anterior column of the spine without instrumentation (posterior instrumentation planned): Spontaneous correction of the scoliosis, restoration of thoracic kyphosis (standing position).

CONCLUSION

Anterior instrumented fusion in AIS is a safe and reliable technique for correction of Lenke type 1 and 5 curves. It provides excellent results in coronal plane correction and especially in restoration of the sagittal profile and apical derotation. Fusion is shorter compared to posterior correction. Pulmonary function is impaired postoperatively, but recovers within two years.

REFERENCES

[1] Schlösser TP, Shah SA, Reichard SJ, Rogers K, Vincken KL, Castelein RM. Differences in early sagittal plane alignment between thoracic and lumbar adolescent idiopathic scoliosis. *Spine J*. 2014;14(2):282-90.
[2] Konieczny MR, Senyurt H, Krauspe R. Epidemiology of adolescent idiopathic scoliosis. *J Child Orthop* 2013;7(1):3–9.
[3] Pehrsson K, Larsson S, Oden A, Nachemson A. Long-term follow-up of patients with untreated scoliosis. A study of mortality, causes of death, and symptoms. *Spine* 1992;17(9):1091-6.

[4] Lenke LG, Betz RR, Harms J, Bridwell KH, Clements DH, Lowe TG, Blanke K. Adolescent idiopathic scoliosis: a new classification to determine extent of spinal arthrodesis. *J Bone Joint Surg Am.* 2001;83-A(8):1169-81.

[5] Dwyer AF, Schafer MF. Anterior approach to scoliosis. Results of treatment in fifty-one cases. *J Bone Joint Surg Br.* 1974;56(2):218-24.

[6] Hsu LC, Zucherman J, Tang SC, Leong JC. Dwyer instrumentation in the treatment of adolescent idiopathic scoliosis. *J Bone Joint Surg Br* 1982;64: 536–41.

[7] Hammerberg KW, Zielke, K. *VDS instrumentation for idiopathic thoracic curvatures. Presented at the Annual Meeting of the American Academy of Orthopedic Surgeons*, Las Vegas 1985.

[8] Harms J, Jeszenszky D, Beele B. Ventral correction of thoracic scoliosis. In Bridwell KH, DeWald RD, eds. *The Textbook of Spinal Surgery,* 2nd ed. Philadelphia:Lippincott-Raven, 1997, pp 611-626.

[9] Kaneda K, Shono Y, Satoh S, Abumi K. Anterior correction of thoracic scoliosis with Kaneda anterior spinal system. A preliminary report. *Spine* 1997;22(12):1358-68.

[10] Halm HF, Liljenqvist U, Niemeyer T, Chan DP, Zielke K, Winkelmann W. Halm-Zielke instrumentation for primary stable anterior scoliosis surgery: operative technique and 2-year results in ten consecutive adolescent idiopathic scoliosis patients within a prospective clinical trial. *Eur Spine J.* 1998;7(5):429-34.

[11] Betz RR, Harms J, Clements DH 3rd, Lenke LG, Lowe TG, Shufflebarger HL, Jeszenszky D, Beele B. Comparison of anterior and posterior instrumentation for correction of adolescent thoracic idiopathic scoliosis. *Spine* 1999;24(3):225–239.

[12] Nambiar M, Yang Y, Liew S, Turner PL, Torode IP. Single- versus dual-rod anterior instrumentation of thoracolumbar curves in adolescent idiopathic scoliosis. *Eur Spine J.* 2016;25(10):3249-3255.

[13] Ruf M, Letko L, Ostrowski G, Merk H. *Langzeitergebnisse nach ventraler Korrektur der idiopathischen Adoleszentenskoliose.* [*Long-term results after ventral correction of idiopathic adolescent scoliosis.*] Presented at: Süddeutscher Orthopädenkongress [South German Orthopedic Congress], Baden-Baden 2014.

[14] Akazawa T, Minami S, Kotani T, Nemoto T, Koshi T, Takahashi K. Health-related quality of life and low back pain of patients surgically treated for scoliosis after 21 years or more of follow-up: comparison among nonidiopathic scoliosis, idiopathic scoliosis, and healthy subjects. *Spine* 2012;37(22):1899-903.

[15] Tis JE, O'Brien MF, Newton PO, Lenke LG, Clements DH, Harms J, Betz RR. Adolescent idiopathic scoliosis treated with open instrumented anterior spinal fusion: five-year follow-up. *Spine* 2010;35(1):64-70.

[16] Sudo H, Ito M, Kaneda K, Shono Y, Takahata M, Abumi K. Long-term outcomes of anterior spinal fusion for treating thoracic adolescent idiopathic scoliosis curves: average 15-year follow-up analysis. *Spine* 2013;38(10):819-26.

[17] Rushton PR, Grevitt MP, Sell PJ. Anterior or posterior surgery for right thoracic adolescent idiopathic scoliosis (AIS)? A prospective cohorts' comparison using radiologic and functional outcomes. *J Spinal Disord Tech.* 2015;28(3):80-8.

[18] Liljenqvist U, Halm H, Bullmann V. Spontaneous lumbar curve correction in selective anterior instrumentation and fusion of idiopathic thoracic scoliosis of Lenke type C. *Eur Spine J.* 2013;22 Suppl 2:S138-48.

[19] Sudo HS, Mayer MM, Kaneda KK, Núñez-Pereira S, Shono SY, Hitzl WH, Iwasaki NI, Koller HK. Maintenance of spontaneous lumbar curve correction following thoracic fusion of main thoracic curves in adolescent idiopathic scoliosis. *Bone Joint J*. 2016;98-B(7):997-1002.

[20] Verma K, Auerbach JD, Kean KE, Chamas F, Vorsanger M, Lonner BS. Anterior spinal fusion for thoracolumbar scoliosis: comprehensive assessment of radiographic, clinical, and pulmonary outcomes on 2-years follow-up. *J Pediatr Orthop*. 2010;30(7):664-9.

[21] Kelly DM, McCarthy RE, McCullough FL, Kelly HR. Long-term outcomes of anterior spinal fusion with instrumentation for thoracolumbar and lumbar curves in adolescent idiopathic scoliosis. *Spine* 2010;35(2):194-8.

[22] Sudo H, Ito M, Kaneda K, Shono Y, Abumi K. Long-term outcomes of anterior dual-rod instrumentation for thoracolumbar and lumbar curves in adolescent idiopathic scoliosis: a twelve to twenty-three-year follow-up study. *J Bone Joint Surg Am*. 2013;95(8):e49.

[23] Delfino R, Pizones J, Ruiz-Juretschke C, Sánchez-Mariscal F, Zúñiga L, Izquierdo E. Selective Anterior Thoracolumbar Fusion in Adolescent Idiopathic Scoliosis: Long-Term Results After 17-Year Follow-Up. *Spine* 2017;42(13):E788-E794.

[24] Parvaresh KC, Osborn EJ, Reighard FG, Doan J, Bastrom TP, Newton PO. Predicting 3D Thoracic Kyphosis Using Traditional 2D Radiographic Measurements in Adolescent Idiopathic Scoliosis. *Spine Deform*. 2017;5(3):159-165.

[25] Lowe TG, Betz R, Lenke L, Clements D, Harms J, Newton P, Haher T, Merola A, Wenger D. Anterior single-rod instrumentation of the thoracic and lumbar spine: saving levels. *Spine* 2003;28(20):S208-16.

[26] Chaloupka R, Repko M, Tichý V, Leznar M, Krbec M. [Comparison of two surgical methods for treatment of idiopathic thoracic scoliosis - anterior versus posterior approaches]. *Acta Chir Orthop Traumatol Cech*. 2012;79(5):422-8.

[27] Newton PO, Marks MC, Bastrom TP, Betz R, Clements D, Lonner B, Crawford A, Shufflebarger H, O'Brien M, Yaszay B; Harms Study Group. Surgical treatment of Lenke 1 main thoracic idiopathic scoliosis: results of a prospective, multicenter study. *Spine* 2013;38(4):328-38.

[28] Bernstein P, Hentschel S, Platzek I, Hühne S, Ettrich U, Hartmann A, Seifert J. Thoracal flat back is a risk factor for lumbar disc degeneration after scoliosis surgery. *Spine J*. 2014;14(6):925-32.

[29] Tao F, Wang Z, Li M, Pan F, Shi Z, Zhang Y, Wu Y, Xie Y. A comparison of anterior and posterior instrumentation for restoring and retaining sagittal balance in patients with idiopathic adolescent scoliosis. *J Spinal Disord Tech*. 2012;25(6):303-8.

[30] Luo M, Wang W, Shen M, Xia L. Anterior versus posterior approach in Lenke 5C adolescent idiopathic scoliosis: a meta-analysis of fusion segments and radiological outcomes. *J Orthop Surg Res*. 2016;11(1):77.

[31] Miyanji F, Nasto LA, Bastrom T, Samdani AF, Yaszay B, Clements D, Shah SA, Lonner B, Betz RR, Shufflebarger HL, Newton PO. A Detailed Comparative Analysis of Anterior Versus Posterior Approach to Lenke 5C Curves. *Spine* 2018;43(5):E285-E291.

[32] Bullmann V, Schulte TL, Schmidt C, et al. Pulmonary function after anterior double thoracotomy approach versus posterior surgery with costectomies in idiopathic thoracic scoliosis. *Eur Spine J* 2013;22:S164–71.

[33] Lee AC1, Feger MA, Singla A, Abel MF Effect of Surgical Approach on Pulmonary Function in Adolescent Idiopathic Scoliosis Patients: A Systemic Review and Meta-analysis. *Spine* 2016;41(22):E1343-E1355.

[34] Ruiz-Juretschke C, Pizones J, Delfino R, Sánchez-Mariscal F, Zúñiga L, Izquierdo E. Long-term Pulmonary Function After Open Anterior Thoracolumbar Surgery in Thoracolumbar/Lumbar Idiopathic Adolescent Scoliosis. *Spine* 2017;42(16):1241-1247.

[35] Ruf M, Letko L, Matis N, Merk HR, Harms J. The Effect of Anterior Mobilisation and Shortening in the Correction of Rigid Idiopathic Thoracic Scoliosis. *Spine* 2013;38(26):E1662-8.

In: Scoliosis: Diagnosis, Classification and Management Options   ISBN: 978-1-53614-464-2
Editors: F. Canavese, A. Andreacchio and H. Xu   © 2018 Nova Science Publishers, Inc.

Chapter 16

POSTERIOR MINIMALLY INVASIVE SURGERY FOR THE TREATMENT OF ADOLESCENT IDIOPATHIC SCOLIOSIS

Charlotte de Bodman[1,*], MD, Anne Tabard-Fougère[2], MSc, Alexandre Ansorgue[2], MD, Nicolas Amirghasemi[2], MD and Romain Dayer[1,2], MD

[1]Pediatric Orthopedics and Traumatology Unit, Lausanne University, Lausanne, Switzerland
[2]Division of Paediatric Orthopedics, Geneva University, Geneva, Switzerland

ABSTRACT

Adolescent idiopathic scoliosis (AIS) represents the most frequent indication for scoliosis surgery at the pediatric age. The current reference treatment for surgery of AIS is spinal instrumentation and fusion through a posterior open approach. The recent available data for AIS suggest that the use of posterior minimally invasive surgery (MIS) technique, using 3 skin incisions and muscle splitting approach, is associated with deformity correction and complication rate equivalent to open posterior spinal fusion, with potential benefits related to a less traumatizing exposure, with low blood loss and diminished length of hospital stay.

Keywords: adolescent idiopathic scoliosis, minimally invasive surgery, muscle-splitting approach

---

[*] Corresponding Author Email: charlotte.launay@chuv.ch.

INTRODUCTION

Adolescent idiopathic scoliosis (AIS) represents the majority (51%) of the indications for scoliosis surgery at the pediatric age [1]. Untreated, this pathology is associated with a normal life expectancy in productive and functional at high-level adults, with a minimal physical impairment other than decreased body satisfaction and back pain [2]. Surgical treatment is usually indicated for scoliosis with major curve exceeding 40 degrees in growing adolescents and 45 degrees in skeletally mature patients [3-5]. The current standard technique for the surgical management of AIS is fusion and instrumentation through posterior approach. Despite reproducible good outcomes with this type of surgery, this standard open posterior approach necessitates extensive muscle dissection and soft-tissue disruption, and it's consequently associated with blood loss, post-operative pain, prolonged recovery, and long lidline scar. In order to try to decrease the approach-related morbidity associated with the conventional posterior approach, a minimally invasive surgery (MIS) technique for posterior spinal fusion has been recently proposed for AIS [6, 7].

INDICATION

The MIS three incisions technique was initially offered to select patients meeting the following criteria [8]:

1) AIS patients
2) Major curve Cobb angle inferior to 70°
3) Flexibility superior to 50% on supine bending films

For the first cases, to be familiar with the deep muscle splitting approach, one single long skin incision can be performed.

However, after a surgeon learning curve of approximately 25 cases in our hands [6], we have been able to offer this procedure to patients with idiopathic curves up to 80°, and we do not take in account curve flexibility in our preoperative evaluation for this technique.

Obesity is not an absolute contra-indication to the technique; however it can render the surgical access more difficult. We have treated patients using the MIS 3 incisions technique with body mass index of up to 32. In patients with morbid obesity, the skin incisions can be extended or even converted to a single long skin incision, while maintaining the deep muscle splitting approach.

SURGICAL TECHNIQUE

Tranexamic acid (TXA) is usually started over 15 minutes after induction of anesthesia with 10mg/kg intravenously, followed by an infusion of 1 mg/kg per hour pre-operatively until wound closure [9]. Cell salvage was systematically used over our first 70 cases, but given the low estimated blood loss encountered over these cases and in agreement with the anesthetic team, we currently do not use it on a routine basis.

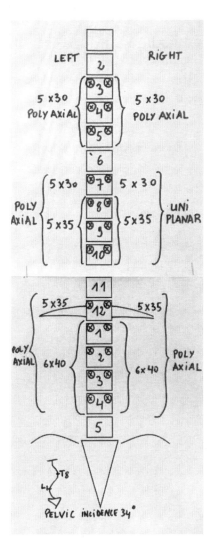

Figure 1. Preoperative planning with levels of instrumentation and fusion, diameter and lenght of pedicle screws to be inserted. The 3 cutaneous incisions will be centered over the 3 segments of instrumentation.

Pre-operative planning is established according these principles (Figure 1): for Lenke type 5 deformity, only one incision was used and all involved vertebrae were instrumented; for all others Lenke types, three incisions were used and two vertebrae were not instrumented.

The patient is installed prone on a radiolucent table, as for a conventional posterior approach. After prepping and draping, fluoroscopy is used to determine the length and localization of skin incisions. Fluoroscopy use is limited to the planning of the skin incisions (Figure 2) [10]. Although a single straight midline incision can be made, three smaller incisions are often more cosmetically appealing to patients. We advise to start the first cases with a single long skin incision, and once the surgeon feel comfortable with the muscle splitting approach and reduction tubes use, to opt for a 3 skin incisions technique. After incision, the skin is then undermined laterally to allow for paramedian extraperiosteal fascial incisions on each side of the spine. A blunt muscle-sparing approach is used down to the facet joints in the lumbar spine, and to the transverse processes in the thoracic spine. Posterior elements are uncovered using electrocoagulation and a small Cobb elevator, from the basis of the lamina to the transverse processes. This is similar to the paraspinal sacrospinalis-splitting approach described by Wiltse for the lumbar spine [11-13] (Figure 3). A small right angle Gelpi retractor helps providing excellent exposure. Once the joint is exposed, wide facetectomies are performed, and the pedicles are cannulated using the free hand technique [14]. We do not routinely use navigation by intraoperative CT scan or by fluoroscopy for the preparation of the pedicles in order to reduce radiation exposure to patients. After cannulation, the pedicles remain localized by the insertion of a cannulated pedicle marker (Figure 4). Prior to the insertion of the pedicle screws, the fusion site is prepared. The facet joints are decorticated using a high-speed burr or an ultrasonic bone scalpel, and bone graft is applied before definitive instrumentation. It consists of a mixture of autograft from the facetectomies and freeze-dried allograft bone.

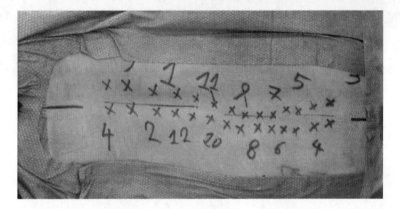

Figure 2. After prepping and draping, the levels of pedicles of the vertebra to be instrumented and fused are marked using fluoroscopy, to allow for planning of the 3 separated skin incisions. The 3 incisions will be made on the median line and centered over the pedicles of the vertebra be instrumented. Right side of the picture: cephalad.

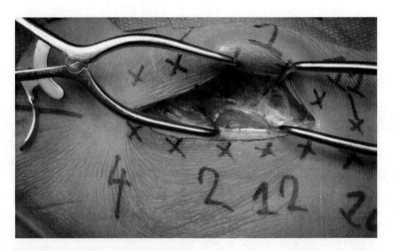

Figure 3. After incision, the skin is undermined laterally to allow for paramedian extraperiosteal fascial incisions on each side of the spine.

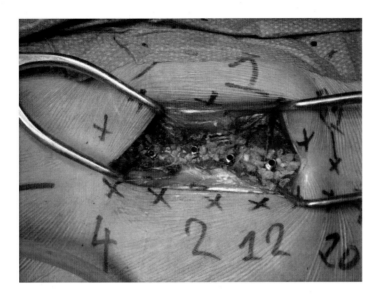

Figure 4. After cannulation, the pedicles remain localized by the insertion of a pedicle marker. Bone graft is applied after decortication with a high-speed burr of the facet joints.

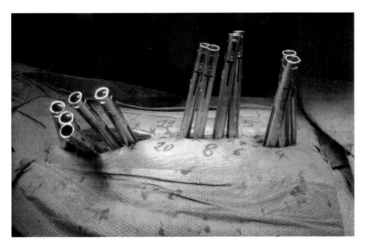

Figure 5. After exchanged pedicle markers using the guide wires, cannulated pedicle screws, already connected to the reduction tubes, are inserted on the convex side.

On an average, three segments are instrumented, one per each skin incision. The intervening facet joints between adjacent skin incisions are left uninstrumented but facetectomies are done by mobilizing precociously skin and soft tissue flaps. These levels are also decorticated and bone graft is laid down before screw placement, in the same way as the other instrumented levels, to promote fusion. Anterioposterior X-ray is taken to confirm adequate position of the cannulated pedicle markers.

Appropriate sizes of cannulated pedicle screws, already connected to reduction tubes, are then inserted on the convex side of the major curve first (Figure 5). They are exchanged with the cannulated pedicle markers using guiding wires. Uniplanar screws are placed in the convexity of the major curve. The remaining screws are polyaxial. Sarwahi et al. proposed to use reduction screws with extended tabs and MIS screws with open connector (reduction tubes) at alternating levels [7, 15]. We prefer to use MIS screws with reduction tubes at every instrumented level. We think this allows for easier insertion of the rod and apical derotation during deformity reduction. Additionally using one tray of instrumentation simplifies the handling and decreases the learning curve of the technique for the scrub nurse team. The MIS 3 incisions technique was primarily developed for the use of pedicle screws. The use of sublaminar bands is theoretically possible, but it is rendered difficult by the use of a paraspinal approach, which does not expose widely the vertebral laminae.

Two 5.5 millimeters diameter cobalt chrome rods are cut to the measured length (one centimeter left at each end of the rod template) (Figure 6) and contoured with the appropriate sagittal profile. The convex side rod is introduced first, passed below the fascia of the cutaneous bridge under direct visualization. A hexagonal wrench is used to control rod rotation (Figure 7). It is inserted from caudal to cephalad using the slots of the reduction tubes [16] (Figure 8). We favor this caudal to cephalad direction for rod insertion because there is no conflict with the head of the patient during the procedure. Conversely some surgeons advocate a cephalad to caudal rod insertion, arguing for increased safety. With a cephalad to caudal rod insertion, the orientation of the overlapping laminae and facets in the thoracic spine tends to prevent an accidental penetration into the spinal canal (7, 15). The rod is first secured using set screws in the extremities. A direct vertebral rotation maneuver is then carried out of the convex-side screws to correct most of the deformity, associated with a gradual spine-to-rod reduction (Figure 9). After derotation, the rod is completely secured using set screws. Pedicle markers on the concave side of the major curve are finally exchanged for pedicle screws. The second concave rod is overcontoured in the sagittal plane to allow for further deformity correction in the transverse plane. It is then also inserted from distal to proximal. Before closure, anteroposterior and lateral X-rays are taken to confirm adequate correction in both planes, and implants length (Figure 10).

In case of intraoperative neuromonitoring alert after insertion of the first corrective rod, the set screws are quickly removed and the rod is disengaged from the head of the pedicles screws. This maneuver is easily and quickly done. It will significantly release the correction of the deformity, without the need to completely remove the rod of its submuscular position.

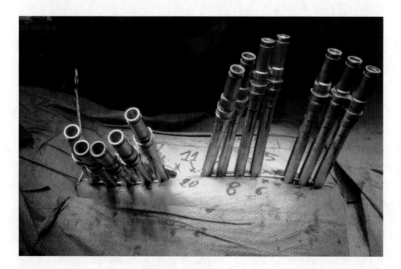

Figure 6. Measure with the rod template of the rod length: 1 centimeter left at each end.

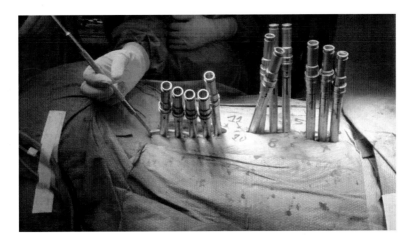

Figure 7. Insertion of the chrome cobalt rod from caudal to cephalad: the convex side rod is introduced first, passed below the fascia of the cutaneous bridge under direct visualization, using a hexagonal wrench.

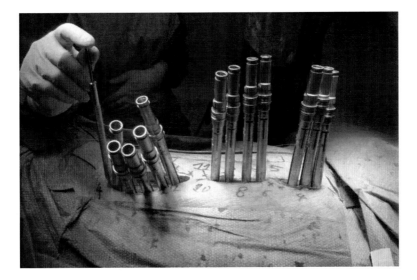

Figure 8. Rod rotation is controlled using the hexagonal wrench, and rod is secured using set screws in the cephalad extremity.

When needed, implants removal can be done using the same approach (3 skin incisions and underlying muscle splitting approach). If the extraction of the rods is difficult after set screws removal, it can be cut at the extremity of the separate incisions to facilitate its removal sequentially though each skin incision. Alternatively, the 3 incisions can be converted into one single skin incision.

Closure is fairly rapid, and is carried out in a layered fashion. Wound was dressed with steristrips with gauze and an occlusive dressing which was not changed during hospital stay. We do not routinely utilize drains.

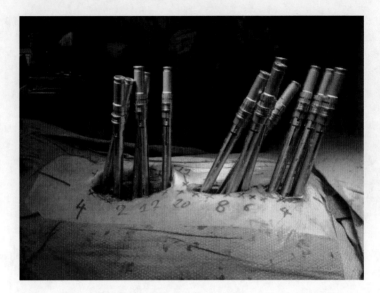

Figure 9. After derotation maneuvers. Note orientation of the lumbar reduction tubes compared to Figure 8.

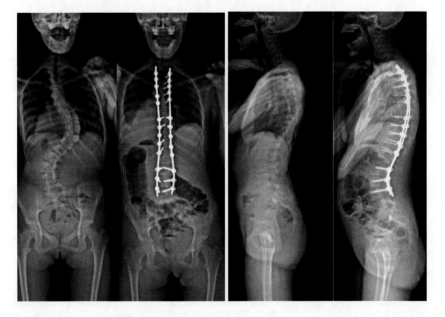

Figure 10. Preoperative and postoperative anteroposterior and lateral x-rays.

RECOVERY PATHWAY

Our postoperative protocol is fairly routine. Patients were prepared before surgery for early discharge. We use accelerated discharge pathway emphasizing early transition to oral pain medications, mobilization with physical therapy 2 times a day, and discharge regardless of return of bowel function. Patients are admitted directly after surgery on general hospital floor.

Postoperative pain management include a morphine PCA until the day after surgery. Then, intravenous pain regimen is switched to an oral one with administration of oral narcotics. Ketorolac is administrated 3 times a day during 2 days.

Patients are mobilized to walk the day after surgery with physical therapy, 2 times a day. Patients must be able to walk up a flight of stairs prior to hospital discharge. With this technique, mean hospital stay is 4.6 days [6].

Patients are transitioned to a regular diet on post-operative day 1.

At two weeks post-op, the dressing is removed and the wound is controlled. They remain out of school for 3 or 4 weeks. Patients can return to swimming or biking 3 months post-op, and to gym class 6 months postop.

ADVANTAGES

MIS could have an additional positive effect of an accelerated discharge pathway on the length of hospital stay (LOS). A shortened hospital stay has many possible benefits including a shorter exposure nosocomial infection [17, 18], a quicker transition to the home setting for patients and for parents with multiple children, earlier return to work for the parents, and lower cost to the healthcare system. With this technique, we reported 4.6 LOS [6] whereas recent data suggest that the LOS for a patient undergoing surgery for AIS is between five and six days [19, 20].

The appearance of the surgical scar seems to be an important factor when considering the patient perception of the outcome of AIS surgery [21, 22]. The only domain that can be significantly improved after surgical correction is patient self-image, while the impact on other domains at long-term follow–up remains unclear. There is a real correlation between patients' expectations and the benefit of surgery, which might favor fusions for moderate curves, mainly for cosmetic reasons.

MIS approach seems also to contribute to a decrease in estimated blood loss [6], probably because of the decreased length of the incision, less extensive soft-tissue dissection and decreased area of subperiosteal exposure. Because of this blood benefit, we now use this splitting approach with one single long skin incision for neuromuscular scoliosis.

LIMITS

Similar to other innovative surgical techniques, our results demonstrate that there is a significant learning curve associated with MIS. This is reflected in the significantly increased overall operative times, blood loss and complications that were seen in the earliest twenty first cases [6] compared with the later cases.

We advise to first improve the experience of the learning surgeon by utilizing MIS technique with one single long skin incision for "easy" AIS curves for example Lenke 1 types, with flexible curve of low magnitude (approx. 50 degrees).

COMPLICATIONS

In our 70 first patients [6] treated with this technique, we reported 11.4% total rate of complications. Early complications rate (4.3%), occurring during the 30 days after surgery, included one subcutaneous hematoma, one deep venous thrombosis and one pulmonary complication. Delayed complications (7.1%) included one superficial wound infection, one suture granuloma and three delayed deep surgical site infections. These three cases needed additional surgery.

Our rate of delayed infection could be attributed to the long operating time due to the learning curve. After the twenty-fifth operated patient, we noticed a clear decrease of the complications rate.

Currently, we have treated more than 130 patients with these technique since June 2014. Our operative time and complications rate are now comparable to those reported with the standard posterior approach.

ADVICES

We insist that everything must be done to reduce the learning curve for a surgeon to treat his patient with this technique. We strongly suggest to start first cases with single (Lenke 1 and Lenke 5) and flexible (more than 50% flexibility index) curves. Moreover, it is better to use a single long skin incision to further diminish operative time. Finally, it is also probably safer to offer this technique to very compliant patients during the beginning of the surgeon experience to minimize the risks due to the learning curve.

REFERENCES

[1] Reames DL, Smith JS, Fu KM, Polly DW, Jr., Ames CP, Berven SH, et al. Complications in the surgical treatment of 19,360 cases of pediatric scoliosis: a review of the Scoliosis Research Society Morbidity and Mortality database. *Spine* (Phila Pa 1976). 2011;36(18):1484-91.

[2] Weinstein S, Dolan LA, Spratt KF, Peterson KK, Spoonamore MJ, Ponseti IV. Health and function of patients with untreated idiopathic scoliosis: a 50-year natural history study. *JAMA*. 2003;289(5):559-67.

[3] Bettany-Saltikov J, Weiss H, Chockalingam N, Taranu R, Srinivas S, Hogg J, et al. Surgical versus non-surgical interventions in people with adolescent idiopathic scoliosis. *Cochrane Database Syst Rev*. 2015;24(4).

[4] Sy N, Bettany-Saltikov J, Moramarco M. Evidence for Conservative Treatment of Adolescent Idiopathic Scoliosis - Update 2015 (Mini-Review). *Curr Pediatr Rev*. 2016;12(1):6-11.

[5] Weinstein SL, Dolan LA, Wright JG, Dobbs MB. Effects of bracing in adolescents with idiopathic scoliosis. *N Engl J Med*. 2013;369(16):1512-21.

[6] de Bodman C, Miyanji F, Borner B, Zambelli PY, Racloz G, Dayer R. Minimally invasive surgery for adolescent idiopathic scoliosis: correction of deformity and perioperative morbidity in 70 consecutive patients. *Bone Joint J.* 2017;99-B(12):1651-7.

[7] Sarwahi V, Wollowick AL, Sugarman EP, Horn JJ, Gambassi M, Amaral TD. Minimally invasive scoliosis surgery: an innovative technique in patients with adolescent idiopathic scoliosis. *Scoliosis.* 2011;6:16.

[8] Sarwahi V, Horn JJ, Kulkarni PM, Wollowick AL, Lo Y, Gambassi M, et al. Minimally Invasive Surgery in Patients with Adolescent Idiopathic Scoliosis: Is it Better than the Standard Approach? A Two Year Follow-Up Study. *Clin Spine Surg.* 2016.

[9] Verma K, Errico T, Diefenbach C, Hoelscher C, Peters A, Dryer J, et al. The relative efficacy of antifibrinolytics in adolescent idiopathic scoliosis. A prospective randomized trial. *J Bone Joint Surg Am.* 2014;96:e80(1-10).

[10] Miyanji F, Samdani A, Ghag A, Marks M, Newton P. Minimally invasive surgery for AIS: en early prospective comparison with standard open surgery. *J Spine.* 2013;001(S5):1-4.

[11] Vialle R, Court C, Khouri N, Olivier E, Miladi L, Tassin JL, et al. Anatomical study of the paraspinal approach to the lumbar spine. *Eur Spine J.* 2005;14(4):366-71.

[12] Wiltse LL. The paraspinal sacrospinalis-splitting approach to the lumbar spine. *Clin Orthop Relat Res.* 1973(91):48-57.

[13] Wiltse LL, Bateman JG, Hutchinson RH, Nelson WE. The paraspinal sacrospinalis-splitting approach to the lumbar spine. *The Journal of bone and joint surgery.* 1968;50(5):919-26.

[14] Kim YJ, Lenke LG, Bridwell KH, Cho YS, Riew KD. Free hand pedicle screw placement in the thoracic spine: is it safe? *Spine.* 2004;29(3):333-42.

[15] Sarwahi V, Horn JJ, Kulkarni PM, Wollowick AL, Lo Y, Gambassi M, et al. Minimally Invasive Surgery in Patients with Adolescent Idiopathic Scoliosis: Is it Better than the Standard Approach? A Two Year Follow-Up Study. *Clin Spine Surg* 2016;29(8):331-40.

[16] Miyanji F, Samdani A, Ghag A, Marks M, Newton PO. Minimally Invasive Surgery for AIS: An Early Prospective Comparison with Standard Open Posterior Surgery. *Journal of Spine.* 2013;S5:001.

[17] Blam OG, Vaccaro AR, Vanichkachorn JS, Albert TJ, Hilibrand AS, Minnich JM, et al. Risk factors for surgical site infection in the patient with spinal injury. *Spine* (Phila Pa 1976). 2003;28(13):1475-80.

[18] Mackenzie WG, Matsumoto H, Williams BA, Corona J, Lee C, Cody SR, et al. Surgical site infection following spinal instrumentation for scoliosis: a multicenter analysis of rates, risk factors, and pathogens. *J Bone Joint Surg Am.* 2013;95(9):800-6, S1-2.

[19] Erickson MA, Morrato E, Campagna E, Elise B, Miller N, Kempe a. Variability in spinal surgery outcomes among children's hospitals in the United States. *J Pediatr Orthop.* 2013;33(1):80-90.

[20] Yoshihara H, Yoneoka D. National trends in spinal fusion for pediatric patients with idiopathic scoliosis: demographics, blood transfusions, and in-hospital outcomes. *Spine* (Phila Pa 1976). 2014;39(14):1144-50.

[21] Kawaguchi Y, Matsui H, Tsuji H. Back muscle injury after posterior lumbar spine surgery. Part 2: Histologic and histochemical analysis in humans. *Spine* (Phila Pa 1976). 1994;19(22):2590-7.

[22] Kim DY, Lee SH, Chung SK, Lee HY. Comparison of multifidus muscle atrophy and trunk extension muscle strength: percutaneous versus open pedicle screw fixation. *Spine* (Phila Pa 1976). 2005;30(1):123-9.

In: Scoliosis: Diagnosis, Classification and Management Options   ISBN: 978-1-53614-464-2
Editors: F. Canavese, A. Andreacchio and H. Xu   © 2018 Nova Science Publishers, Inc.

Chapter 17

PRE- AND POSTOPERATIVE SAGITTAL ALIGNMENT IN PATIENTS WITH ADOLESCENT IDIOPATHIC SCOLIOSIS

Mehmet Çetinkaya[1], MD, Ali Eren[2], MD and Alpaslan Senkoylu[3],*, MD

[1]Erzincan University Mengucek Gazi Training and Research Hospital, Department of Orthopaedics and Traumatology, Erzincan, Turkey
[2]Gümüşhane Kelkit Devlet Hastanesi, Gümüşhane, Turkey
[3]Gazi University School of Medicine, Department of Orthopaedics and Traumatology, Besevler, Ankara, Turkey

ABSTRACT

The goal of the surgical treatment of adolescent idiopathic scoliosis (AIS) should be a stable construct that protects the deformity correction in all sagittal, coronal and axial planes until achieving the solid fusion. A balanced posture is needed to minimize the energy expenditure during the mobilization of the patient, which diminishes when the pelvis and the spine are misaligned. Considerable number studies have been undertaken to understand the normal anatomy of the global sagittal alignment of which the sound knowledge is one of the key points when evaluating the patients and deciding to surgery. Moreover, numerous studies have shown that the appropriate correction of the scoliotic deformity is substantial with minimal loss of correction at mid and long-term follow-ups that results in significant improvement in the quality of life for the patient and maintaining the satisfaction of both the patient and parents, which entails correcting the deformity in all three planes. Therefore, in addition to the coronal balance, the sagittal alignment of the thoracolumbar and cervical spine and the spinopelvic sagittal parameters should be carefully assessed in patients with AIS undergoing surgery.

Keywords: adolescent idiopathic scoliosis, sagittal alignment, spinopelvic parameters, surgery

---

* Corresponding Author Email: drsenkoylu@gmail.com.

1. INTRODUCTION

The goal of the surgical treatment of adolescent idiopathic scoliosis (AIS) should be to constitute a stable construct that protects the deformity correction in all sagittal, coronal and axial planes until achieving the solid fusion [1]. Numerous studies have shown that the appropriate correction of the scoliotic deformity is substantial with minimal loss of correction at mid and long-term follow-ups which results in significant improvement in the quality of life of the patient and satisfaction of both the patient and his/her parents. However, this could be succeeded only by correcting the deformity thoroughly in all three planes [2-5]. Therefore, in addition to the coronal balance, the interest in the sagittal alignment of the thoracolumbar and cervical spine and the spinopelvic sagittal parameters of the patients with AIS is growing every day [6].

2. GLOBAL SAGITTAL BALANCE IN ADOLESCENT IDIOPATHIC SCOLIOSIS

A balanced posture is needed to minimize the energy expenditure during the mobilization of the patient. However, it deteriorates when the pelvis and the spine are misaligned. Recently, considerable efforts have been undertaken to understand the normal anatomy of the global sagittal alignment of which the sound knowledge is one of the key points when evaluating the patients and deciding to surgery.

AIS patients typically have relative lordosis of the thoracic spine additional to the coronal deformity which should be addressed intra-operatively. Therefore, the primary purpose of the surgery should be to achieve a balanced spine in all three planes [7]. The flattened sagittal contours are accompanied by the abnormal spinopelvic balance and abnormal pelvic morphology which are common in AIS [8]. Besides the thoracic, lumbar, and the spinopelvic region, despite being neglected by most studies, several authors have already pointed out the changes also in cervical lordosis (CL) [1, 9, 10].

The global sagittal balance is widely believed to be constituted by the harmony of the curves of the spine. However, there are also authors who believe that the thoracic kyphosis (TK) and lumbar lordosis in AIS patients do not influence each other in contrast with the normal adults. According to an opinion, since the TK is mostly in the normal ranges for scoliotic curves (other than thoracic ones), it can be assumed that the TK is affected mainly by the distorted shape and orientation of the discs and vertebrae in AIS with thoracic curves [11]. This study also commented that the absence of a significant relationship between the TK and the LL, except for the thoracolumbar curves, further supports this hypothesis. Vedantam et al. also found no correlation between TK and LL in adolescents without spinal pathology while a significant relationship was found in adults [12]. However, the vast majority of the studies in the literature confirm this significant correlation between TK and LL for both normal adults and scoliotic patients. Therefore, the influence of the spinal deformity on the TK and a potential correlation between TK and LL must be considered in all efforts to reconstitute the normal standing sagittal posture in dealing with the growing spine of adolescents [11].

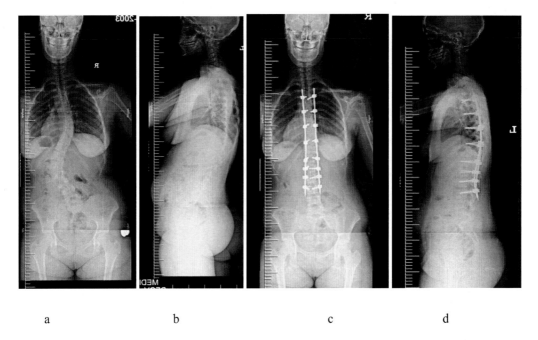

a   b   c   d

Figure 1. A 12-year-old girl with Lenke Type 6C curve (a). Preoperative lateral x-ray examination (b) shows a thoracolumbar junctional kyphosis which compensated by thoracic hypokyphosis. Both main thoracic and thoracolumbar curves were included in fusion, thoracic kyphosis restored and the sagittal alignment was corrected. X-ray examinations revealed that the correction was still maintained at the postoperative 24-month follow-up (c, d).

The normal ranges of the TK have also yet to be elucidated, and the clinically significant and relevant highest and lowest thresholds should be determined. The Lenke classification assumes the TK between 10-40° as normal while some others consider 10-20° as mild hypokyphosis [13, 14]. Another debate in normal sagittal alignment is the unknown effects of the postoperative hypokyphosis in the long-term follow-ups according to the patient-reported outcomes. Ohrt-Nissen et al. commented that the postoperative hypokyphosis is unlikely to affect the patients' quality of life at early and mid-term follow-ups since the AIS patients exhibit a range of compensatory mechanism and rarely become decompensated [8, 10, 15, 16]. However, it was shown by several studies that an optimal sagittal profile is essential to avoid pain and disability in adult patients [17, 18] (Figure 1).

3. SPINOPELVIC ALIGNMENT AND LENKE 5 CURVES IN ADOLESCENT IDIOPATHIC SCOLIOSIS

The Lenke 5 curves have special characteristics of spinopelvic morphology and should be evaluated more carefully than the isolated thoracic curves. There are a couple of studies giving point to these patients and investigating the characteristics of Lenke 5 curves. We found that the anterior instrumentation and spinal fusion as a good treatment of choice in order to maintain lumbar lordosis. However, Cobb's angle measurement might be decreased in mid-term due to graft resorption and disc settlement [19-21]. Yang et al. stated that they found a special sagittal profile related to a horizontal sacrum [22]. Roussouly et al. classified the PT as following;

anteverted, normal, and retroverted with regard to the PT angle ranges [23]. They considered the pelvis as anteverted when PT is less than 20% of PI/2, normal between 20% of PI/2 and 80% of PI/2, and retroverted over 80% of PI/2. According to this classification, almost half of the patients in the study of Yang et al. were found to have an anteverted pelvis, but none of them revealed a retroverted one. They added that the PT was relatively lower than the normal population (regarding their PI) which results in more horizontally aligned sacrum. They also found that the significantly related factors of low PT measurements were lowest instrumented vertebra (LEV) and PI. The rate of the anteverted pelvis was 31% in patients with LEV at L3 while it was 67% in those with LEV at L5.

A retroverted pelvis is assumed to be a compensation mechanism of an anteriorly displaced gravity axis [24, 25]. Similarly, anteriorly shifted pelvic tilt in the Lenke 5 patients should be the same mechanism to compensate their posteriorly shifted gravity axis. The rotational component of these thoracolumbar/lumbar (TL/L) curves results in rotated vertebrae above the curve that brings out the reduction of the segmental LL (upper LL ↓) [11, 24, 26]. This phenomenon is believed to be the reason for working compensatory mechanism by tilting anteriorly to compensate the posteriorly shifted center of gravity. Since the SS cannot be a negative number, the PI plays a role as a determinator for the capacity of the compensation potential by pelvic anterior or posterior tilt [27, 28]. A secondary compensatory mechanism is the increased lower lumbar segment lordosis (lower LL ↑) associated with the anterior tilt of the pelvis (SS ↑ , PT ↓) [22]. In addition to the reduced PT, the reduced lumbar flexibility because of the lumbar vertebrae involved in the lumbar curve is the second reason for the limited compensatory potential for the posteriorly shifted gravity axis [22]. Following the corrective surgery, the sagittal spinopelvic alignment changes obviously by manifesting adjustment in LL (upper LL ↑ , lower LL ↓) and the increase in PT. In the study of Yang et al. the mean increase in PT was 6.3° with a consequent decrease in SS, which was in agreement with the literature [11, 22, 23]. They reported that 61% of the patients with anteverted pelvis had been corrected to normal pelvis tilt after surgery and suggested that surgeons should pay attention to increase the upper LL and decrease the lower LL by pre-bending the rods to revert the pelvic ante-version in Lenke 5 curves.

Yang et al. found that the critical point of the PI may be 39° (median of patients' PI values) for being able to correct the anteverted pelvis [22]. The pelvic ante-version generally develops in patients with very low PI, and it would be very hard to correct in those with much lower PI. They also found that although patients with a preoperative anteverted pelvis had a smaller pre- and postoperative PI than those with the normal pelvis, they had larger LL and a larger lower LL after the surgery. The importance of a larger LL, especially the lower LL, is that it makes difficult to correct an anteverted pelvis. Therefore, the key point to provide a normal pelvis alignment is to adjust the LL in accordance with the PI.

The pelvic morphology measured by the pelvic incidence (PI) angle tends to increase from childhood to adolescence before stabilizing in the adulthood. It is most likely to maintain an adequate sagittal balance in view of the physiologic and morphologic changes developing during the growth [29].

The PI angle is the most widely used parameter giving information about the sacropelvic orientation, and it is calculated by summing the pelvic tilt (PT) angle and the sacral slope (SS). The higher the PI angle, the greater the ability of pelvic compensation of the sagittal imbalance. Ohrt-Nissen et al. concluded that adolescents affected by scoliosis are more or less in an ideal condition of PT which means they do not have enough compensatory potential that can be gained with surgery [8].

The choice of LIV was another critical factor related to an unimproved postoperative pelvic sagittal alignment in the study of Yang et al. [22]. They stated that the rate of recovery of the anteverted pelvis was 100% when the LIV was L3 and 25% when the LIV was L5. According to these results, it was the most difficult condition to be recovered when the fusion level was extended to L5. This can be explained by the loss of compensatory potential of the uninstrumented LL below the LL within fusion [30-32].

The sagittal alignment of the thoracolumbar region is related to the sagittal alignment of the pelvis, which differs individually [33, 34]. A small pelvic incidence comes with a small lumbar lordosis and flat back while a large pelvic incidence comes with large lumbar lordosis and thoracic kyphosis [35]. Somewhat postural compensation can be achieved depending on the spinopelvic configuration once the thoracolumbar imbalance has developed. Compensation mechanism has been described previously and involve the pelvic retroversion and knee flexion as key factors when analyzing the anterior imbalance. This misalignment can be recognized by an increased pelvic tilt, which is correlated with the sacral vertical axis (SVA), PI, and LL [17, 36, 37].

4. CERVICAL SAGITTAL ALIGNMENT IN ADOLESCENT IDIOPATHIC SCOLIOSIS

The impact of sagittal alignment on long-term outcomes of instrumented and mobile segments and the impact of sagittal thoracolumbar alignment on health-related quality of life in patients with scoliosis who underwent deformity correction have been shown previously [33, 38-40]. Understanding the characteristics of the deformity from occiput to coccyx is crucial to improve the surgical treatment and short and long-term follow-up outcomes and to correct not only the coronal deformity, also the axial and sagittal deformities. As a result of this requirement, the influence of the main deformity on the thoracolumbar region, cervical region, and the spinopelvic region is investigated by a few studies [6, 41, 42]. However, most authors do not differentiate between radiographic cervical morphologies (lordotic, straight, kyphotic, sigmoid-shaped) before surgery [43, 44], which may be secondary to thoracolumbar deformity and adaptive changes [34].

New studies are now focusing on the change in cervical sagittal alignment (CSA) following the surgery [45-48]. Several studies have found a strong correlation between the TK and the CSA [42, 49]. We have found by a retrospective study that less cervical kyphosis was seen in Lenke 5 and 6, and greater cervical kyphosis in Lenke 1, 2 and 3 curves (50). Nevertheless, this was a sort of compensation of thoracic alignment postoperatively, and this compensation mechanism has obviously neutralized the global sagittal alignment [47, 51]. Another study found the correlation between the CSA and T2 sagittal tilt [45]. There are some studies emphasizing the importance and the effect of CSA on health-related quality of life (HRQOL) in patients with spinal deformity, particularly in adults [52-54]. However, there is no consensus among authors yet in threshold values of CL angles for operated patients with AIS. Some studies suggested that patients with CL of 20° or lower are more susceptible to cervical disorders and pain. If the CL is lower than 0°, the cervical disorders becomes more severe [55].

These patients are also pronounced to have a significantly higher frequency of progression in age-related cervical spine degeneration at the long-term follow-up.

Although a clear relationship between CL and TK does not still exist, appropriate thoracic sagittal alignment, which leads to also an improvement in CL [6, 41], seems crucial for satisfactory outcomes postoperatively [56, 57]. The cervical realignment following the kyphosis restoration was previously described very well [6, 41, 42, 58], and Charles et al. classified the cervical lordosis shape in 5 types; Type 1: C2–C6 lordosis ≤ − 20°, Type 2: C2–C6 lordosis between −19° and 0° appearing as straight cervical spine, Type 3: C2–C6 lordosis more than 0° appearing as kyphotic cervical spine, Type 4: Sigmoid-shaped cervical spine with cranial lordosis and caudal kyphosis, and Type 5: Sigmoid-shaped cervical spine with cranial kyphosis and caudal lordosis [34]. The alignment of the cervical region is analyzed with the following parameters; C0-C2 and C2-C6 lordosis, T1 slope, chin-brow vertical angle (CBVA), C2 and C7 plumb lines [42, 44, 59, 60] (Figure 2). Charles et al. stated that the cervical alignment is likely to result from the extent of the cranial thoracic kyphosis in sigmoid types and that the adaptive changes occur at C7 and C2 by anterior-posterior shifts adjacent to the instrumented thoracolumbar spine [38]. However, the C2 and C7 plumb lines should also be considered in adjusting the sagittal balance when planning surgery for scoliosis. The Δ sagittal vertical axis of C2 and C7 is reported to be ranging between 10 and 17 mm [59-61], and the C7 plump line reported to move usually backward from childhood to adulthood where it stabilizes and may move forward following the degenerative changes with older ages [29].

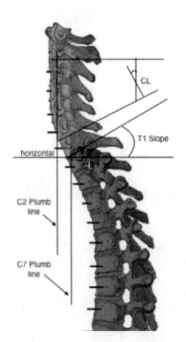 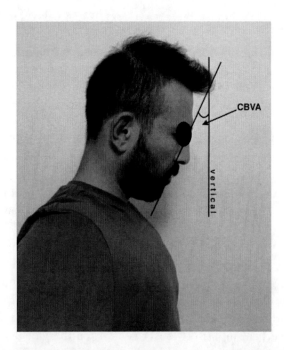

Figure 2. The demonstration of the cervical lordosis angle, T1 slope angle, C2 plumb line, C7 plumb line (A), and chin-brow vertical line angle (B). CL: Cervical lordosis, CBVA: Chin-brow vertical angle.

The normal average values of CL for normal adults are reported between -6° to -22°, which is usually measured between C2-C6 or C2-C7, and the lordosis is reported to increase with age [59, 60, 62]. Secondary to scoliosis, vertebral rotation and anterior and lateral translation of thoracic vertebrae result in hypokyphosis, and it is known that TK and CL are related to each other in AIS [6, 41, 42]. Hilibrand et al. found that 89% of 38 patients had a lordosis more than -5° with an average of 6°. Hwang et al. found that 38 of 16 patients had kyphosis of 13°. Canavese et al. found an average kyphosis of 4° and average lordosis more than -20° in 84% of 32 patients. Ilharreborde et al. found that 79% of 49 patients presented an average kyphosis of 11.2° which was correlated with thoracic kyphosis angle less than 20° [6, 41, 42, 58].

The sagittal alignment of the cervicothoracic junction also changes with the deformity correction in the thoracic region in a similar manner with the lumbopelvic region and includes modification of the head position and cervical alignment. It is another key point for cervical alignment which is neglected by most authors while evaluating the cervical and thoracic sagittal profile [34]. An increased T1 slope may trigger increased CL which is a compensatory mechanism of the cervical region to position the head for sustaining horizontal gaze [59, 61-63]. The T1 sagittal inclination is further related to thoracic kyphosis, which may influence each other [43, 63]. One of the most devastating results of scoliosis deformity correction surgery is the proximal junctional kyphosis (PJK), of which prevalence is reported to be as high as 27% in the literature [64, 65]. An increased T1-T4 kyphosis was reported to be correlated with a compensatory increased T1 slope and C2-T1 lordosis, however, the PJK was fortunately not linked to specific sagittal alignment types pre- and postoperatively [34]. In the light of the aforementioned data, the question is that how much slope angle should the surgeon aim for the T1 vertebra during the surgery for a desired cervical sagittal alignment. Instead of using the T1 slope angle as a guide, Yagi et al. suggested the T2 sagittal tilt and stated that the T2 tilt suggested a strong positive association with CL. They also reported that CL was closely related to the global sagittal balance rather than the TK according to the finding of the importance of the T2 sagittal tilt [45]. Nevertheless, despite the significant increase of cervical lordosis with all efforts of the surgeons, Yagi et al. stated that 85% of their patients still had a kyphotic or less lordotic cervical spine after the corrective surgery.

The relationship between the LL and CL represents a more complicated issue to interpret than the relationship between TK and CL. According to the study by Roussouly et al, CL improved and correlated with the amount of gained LL [66]. This study also commented that an increase of lordosis within the instrumented lumbar segments could improve cervical lordosis, however, thoracic correction and the cranial extent of the instrumentation additionally influence the cervical alignment.

Although the sagittal balance should be evaluated globally from occiput to coccyx, the TK and LL are usually compensated by each other, whereas when the thoracic and lumbar region are both instrumented, the compensation mechanisms in the cervical and spinopelvic regions become more significant which was mentioned previously by Yang et al. [67]. Another debate about the cervical realignment following the correction of the scoliosis is whether the UIV influence on the CSA. Yanik et al. reported that the UIV did not affect the CSA in their study including 55 patients with Lenke 3C or 6C deformity [51]. They attributed the decreased CL mainly to the decrease in T5-T12 kyphosis and T1 slope angle, therefore they recommended extending the fusion to the appropriate upper level to avoid the risk of cervical kyphosis.

Charles et al. stated that proximal thoracic kyphosis was one of the factors influencing the CL [34]. However, it was the decrease in T5-T12 kyphosis that caused loss of CL according to the study of Yanik et al. [51]. They also concluded that T1-T5 kyphosis did not change significantly after the surgery. Because of the hypokyphotic effect of pedicle screws on the thoracic area, the patients with cervical kyphosis remained kyphotic in the cervical region also postoperatively, and some of the patients without cervical kyphosis also developed kyphosis in the cervical region after the surgery in their study. They also stated that the more the coronal deformity was corrected, the more hypokyphosis developed in the thoracic region. Therefore, one has to decide between correcting the coronal deformity better which is the main deformity seen by the patient when he/she looks at himself/herself in the mirror and leaving some degree of coronal deformity, thus aligning the spine in normal ranges in the sagittal plane.

The relationship between the thoracolumbar and cervical alignment still less understood, and it may have a clinical impact on functional outcomes which is not evidenced yet [34]. The influence of thoracic curves leading to hypokyphosis on cervical alignment has been emphasized before [68, 69]. The cervical lordosis (CL) is said to decrease and lead to straight, kyphotic, or sigmoid cervical shapes subsequently [70].

5. PEDICLE SCREW CONSTRUCTS AND SAGITTAL BALANCE IN ADOLESCENT IDIOPATHIC SCOLIOSIS

A recent meta-analysis showed that the PS constructs had less power in maintaining the normal TK than the hook-and-wire constructs and underlined the hypokyphotic effects of pedicle screws [3, 71, 72]. It is also known that reverting a smaller preoperative TK to normal ranges is very difficult with traditional pedicle screw constructs [29]. The major factor that affects restoring the sagittal profile has been suggested to be the insertion and appropriately contouring of the rods. Additionally, it is widely believed that increasing the strength of the rod can reduce intraoperative flattening, thus can ensure retention of the shape of the pre-contoured rod [73, 74]. However, Prince et al. found no evidence in their study, in which they reviewed more than 1100 patients, supporting the opinion that increasing the rod strength improves TK [75]. Monazzam et al. also emphasized the same findings and added that the restoration of normal TK is primarily ensured by surgical technique [14].

Subsequently, PS constructs were developed to restore better alignment and to correct the deformity further for more satisfactory outcomes for the patients and their parents. In a study made by Ohrt-Nissen et al. modified, hybrid, and standard PS constructs were compared to each other. They found that the standard constructs were not sufficient as the modified and hybrid constructs in achieving the restoration of normal sagittal alignment [8]. There was only 1 patient with hypokyphosis postoperatively out of 69 modified and hybrid constructs while there were 12 patients of those out of 70 standard constructs. Furthermore, modified and hybrid constructs corrected not only the hypokyphosis but also the hyperkyphosis of the patients. Ohrt-Nissen et al. also stated that increased rigidity of the rods may have a negative effect on the sagittal profile as it can be technically challenging to achieve sufficient kyphosis of the rod while ensuring correct rod insertion and at the same time correcting the coronal deformity. In another study using a computerized model and supporting this study, it was showed that the use of rods with a small-diameter transition at the most cranial level results in decreased stress at the proximal junction, and it was added that this may have an effect on the sagittal profile in a clinical setting [76].

Other points of issue are the screw density and its hypokyphotic effects. There has been no high evidence supporting this hypothesis in the literature yet [3, 71, 72, 77-79]. However, low-density constructs seem to be effective enough for restoring alignment in all three planes (Figure 3).

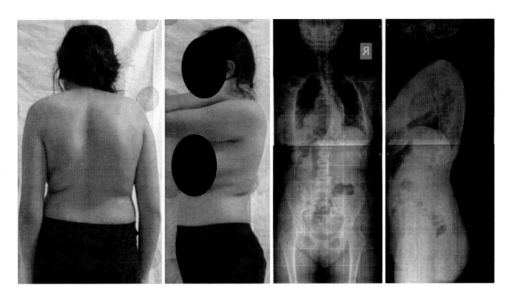

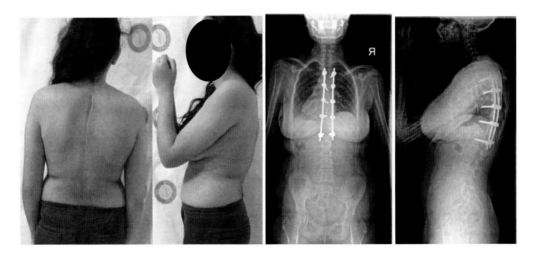

Figure 3. A 13-year-old girl suffered from AIS classified as Lenke Type-1A. Selective thoracic fusion was done with a low-intensity pedicle screw construct. Postoperative one-year follow-up x-rays revealed a very good deformity correction and its maintenance with low screw density strategy.

Today, the desired constructions are being mostly achieved through a posterior-only approach with pedicle screws (PS). However, several studies stated that PS constructs are not efficient enough in restoring the thoracic sagittal profile to a normal range [3, 71, 72]. Legarreta et al. apparently emphasized that independent of the used surgical technique for correction, the cervical spine had a tendency to decompensate and acquire a kyphotic profile. They also added that the constructs based on pedicle screws have rather stronger hypokyphotic effects on the thoracic spine, especially in cases with the upper instrumented vertebra (UIV) above the T4 level [10]. Tao et al. reported that anterior solid screw instrumentation resulted in shorter fusion segments while providing better sagittal alignment and quality of life when compared to posterior pedicle screw instrumentation in patients with Lenke 5 AIS, however, he also added that there is no data showing pre- or postoperative difference in lumbar lordosis has the ability to improve quality of life [80]. According to the study of Pesenti et al, the subliminal bands were even efficient for both coronal and sagittal plane deformity correction [81]. They also concluded that the restoration of the normal thoracic kyphosis was followed by an adaptation of the adjacent curvatures with improved cervical lordosis and lumbar lordosis.

6. STF VERSUS NSTF IN ADOLESCENT IDIOPATHIC SCOLIOSIS

One debate in the sagittal deformity may be the differences between the selective thoracic fusion (STF) and non-selective thoracic fusion (NSTF) for Lenke 1 curves. A study by Celestre et al. has explained this question very well already [82]. They reported in their study with Lenke 1C curves that, as reported previously in the literature, the residual thoracolumbar/lumbar scoliosis was less in the NSTF group and more lumbar motion segments can be preserved with STF which may be associated with increased thoracic and thoracolumbar kyphosis compared to NSTF. They commented that the thoracolumbar kyphosis may be compensated with the pelvic sagittal realignment, however, thoracic kyphosis cannot be realigned since this region is involved in the fusion. This can be beneficial for these AIS patients by avoiding hypokyphotic alignment of the thoracic region and hypokyphotic effects of pedicle screws. Another risk of NSTF for sagittal balance is the instrumentation of the lumbar region, thus preventing the compensatory mechanisms of the lumbar region to constitute the new sagittal balance following the instrumentation of the thoracic region. If the LL is overcorrected with NSTF, posterior shift of the fusion mass and expose to junctional syndromes and poor functional outcomes in this particular patients may develop [83].

7. THE HEREDITARY IN KYPHOSIS COMPONENT OF ADOLESCENT IDIOPATHIC SCOLIOSIS

The hereditary in the sagittal spinal profile of scoliotic children was also investigated. Janssen et al. reported that the fathers of those children were also found to have significantly flatter sagittal spinal profile than the fathers of non-scoliotic children [84]. Although it is widely known that scoliotic mothers have an increased risk of having a scoliotic child, Janssen et al. showed that the sagittal component of the children's scoliotic deformity come from their fathers.

The sagittal profile of the patients may change between races. Long et al. have already shown that the race may influence an individual's spinopelvic morphology and added that the evaluation of the thoracolumbar sagittal morphology of a patient with AIS is crucial for surgical planning to provide a normal sagittal balance postoperatively [85]. Actually, the sagittal profile may change between each individual, therefore, postoperative sagittal characteristics should be adjusted following a detailed evaluation of the patient's global sagittal profile.

When a patient with AIS has a thoracic hyperkyphosis instead of hypokyphosis, a neural axis abnormality should be sought elaborately. Lee et al. found in their magnetic resonance imaging study with 378 consecutive AIS patients that thoracic hyperkyphosis was significantly associated with neural axis abnormalities [86]. Several other studies also reported similar findings in their studies [87-91]. Furthermore, Davids et al. reported that patients with presumed AIS have lesions in the central nervous system when the sagittal thoracic alignment is >20° of kyphosis [89].

CONCLUSION

Despite the increase in focus on sagittal alignment in patients with AIS, the clinical significance of the thoracic hypokyphosis is still unclear and has yet to be dissolved. The clarification of the unknown points of the sagittal characteristics of AIS needs to provide and start from sound mainstays. Therefore, the authors struggled to exhibit the changes in curvatures with the correction of AIS deformity to prevent undesired sagittal balance postoperatively. However, to understand and interpret these unknown data, the normal parameters of the sagittal alignment are required to be clarified. However, even the normal thoracic kyphosis has no consensus among authors. Lenke et al. explained the hypokyphosis as <10° while Monazzam et al. as <20° [13, 14]. Moreover, whether the sagittal alignment after the surgery is important in the short-term and long-term follow-ups, whether it influences the durability of the instruments, how much thoracic kyphosis should be provided, or whether the gained normal kyphosis with surgery provides better clinical outcomes have remained unclear. Besides, whether the focus increasing toward sagittal balance is relevant or not is not discussed by the authors yet. Nevertheless, despite all these unknowns, it seems that authors should constitute the normal spinal curvatures if possible until the spine masters found new evidence-based data explaining what to do.

REFERENCES

[1] de Kleuver M, Lewis SJ, Germscheid NM, Kamper SJ, Alanay A, Berven SH et al. Optimal surgical care for adolescent idiopathic scoliosis: an international consensus. *Eur Spine J* 2014; 23:2603-18.

[2] Haher TR, Gorup JM, Shin TM, Homel P, Merola AA, Grogan DP et al. Results of the Scoliosis Research Society instrument for evaluation of surgical outcome in adolescent idiopathic scoliosis. A multicenter study of 244 patients. *Spine (Phila Pa 1976)* 1999; 24:1435-40.

[3] Rushton PR, Grevitt MP. What is the effect of surgery on the quality of life of the adolescent with adolescent idiopathic scoliosis? A review and statistical analysis of the literature. *Spine (Phila Pa 1976)* 2013; 38:786-94.

[4] Ghandehari H, Mahabadi MA, Mahdavi SM, Shahsavaripour A, Seyed Tari HV, Safdari F. Evaluation of Patient Outcome and Satisfaction after Surgical Treatment of Adolescent Idiopathic Scoliosis Using Scoliosis Research Society-30. *Arch Bone Jt Surg* 2015; 3:109-13.

[5] Ng BK, Chau WW, Hui CN, Cheng PY, Wong CY, Wang B et al. HRQoL assessment by SRS-30 for Chinese patients with surgery for Adolescent Idiopathic Scoliosis (AIS). *Scoliosis* 2015; 10:S19.

[6] Ilharreborde B, Vidal C, Skalli W, Mazda K. Sagittal alignment of the cervical spine in adolescent idiopathic scoliosis treated by posteromedial translation. *Eur Spine J* 2013; 22:330-7.

[7] Newton PO, Fujimori T, Doan J, Reighard FG, Bastrom TP, Misaghi A. Defining the "Three-Dimensional Sagittal Plane" in Thoracic Adolescent Idiopathic Scoliosis. *J Bone Joint Surg Am* 2015; 97:1694-701.

[8] Ohrt-Nissen S, Dragsted C, Dahl B, Ferguson JAI, Gehrchen M. Improved restoration of thoracic kyphosis using a rod construct with differentiated rigidity in the surgical treatment of adolescent idiopathic scoliosis. *Neurosurg Focus* 2017; 43:E6.

[9] Crawford AH, Lykissas MG, Gao X, Eismann E, Anadio J. All-pedicle screw versus hybrid instrumentation in adolescent idiopathic scoliosis surgery: a comparative radiographical study with a minimum 2-Year follow-up. *Spine (Phila Pa 1976)* 2013; 38:1199-208.

[10] Legarreta CA, Barrios C, Rositto GE, Reviriego JM, Maruenda JI, Escalada MN et al. Cervical and thoracic sagittal misalignment after surgery for adolescent idiopathic scoliosis: a comparative study of all pedicle screws versus hybrid instrumentation. *Spine (Phila Pa 1976)* 2014; 39:1330-7.

[11] La Maida GA, Zottarelli L, Mineo GV, Misaggi B. Sagittal balance in adolescent idiopathic scoliosis: radiographic study of spino-pelvic compensation after surgery. *Eur Spine J* 2013; 22 Suppl 6:S859-67.

[12] Vedantam R, Lenke LG, Keeney JA, Bridwell KH. Comparison of standing sagittal spinal alignment in asymptomatic adolescents and adults. *Spine (Phila Pa 1976)* 1998; 23:211-5.

[13] Lenke LG, Betz RR, Harms J, Bridwell KH, Clements DH, Lowe TG et al. Adolescent idiopathic scoliosis: a new classification to determine extent of spinal arthrodesis. *J Bone Joint Surg Am* 2001; 83-A:1169-81.

[14] Monazzam S, Newton PO, Bastrom TP, Yaszay B, Harms Study G. Multicenter Comparison of the Factors Important in Restoring Thoracic Kyphosis During Posterior Instrumentation for Adolescent Idiopathic Scoliosis. *Spine Deform* 2013; 1:359-64.

[15] Arlet V, Ouellet JA, Shilt J, Shen FH, Wood K, Chan D et al. Subjective evaluation of treatment outcomes of instrumentation with pedicle screws or hybrid constructs in Lenke Type 1 and 2 adolescent idiopathic scoliosis: what happens when judges are blinded to the instrumentation? *Eur Spine J* 2009; 18:1927-35.

[16] Bennett JT, Hoashi JS, Ames RJ, Kimball JS, Pahys JM, Samdani AF. The posterior pedicle screw construct: 5-year results for thoracolumbar and lumbar curves. *J Neurosurg Spine* 2013; 19:658-63.

[17] Roussouly P, Nnadi C. Sagittal plane deformity: an overview of interpretation and management. *Eur Spine J* 2010; 19:1824-36.

[18] Hallager DW, Hansen LV, Dragsted CR, Peytz N, Gehrchen M, Dahl B. A Comprehensive Analysis of the SRS-Schwab Adult Spinal Deformity Classification and Confounding Variables: A Prospective, Non-US Cross-sectional Study in 292 Patients. *Spine (Phila Pa 1976)* 2016; 41:E589-97.

[19] Le Huec JC, Lesprit E, Delavigne C, Clement D, Chauveaux D, Le Rebeller A. Tricalcium phosphate ceramics and allografts as bone substitutes for spinal fusion in idiopathic scoliosis as bone substitutes for spinal fusion in idiopathic scoliosis: comparative clinical results at four years. *Acta Orthop Belg* 1997; 63:202-11.

[20] Senkoylu A, Luk KD, Wong YW, Cheung KM. Prognosis of spontaneous thoracic curve correction after the selective anterior fusion of thoracolumbar/lumbar (Lenke 5C) curves in idiopathic scoliosis. *Spine J* 2014; 14:1117-24.

[21] Zhang Y, Lin G, Zhang J, Guo J, Wang S, Yang Y et al. Radiographic evaluation of posterior selective thoracolumbar or lumbar fusion for moderate Lenke 5C curves. *Arch Orthop Trauma Surg* 2017; 137:1-8.

[22] Yang X, Liu L, Song Y, Zhou C, Zhou Z, Wang L et al. Pre- and postoperative spinopelvic sagittal balance in adolescent patients with lenke type 5 idiopathic scoliosis. *Spine (Phila Pa 1976)* 2015; 40:102-8.

[23] Roussouly P, Labelle H, Rouissi J, Bodin A. Pre- and post-operative sagittal balance in idiopathic scoliosis: a comparison over the ages of two cohorts of 132 adolescents and 52 adults. *Eur Spine J* 2013; 22 Suppl 2:S203-15.

[24] Hong JY, Suh SW, Modi HN, Hur CY, Yang JH, Song HR. Correlation of pelvic orientation with adult scoliosis. *J Spinal Disord Tech* 2010; 23:461-6.

[25] Schuller S, Charles YP, Steib JP. Sagittal spinopelvic alignment and body mass index in patients with degenerative spondylolisthesis. *Eur Spine J* 2011; 20:713-9.

[26] Clement JL, Geoffray A, Yagoubi F, Chau E, Solla F, Oborocianu I et al. Relationship between thoracic hypokyphosis, lumbar lordosis and sagittal pelvic parameters in adolescent idiopathic scoliosis. *Eur Spine J* 2013; 22:2414-20.

[27] Barrey C, Jund J, Noseda O, Roussouly P. Sagittal balance of the pelvis-spine complex and lumbar degenerative diseases. A comparative study about 85 cases. *Eur Spine J* 2007; 16:1459-67.

[28] Barrey C, Roussouly P, Le Huec JC, D'Acunzi G, Perrin G. Compensatory mechanisms contributing to keep the sagittal balance of the spine. *Eur Spine J* 2013; 22 Suppl 6:S834-41.

[29] Fletcher ND, Hopkins J, McClung A, Browne R, Sucato DJ. Residual thoracic hypokyphosis after posterior spinal fusion and instrumentation in adolescent idiopathic scoliosis: risk factors and clinical ramifications. *Spine (Phila Pa 1976)* 2012; 37:200-6.

[30] Ghiselli G, Wang JC, Hsu WK, Dawson EG. L5-S1 segment survivorship and clinical outcome analysis after L4-L5 isolated fusion. *Spine (Phila Pa 1976)* 2003; 28:1275-80; discussion 80.

[31] Rinella A, Bridwell K, Kim Y, Rudzki J, Edwards C, Roh M et al. Late complications of adult idiopathic scoliosis primary fusions to L4 and above: the effect of age and distal fusion level. *Spine (Phila Pa 1976)* 2004; 29:318-25.

[32] Tanguay F, Mac-Thiong JM, de Guise JA, Labelle H. Relation between the sagittal pelvic and lumbar spine geometries following surgical correction of adolescent idiopathic scoliosis. *Eur Spine J* 2007; 16:531-6.

[33] Schwab FJ, Blondel B, Bess S, Hostin R, Shaffrey CI, Smith JS et al. Radiographical spinopelvic parameters and disability in the setting of adult spinal deformity: a prospective multicenter analysis. *Spine (Phila Pa 1976)* 2013; 38:E803-12.

[34] Charles YP, Sfeir G, Matter-Parrat V, Sauleau EA, Steib JP. Cervical sagittal alignment in idiopathic scoliosis treated by posterior instrumentation and in situ bending. *Spine (Phila Pa 1976)* 2015; 40:E419-27.

[35] Roussouly P, Gollogly S, Berthonnaud E, Dimnet J. Classification of the normal variation in the sagittal alignment of the human lumbar spine and pelvis in the standing position. *Spine (Phila Pa 1976)* 2005; 30:346-53.

[36] Le Huec JC, Charosky S, Barrey C, Rigal J, Aunoble S. Sagittal imbalance cascade for simple degenerative spine and consequences: algorithm of decision for appropriate treatment. *Eur Spine J* 2011; 20 Suppl 5:699-703.

[37] Schwab F, Ungar B, Blondel B, Buchowski J, Coe J, Deinlein D et al. Scoliosis Research Society-Schwab adult spinal deformity classification: a validation study. *Spine (Phila Pa 1976)* 2012; 37:1077-82.

[38] Clement JL, Chau E, Kimkpe C, Vallade MJ. Restoration of thoracic kyphosis by posterior instrumentation in adolescent idiopathic scoliosis: comparative radiographic analysis of two methods of reduction. *Spine (Phila Pa 1976)* 2008; 33:1579-87.

[39] Smith JS, Klineberg E, Schwab F, Shaffrey CI, Moal B, Ames CP et al. Change in classification grade by the SRS-Schwab Adult Spinal Deformity Classification predicts impact on health-related quality of life measures: prospective analysis of operative and nonoperative treatment. *Spine (Phila Pa 1976)* 2013; 38:1663-71.

[40] Terran J, Schwab F, Shaffrey CI, Smith JS, Devos P, Ames CP et al. The SRS-Schwab adult spinal deformity classification: assessment and clinical correlations based on a prospective operative and nonoperative cohort. *Neurosurgery* 2013; 73:559-68.

[41] Hilibrand AS, Tannenbaum DA, Graziano GP, Loder RT, Hensinger RN. The sagittal alignment of the cervical spine in adolescent idiopathic scoliosis. *J Pediatr Orthop* 1995; 15:627-32.

[42] Hwang SW, Samdani AF, Tantorski M, Cahill P, Nydick J, Fine A et al. Cervical sagittal plane decompensation after surgery for adolescent idiopathic scoliosis: an effect imparted by postoperative thoracic hypokyphosis. *J Neurosurg Spine* 2011; 15:491-6.

[43] Ohara A, Miyamoto K, Naganawa T, Matsumoto K, Shimizu K. Reliabilities of and correlations among five standard methods of assessing the sagittal alignment of the cervical spine. *Spine (Phila Pa 1976)* 2006; 31:2585-91; discussion 92.

[44] Yu M, Silvestre C, Mouton T, Rachkidi R, Zeng L, Roussouly P. Analysis of the cervical spine sagittal alignment in young idiopathic scoliosis: a morphological classification of 120 cases. *Eur Spine J* 2013; 22:2372-81.

[45] Yagi M, Iizuka S, Hasegawa A, Nagoshi N, Fujiyoshi K, Kaneko S et al. Sagittal Cervical Alignment in Adolescent Idiopathic Scoliosis. *Spine Deform* 2014; 2:122-30.

[46] Youn MS, Shin JK, Goh TS, Kang SS, Jeon WK, Lee JS. Relationship between cervical sagittal alignment and health-related quality of life in adolescent idiopathic scoliosis. *Eur Spine J* 2016; 25:3114-9.

[47] Wang L, Liu X. Cervical sagittal alignment in adolescent idiopathic scoliosis patients (Lenke type 1-6). *J Orthop Sci* 2017; 22:254-9.

[48] Zhao J, Chen Z, Yang M, Li G, Zhao Y, Li M. Does spinal fusion to T2, T3, or T4 affects sagittal alignment of the cervical spine in Lenke 1 AIS patients: A retrospective study. *Medicine (Baltimore)* 2018; 97:e9764.

[49] Hiyama A, Sakai D, Watanabe M, Katoh H, Sato M, Mochida J. Sagittal alignment of the cervical spine in adolescent idiopathic scoliosis: a comparative study of 42

adolescents with idiopathic scoliosis and 24 normal adolescents. *Eur Spine J* 2016; 25:3226-33.
[50] Guler UO, Ozalay M, Eyvazov K, Senkoylu A, Beyaz S, Sagittal Cervical Compensation in Adolescent Idiopathic Scoliosis, in *Global Spine Congress*. 2017.
[51] Yanik HS, Ketenci IE, Erdem S. Cervical Sagittal Alignment in Extensive Fusions for Lenke 3C and 6C Scoliosis: The Effect of Upper Instrumented Vertebra. *Spine (Phila Pa 1976)* 2017; 42:E355-E62.
[52] Protopsaltis TS, Scheer JK, Terran JS, Smith JS, Hamilton DK, Kim HJ et al. How the neck affects the back: changes in regional cervical sagittal alignment correlate to HRQOL improvement in adult thoracolumbar deformity patients at 2-year follow-up. *J Neurosurg Spine* 2015; 23:153-8.
[53] Iyer S, Nemani VM, Nguyen J, Elysee J, Burapachaisri A, Ames CP et al. Impact of Cervical Sagittal Alignment Parameters on Neck Disability. *Spine (Phila Pa 1976)* 2016; 41:371-7.
[54] Scheer JK, Passias PG, Sorocean AM, Boniello AJ, Mundis GM, Jr., Klineberg E et al. Association between preoperative cervical sagittal deformity and inferior outcomes at 2-year follow-up in patients with adult thoracolumbar deformity: analysis of 182 patients. *J Neurosurg Spine* 2016; 24:108-15.
[55] McAviney J, Schulz D, Bock R, Harrison DE, Holland B. Determining the relationship between cervical lordosis and neck complaints. *J Manipulative Physiol Ther* 2005; 28:187-93.
[56] Lee SM, Suk SI, Chung ER. Direct vertebral rotation: a new technique of three-dimensional deformity correction with segmental pedicle screw fixation in adolescent idiopathic scoliosis. *Spine (Phila Pa 1976)* 2004; 29:343-9.
[57] Vallespir GP, Flores JB, Trigueros IS, Sierra EH, Fernandez PD, Olaverri JC et al. Vertebral coplanar alignment: a standardized technique for three dimensional correction in scoliosis surgery: technical description and preliminary results in Lenke type 1 curves. *Spine (Phila Pa 1976)* 2008; 33:1588-97.
[58] Canavese F, Turcot K, De Rosa V, de Coulon G, Kaelin A. Cervical spine sagittal alignment variations following posterior spinal fusion and instrumentation for adolescent idiopathic scoliosis. *Eur Spine J* 2011; 20:1141-8.
[59] Ames CP, Blondel B, Scheer JK, Schwab FJ, Le Huec JC, Massicotte EM et al. Cervical radiographical alignment: comprehensive assessment techniques and potential importance in cervical myelopathy. *Spine (Phila Pa 1976)* 2013; 38:S149-60.
[60] Park MS, Moon SH, Lee HM, Kim SW, Kim TH, Lee SY et al. The effect of age on cervical sagittal alignment: normative data on 100 asymptomatic subjects. *Spine (Phila Pa 1976)* 2013; 38:E458-63.
[61] Knott PT, Mardjetko SM, Techy F. The use of the T1 sagittal angle in predicting overall sagittal balance of the spine. *Spine J* 2010; 10:994-8.
[62] Park JH, Cho CB, Song JH, Kim SW, Ha Y, Oh JK. T1 Slope and Cervical Sagittal Alignment on Cervical CT Radiographs of Asymptomatic Persons. *J Korean Neurosurg Soc* 2013; 53:356-9.
[63] Scheer JK, Tang JA, Smith JS, Acosta FL, Jr., Protopsaltis TS, Blondel B et al. Cervical spine alignment, sagittal deformity, and clinical implications: a review. *J Neurosurg Spine* 2013; 19:141-59.

[64] Kim YJ, Lenke LG, Bridwell KH, Kim J, Cho SK, Cheh G et al. Proximal junctional kyphosis in adolescent idiopathic scoliosis after 3 different types of posterior segmental spinal instrumentation and fusions: incidence and risk factor analysis of 410 cases. *Spine (Phila Pa 1976)* 2007; 32:2731-8.

[65] Hollenbeck SM, Glattes RC, Asher MA, Lai SM, Burton DC. The prevalence of increased proximal junctional flexion following posterior instrumentation and arthrodesis for adolescent idiopathic scoliosis. *Spine (Phila Pa 1976)* 2008; 33:1675-81.

[66] Roussouly P, Gollogly S, Noseda O, Berthonnaud E, Dimnet J. The vertical projection of the sum of the ground reactive forces of a standing patient is not the same as the C7 plumb line: a radiographic study of the sagittal alignment of 153 asymptomatic volunteers. *Spine (Phila Pa 1976)* 2006; 31:E320-5.

[67] Yang M, Yang C, Chen Z, Wei X, Chen Y, Zhao J et al. Lumbar Lordosis Minus Thoracic Kyphosis: Remain Constant in Adolescent Idiopathic Scoliosis Patients Before and After Correction Surgery. *Spine (Phila Pa 1976)* 2016; 41:E359-63.

[68] Vaz G, Roussouly P, Berthonnaud E, Dimnet J. Sagittal morphology and equilibrium of pelvis and spine. *Eur Spine J* 2002; 11:80-7.

[69] Berthonnaud E, Dimnet J, Roussouly P, Labelle H. Analysis of the sagittal balance of the spine and pelvis using shape and orientation parameters. *J Spinal Disord Tech* 2005; 18:40-7.

[70] Mac-Thiong JM, Berthonnaud E, Dimar JR, 2nd, Betz RR, Labelle H. Sagittal alignment of the spine and pelvis during growth. *Spine (Phila Pa 1976)* 2004; 29: 1642-7.

[71] Yilmaz G, Borkhuu B, Dhawale AA, Oto M, Littleton AG, Mason DE et al. Comparative analysis of hook, hybrid, and pedicle screw instrumentation in the posterior treatment of adolescent idiopathic scoliosis. *J Pediatr Orthop* 2012; 32:490-9.

[72] Cao Y, Xiong W, Li F. Pedicle screw versus hybrid construct instrumentation in adolescent idiopathic scoliosis: meta-analysis of thoracic kyphosis. *Spine (Phila Pa 1976)* 2014; 39:E800-10.

[73] Lamerain M, Bachy M, Delpont M, Kabbaj R, Mary P, Vialle R. CoCr rods provide better frontal correction of adolescent idiopathic scoliosis treated by all-pedicle screw fixation. *Eur Spine J* 2014; 23:1190-6.

[74] Liu H, Li Z, Li S, Zhang K, Yang H, Wang J et al. Main thoracic curve adolescent idiopathic scoliosis: association of higher rod stiffness and concave-side pedicle screw density with improvement in sagittal thoracic kyphosis restoration. *J Neurosurg Spine* 2015; 22:259-66.

[75] Prince DE, Matsumoto H, Chan CM, Gomez JA, Hyman JE, Roye DP, Jr. et al. The effect of rod diameter on correction of adolescent idiopathic scoliosis at two years follow-up. *J Pediatr Orthop* 2014; 34:22-8.

[76] Cahill PJ, Wang W, Asghar J, Booker R, Betz RR, Ramsey C et al. The use of a transition rod may prevent proximal junctional kyphosis in the thoracic spine after scoliosis surgery: a finite element analysis. *Spine (Phila Pa 1976)* 2012; 37:E687-95.

[77] Sudo H, Abe Y, Kokabu T, Ito M, Abumi K, Ito YM et al. Correlation analysis between change in thoracic kyphosis and multilevel facetectomy and screw density in main thoracic adolescent idiopathic scoliosis surgery. *Spine J* 2016; 16:1049-54.

[78] Delikaris A, Wang X, Boyer L, Larson AN, Ledonio CGT, Aubin CE. Implant Density at the Apex is More Important than Overall Implant Density for 3D Correction in

Thoracic Adolescent Idiopathic Scoliosis Using Rod Derotation and En Bloc Vertebral Derotation Technique. *Spine (Phila Pa 1976)* 2017.

[79] Luo M, Wang W, Shen M, Luo X, Xia L. Does higher screw density improve radiographic and clinical outcomes in adolescent idiopathic scoliosis? A systematic review and pooled analysis. *J Neurosurg Pediatr* 2017; 19:448-57.

[80] Tao F, Wang Z, Li M, Pan F, Shi Z, Zhang Y et al. A comparison of anterior and posterior instrumentation for restoring and retaining sagittal balance in patients with idiopathic adolescent scoliosis. *J Spinal Disord Tech* 2012; 25:303-8.

[81] Pesenti S, Chalopin A, Peltier E, Choufani E, Ollivier M, Fuentes S et al. How Sublaminar Bands Affect Postoperative Sagittal Alignment in AIS Patients with Preoperative Hypokyphosis? Results of a Series of 34 Patients with 2-Year Follow-Up. *Biomed Res Int* 2016; 2016:1954712.

[82] Celestre PC, Carreon LY, Lenke LG, Sucato DJ, Glassman SD. Sagittal Alignment Two Years After Selective and Nonselective Thoracic Fusion for Lenke 1C Adolescent Idiopathic Scoliosis. *Spine Deform* 2015; 3:560-5.

[83] Vidal C, Mazda K, Ilharreborde B. Sagittal spino-pelvic adjustment in severe Lenke 1 hypokyphotic adolescent idiopathic scoliosis patients. *Eur Spine J* 2016; 25:3162-9.

[84] Janssen MM, Vincken KL, van Raak SM, Vrtovec T, Kemp B, Viergever MA et al. Sagittal spinal profile and spinopelvic balance in parents of scoliotic children. *Spine J* 2013; 13:1789-800.

[85] Yong Q, Zhen L, Zezhang Z, Bangping Q, Feng Z, Tao W et al. Comparison of sagittal spinopelvic alignment in Chinese adolescents with and without idiopathic thoracic scoliosis. *Spine (Phila Pa 1976)* 2012; 37:E714-20.

[86] Lee CS, Hwang CJ, Kim NH, Noh HM, Lee MY, Yoon SJ et al. Preoperative Magnetic Resonance Imaging Evaluation in Patients with Adolescent Idiopathic Scoliosis. *Asian Spine J* 2017; 11:37-43.

[87] Ferguson RL, DeVine J, Stasikelis P, Caskey P, Allen BL, Jr. Outcomes in surgical treatment of "idiopathic-like" scoliosis associated with syringomyelia. *J Spinal Disord Tech* 2002; 15:301-6.

[88] Ouellet JA, LaPlaza J, Erickson MA, Birch JG, Burke S, Browne R. Sagittal plane deformity in the thoracic spine: a clue to the presence of syringomyelia as a cause of scoliosis. *Spine (Phila Pa 1976)* 2003; 28:2147-51.

[89] Davids JR, Chamberlin E, Blackhurst DW. Indications for magnetic resonance imaging in presumed adolescent idiopathic scoliosis. *J Bone Joint Surg Am* 2004; 86-A:2187-95.

[90] Richards BS, Sucato DJ, Johnston CE, Diab M, Sarwark JF, Lenke LG et al. Right thoracic curves in presumed adolescent idiopathic scoliosis: which clinical and radiographic findings correlate with a preoperative abnormal magnetic resonance image? *Spine (Phila Pa 1976)* 2010; 35:1855-60.

[91] Diab M, Landman Z, Lubicky J, Dormans J, Erickson M, Richards BS et al. Use and outcome of MRI in the surgical treatment of adolescent idiopathic scoliosis. *Spine (Phila Pa 1976)* 2011; 36:667-71.

In: Scoliosis: Diagnosis, Classification and Management Options ISBN: 978-1-53614-464-2
Editors: F. Canavese, A. Andreacchio and H. Xu © 2018 Nova Science Publishers, Inc.

Chapter 18

POSTOPERATIVE SHOULDER IMBALANCE (PSI) AND ADDING-ON PHENOMENON

*Ismail Daldal[1], Erdem Aktas[2] and Alpaslan Senkoylu[3],***

[1]Sakarya University Research and Training Hospital,
Department of Orthopaedics and Traumatology, Sakarya, Turkey
[2]TOBB University of Economics and Technology, Faculty of Medicine,
Department of Orthopaedics and Traumatology, Ankara, Turkey
[3]Gazi University, Department of Orthopaedics and Traumatology,
Besevler, Ankara, Turkey

ABSTRACT

Scoliosis is a three-dimensional spinal deformity involving axial-plane rotation, lateral curvature in the coronal plane, and alteration of the sagittal spinal profile. Surgical treatment is still considered the definitive treatment option for patients with severe scoliosis. Spine surgeons universally aim to fuse the smallest number of motion segments necessary to create a satisfactory balance of the trunk, shoulders, neck and pelvis. Several conditions militate in favor of fusing more segments, rather than fewer: we address two of them: post-operative shoulder imbalance (PSI), and the adding-on phenomenon (AO).

The definition of PSI remains controversial. Cosmetic shoulder balance is a major concern for patients with scoliosis, although surgeons are commonly more concerned with radiological shoulder balance. No consensus exists on the incidence of, or risk factors for, PSI. Additional research is needed to reveal PSI risk factors and quantify its incidence.

Although the clinical implications of AO remain unclear, decompensation of coronal balance can lead to unfavorable radiological and clinical outcomes, which may require revision surgery. Extension of the primary curve, disc wedging, and degenerative changes may necessitate extending the fusion distally.

The radiological and clinical parameters mentioned throughout this chapter will help deformity surgeons to identify the onset of AO. Meticulous preoperative planning and adequate surgical technique is mandatory to achieve a balanced spine and prevent AO in high-risk patients with adolescent idiopathic scoliosis. If it occurs regardless, there are still treatment options available, and we will review some of these here.

---

* Corresponding Author Email: drsenkoylu@gmail.com.

Keywords: scoliosis, adding-on phenomenon, shoulder, posterior instrumented fusion

INTRODUCTION

Adolescent idiopathic scoliosis (AIS) is a three-dimensional spinal deformity involving axial-plane rotation, lateral curvature in the coronal plane, and alteration of the sagittal spinal profile. Surgical treatment is still considered the definitive treatment option for patients with severe scoliosis [1, 2]. Spine surgeons universally aim to fuse the smallest number of motion segments necessary to create a satisfactory balance of the trunk, shoulders, neck and pelvis. Several conditions militate in favor of fusing more segments, rather than fewer: we address two of them: post-operative shoulder imbalance (PSI), and the adding-on phenomenon (AO).

POSTOPERATIVE SHOULDER IMBALANCE

In a normal, healthy individual, shoulder, trunk, and pelvis are balanced and symmetrical. However, Akel et al. [3] reported that adolescents presenting to pediatric outpatient clinics without any musculoskeletal pathology often do not have symmetrical shoulder levels. In their study, radiological and clinical evaluation of healthy adolescents revealed that 28% of individuals had a difference in shoulder height of more than 10 mm, and healthy adolescents may have up to a 27-mm difference between their shoulders without a change in body-image perception.

Diagnosis

In the radiological evaluation of shoulder balance, coracoid height difference (CHD), clavicular angle (CA), clavicle-rib cage intersection difference (CRID), T1 tilt, and clavicular tilt angle difference (CTAD) can be measured on anteroposterior radiographs as described by Bagó. [4] CHD is the measured height difference between the coracoid processes. CA is the angle between the horizontal plane and a line intersecting the highest points of both clavicles. Clavicular tilt angle is the angle between the horizontal plane and the line bisecting the proximal ends of both clavicles. The difference between these two clavicular tilt angles represents CTAD. Lastly, CRID represents the height difference between the horizontal lines passing through the point where the superior border of the clavicle intersects the outer edge of the second rib. All these measurements are depicted in Figure 1.

Qiu et al. [5] demonstrated that a discrepancy often exists between radiographic shoulder imbalance and cosmetic shoulder imbalance in AIS patients with double-thoracic curves. Wang et al. [6] reported that CHD, CRID, CA, and radiographic shoulder height (RSH) all have good correlation with clinical shoulder height. They also demonstrated that neck tilt is a distinct clinical entity from shoulder imbalance.

PSI has an influence on patients' appearance and satisfaction after correction surgery. Therefore, achieving good shoulder symmetry is one of the most important measurements of success in scoliosis surgery. Kuklo et al. [7] defined "balanced" shoulders in AIS patients as a side-to-side height difference on clinical examination of less than 10 mm. Furthermore, some authors have reported that postoperative shoulder balance is significantly different between patients with and without truncal shift, probably due to its function as a shoulder-leveling mechanism, and that postoperative unilateral shoulder elevation more than 20 mm is a potential cause of dissatisfaction [8].

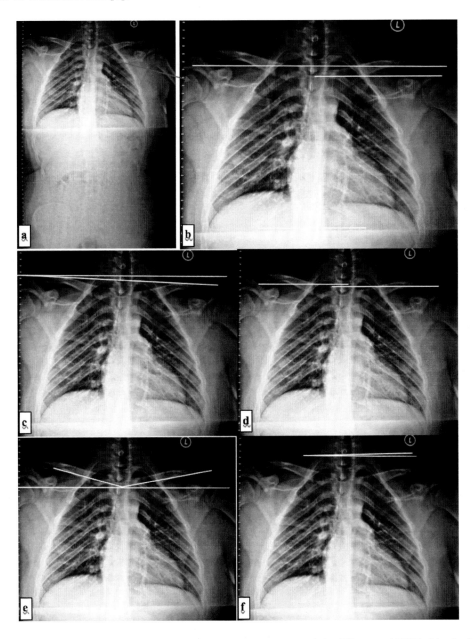

Figure 1. Radiological evaluation of shoulder balance. Coracoid height difference (CHD) (**b**), clavicular angle (CA) (**c**), clavicle-rib cage intersection difference (CRID) (**d**), clavicular tilt angle difference (CTAD) (**e**) and T1 tilt (**f**).

Risk Factors and Incidence

There is no consensus on the incidence of PSI in patients with scoliosis after deformity treatment or on the risk factors for PSI. According to a meta-analysis [9], when using RSH asymmetry ≥ 10 mm as the criterion for PSI, preoperative lumbar curve (LC), postoperative RSH, and correction magnitude of the main thoracic curve are primary risk factors for PSI. Age, Risser sign, sex, preoperative flexibility, and preoperative thoracic curve were not found to be risk factors for PSI. However, Lee et al. [10] reported that Risser sign is a risk factor for PSI. They posited that patients who have higher Risser grades are more likely to develop PSI because the more mature the skeleton, the more rigid the scoliotic curves.

According to a recently published meta-analysis [9], LC is the only preoperative risk factor for PSI, but this report is inconsistent with some other studies [11, 12]. Yazsay et al. [13] reported that preoperative LC angles are a significant predictor of postoperative shoulder balance. The association between preoperative LC and other factors affecting PSI could mediate the role of preoperative LC in predicting PSI.

It is widely accepted that inappropriate proximal-fusion–level selection can result in poor outcomes, including shoulder imbalance. PSI concerns are more critical for Lenke type 2 and 4 deformities in which the proximal thoracic (PT) curve is structural. Studies done by the Lenke and Suk groups [14, 15] led them to recommend that if the PT curve is greater than 30°, and greater than 20° on bending radiographs, both the PT and main thoracic (MT) curves should be fused (Figure 2). However, some reports suggested a non-fusion strategy for PT curves between 35° and 45° because of the possibility of spontaneous correction of such curves [16, 17].

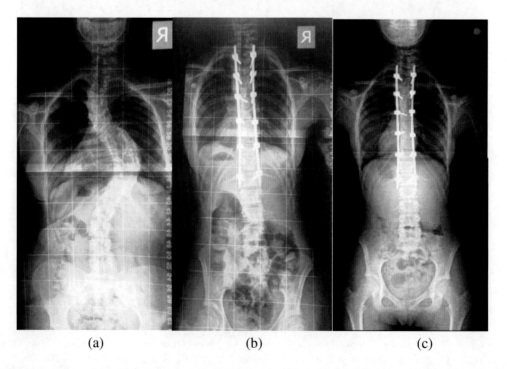

(a) (b) (c)

Figure 2. Selective thoracic fusion has been performed in a 14 year-old AIS patient with Lenke Type-2 curve (a). Proximal thoracic curve was also included to fusion (b). There is no decompensation in 18-month follow-up.

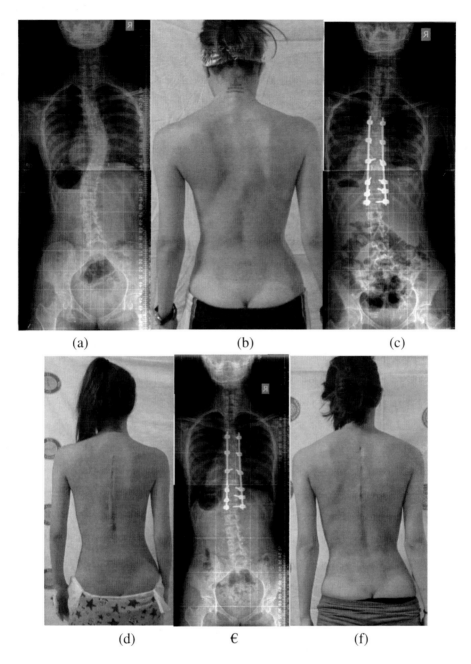

Figure 3. Selective thoracic fusion has been performed in a 16 year-old AIS patient with Lenke Type-1 curve (a, b). Early postoperative x-ray and clinical picture revealed left shoulder elevation (c, d) which spontaneously improved postoperative 6. month follow-up examination (e, f).

Lee et al. [10] found that the postoperative PT-curve/MT-curve ratio might also be an important factor for the onset of PSI. They aimed to serially demonstrate postoperative changes in shoulder imbalance and identify risk factors for PSI in Lenke Type 2 double-thoracic curves. They also reported that PSI is correlated with a higher Risser grade and a larger postoperative proximal wedge angle (PWA) (PWA is defined as the angle of coronal wedging in the first disc space above the highest instrumented vertebra) as well as with the PT-curve/MT-curve ratio.

The incidence of PSI varies widely in different studies. Menon et al. [18] reported 5.1%; a meta-analysis [9] reported the pooled incidence in all types of scoliosis was 25%; Smyrnis et al. showed 57.1%. [8]

Another important consideration is the timing of the evaluation for PSI. In some of cases, shoulders are not level in the early postoperative period, probably due to pain. Later, shoulders may become level spontaneously (Figure 3). Thus, a surgeon should wait several months before considering a remedial operation.

Prevention

Although numerous studies have been conducted regarding this issue, there is still no solution for preventing shoulder imbalance in adolescent AIS surgery. Nevertheless, a few tips and tricks based on current literature and experience are available.

If a patient has a structural PT curve (i.e., Lenke Type 2 or 4 curvature, or kyphosis between vertebral levels T2 and T6), T2 or T3 should be considered as the upper instrumented vertebra (UIV) (Figure 2). Another indication for including the PT curve in the surgery might be preoperative left shoulder elevation (Figure 4).

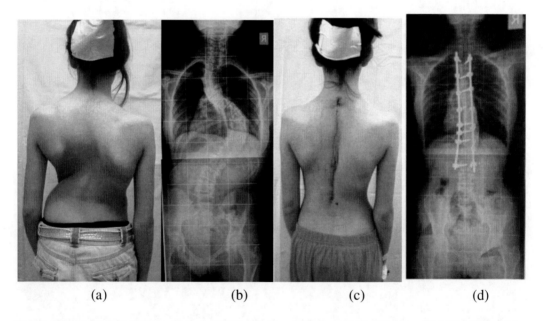

(a) (b) (c) (d)

Figure 4. Posterior spinal fusion between T2-L2 has been performed in a 13 year-old AIS patient with Lenke Type-4 curve (a, b). Preoperatively, she has an obvious left shoulder elevation which improved postoperatively (c, d).

Many studies relate T1 tilt to shoulder balance. A positive T1 tilt, high on the left side, is an indication for including the PT curve in the fusion, in order to prevent deterioration of shoulder imbalance. However, in a recent study Luhmann et al. analyzed preoperative and postoperative radiographic shoulder measurements of 618 AIS patients to identify whether T1 tilt could be used as an intraoperative indicator for shoulder balance determination.

Interestingly, they found that T1 tilt cannot be used as an intraoperative indicator for preventing shoulder imbalance in structural PT curves. [19]

Does a surgically level upper thoracic spine mean balanced shoulders postoperatively? Amir et al. found that trapezial prominence is affected by T1 via the first rib. Nevertheless, leveling the upper thoracic spine is not an assurance of clinically well-balanced shoulders. [20] Similarly, correction of trapezial prominence was found to be more predictable when compared with CA [21].

All this ultimately proves our initial point: the ideal means for preventing shoulder imbalance following AIS surgery are, regrettably, still not clear enough.

THE ADDING-ON PHENOMENON

The main goal of surgical treatment in AIS is to achieve optimal correction of scoliosis while preventing postoperative progression and preserving flexibility of the lumbar spine.

Although to date various definitions have been proposed regarding AO, the entity can be defined as: postoperative progression of the curve below the lowest level of spinal fusion instrumentation. Studies reveal that AO is characterized by several parameters [22-24].

1. Progression of the primary Cobb angle below the level of instrumentation, visualized as an increase in disc angulation distal to the instrumentation;
2. Increase in the number of vertebrae in the measured curve either proximally or distally, combined with a curve increase of more than 5 degrees compared to the first postoperative radiograph;
3. Increase of more than 5 degrees in the narrowing of the first vertebra below instrumentation;
4. Deviation of more than 5 mm in the lowest instrumented vertebrae (LIV) from the central sacral vertical line (CSVL); and/or
5. Increase of more than 10 mm in the deviation of the first vertebra below the LIV from the CSVL at 2-year follow-up.

Incidence

The incidence of AO as reported in the literature ranges widely. Lehman has reported 2%, while Matsumoto estimates 18.8%, Suk 33.3% and Wang 51.1%. [25–28] This could be due to the higher incidence of distal AO reported in certain types of AIS: Schlechter et al. [22] have reported an incidence rate of up to 13% for distal AO in Lenke 1A and 2A scoliosis (King III and King IV) patients, in whom the single thoracic curves with the compensatory lumbar curves do not cross the midline.

Diagnosis

Diagnosis of the onset of AO is crucial. There are several relevant diagnostic radiographical parameters defined in the literature to determine the onset of AO [29]:

1. Increase in the lumbar Cobb angle;
2. Deviation of the LIV by more than 5 mm from the CSVL;
3. Increase in the number of vertebrae included in the curve, a minimum of 1 year postoperatively; and
4. Increase in the narrowing of the first vertebra below instrumentation (LIV+1) exceeding 5 degrees.

Sponseller et al. reported [23] a mean Cobb angle increase of 7.3° in scoliosis patients treated with posterior fusion. Similarly, Schlechter et al. described 52 patients, among a total of 407 patients, with distal AO who had a mean postoperative 7.4° increase in thoracic Cobb angle [22].

Risk Factors and Prevention

Although the pathophysiology of AO is clearly multifactorial, there are certain risk factors and related conditions that affect the incidence of adding-on:

1. Maturity and/or age at surgery;
2. Preoperative Cobb angle;
3. Degrees of correction achieved;
4. Deformity progression;
5. Inappropriate selection of LIV;
6. The stable vertebra-lowest instrumented vertebra (SV-LIV) gap difference (the gap difference is defined as the numerical value of the related vertebrae. e.g., the SV-LIV gap difference is 2 where SV is L2 and LIV is T12);
7. The neutral vertebra (NV)-LIV gap difference;
8. The lower end vertebra (EV)-LIV gap difference; and
9. Preoperative deviation of LIV+1 from CSVL

Appropriate selection of the LIV is critical to prevent AO. If the extent of fusion is too short distally, there is a high chance the distal curve will progress, leading to AO [9]. LIV selection is also important to maintenance of the correction achieved and preservation of growth potential and lumbar spine mobility. Although more detailed recent classification systems can help guide deformity surgeons to make the ideal selection of LIV and fusion levels, LIV selection still remains highly variable in practice. Especially in Lenke 1A type scoliosis, the selection of LIV is highly correlated with the presence of AO [14, 30-33].

Measurement of LIV+1 deviation from CSVL on the preoperative standing anteroposterior radiograph can guide surgeons to predict whether or not a patient will develop distal AO after surgery. The patient is likely to develop distal AO if LIV+1 deviation from CSVL is more than 10 mm.

Wang You et al. reported [28] that selecting the first vertebra below the lower-end vertebra (EV+1) and/or the first vertebra in the cephalad direction from the sacrum whose deviation from the center sacral vertical line was more than 10 mm (DV) as the LIV yielded the best outcomes. In all cases evaluated, at least one vertebra was required to be added distally to the intended fusion length. Unacceptable outcomes were reported when the EV was used as the LIV.

Suk et al. suggested focusing on the NV [27]. They concluded that there was an increased risk of AO when LIV was proximal to the NV by more than 2 vertebrae. They also recommend that if the NV is located less than 2 levels from the EV, fusion may be extended to the NV. In another study, Ni et al. recommended that the choice of LIV can be based on an evaluation of the flexibility of the intervertebral discs on anteroposterior roentgenograms [34]. Lakhal et al. used the same criteria to select LIV and also considered the degree and reducibility of the lumbar curve. The lumbar curve was not instrumented if it was less than 45 degrees and could be reduced by more than 50%. They concluded that in Lenke 1 scoliosis, the choice of LIV based on this analysis of coronal and sagittal range of motion prevents AO [35].

Other strategies for determining LIV are; (1) choosing the EV as the LIV; (2) choosing the first vertebra below the EV as the LIV; (3) choosing the DV as the LIV.

In a study conducted by Wang You et al., AO patients experienced a spontaneous lumbar curve correction correlated with selective thoracic fusion. Although the LIV+1 vertebra was not instrumented, their mean deviation from CSVL was shown to be decreased by 16.2 mm after surgery. This finding can be plainly stated as: selective thoracic fusion also corrected the lumbar curves to some extent, in addition to the thoracic curves. However, there was a later loss of this lumbar curve correction. Deviation of LIV+1 was reported to be increased by 11.8 mm at 1-year follow-up. There was a 73% loss of the spontaneous lumbar curve correction. In light of these findings they concluded that, if the instrumentation is too short distally to maintain this spontaneous correction, there is a high likelihood of lumbar vertebral correction loss, and the lumbar vertebrae will gradually move back to their previous locations [28].

Yang et al. concluded that number of non-fused segments and posterior Cobb angle of the lumbar curve were two important factors affecting the occurrence of AO in Lenke 1 and 2 AIS patients [36]. The authors also pointed out that this phenomenon was influenced more by skeletal immaturity, shoulder imbalance and the increase of the LIV-CSVL distance by more than 10 mm in the postoperative period.

Cho et al. emphasized different parameters, including: L4 vertebral tilt; preoperative thoracic and lumbar curves; and coronal flexibility [37]. They concluded that two variables were significant predictive factors for the development of adding-on: age and Risser stage. Based on the laterality of L4 tilt, Miyanji et al. identified two subtypes of Lenke 1A curve patterns, Lenke 1A-L and 1A-R, and concluded that they behave differently [38].

They evaluated distal AO and associated risk factors in Lenke 1A-L and 1A-R curve patterns and reported that compared to Lenke 1A-L curves, Lenke 1A-R curves are twice as likely to manifest adding-on. Thus, they recommend choosing a LIV such as the last substantially touched vertebra (LSTV) or the NV.

Xu et al. included all types of Lenke AIS patients and classified the region between the CSVL and LIV pedicle into three types (A, B, or C) depending on whether the CSVL touched the LIV pedicle. In Touch Type A, the LIV pedicle did not touch the CSVL, indicating that the LIV deviates markedly from the centerline of the body. They found that the AO incidence of patients with an LIV classed as Touch Type A was as high as 58% [39]. They stated that Touch Type classification is an important risk factor, highly correlated with the incidence of AO, and that the best LIV choice to preserve lumbar activity as much as possible is one that is Touch Type C. They observed no significant difference in terms of SRS-22 scores between their Touch-Type–C group and the control group.

In their series, Matsumoto et al. investigated distal AO in Lenke 1A curve patterns and reported an 18.8% incidence of adding-on. When they investigated the difference between the

LIV and the EV, NV, SV, and last touched vertebra (LTV), two significant factors were identified as predictive of AO: relationship of the LIV to the LTV; and apical translation of the main thoracic curve immediately after surgery. AO was reported as 6.7 times more likely with a LIV proximal to the LTV. To prevent postoperative AO, they recommended the LIV be extended to or beyond the LTV [26]. Similarly, Cao et al. reported AO to be significantly higher in patients with a LIV proximal to the LTV and concluded that the selection of LIV substantially influences the development of AO, especially in Lenke 2A curvatures [40].

Murphy et al. emphasized the importance of three preoperative predictors of AO. These were: (1) fusing short of the LSTV; (2) Risser stage 0; and (3) preoperative C7–CSVL distance of less than 2 cm. They reported that the rate of AO increases with the number of predictors present. The risk can be as high as 80% when all three risk factors are present. When correcting spinal deformities in AIS, parameters such as LSTV, SV, NV, and EV should be considered thoroughly to determine the most appropriate LIV, since fusing short of the LSTV, especially in a skeletally immature patient, prominently increases the risk of AO [41].

Cao et al. [12] studied the association of postoperative shoulder balance with AO in Lenke Type II AIS and pointed out that shoulder balance also has an impact on AO. Similarly, Shigematsu et al. emphasized the importance of a balanced shoulder level, truncal shift, and listing, and presumed that the distal AO may be a compensatory mechanism. They postulated that the shape of the fusion mass was associated with this compensatory mechanism. Their findings suggest that a residual fusion-mass shift greater than 20 mm is strongly associated with distal AO. They recommended preoperative fulcrum-bending radiographs to guide deformity surgeons to select the appropriate fusion levels, and thus predictably attain a postoperative fusion-mass shift of less than 20 mm [42].

Treatment

AO may become a frustrating problem not only for the patient and parents, but also for the surgeon. Treatment options can be conceptualized as swinging over wide range, with observation on one end of the pendulum's arc, and surgical treatment on the other end. Once AO is identified, surgeons should evaluate patients' SRS-22 scores, together with full-length spinal X-rays, and inform the patient and parents about the natural history of AO after AIS surgery. Sometimes, X-rays may not correlate with the clinical appearance of the patient. Thus, some patients with moderate or even severe curvatures are well balanced and do not decompensate clinically (Figure 5). In this situation, surgical treatment is not necessary in non-progressive curves.

However, if the patient has a clinically significant waistline asymmetry or truncal shift, extension of the fusion and instrumentation should be considered (Figure 6a, b). Once surgical intervention is decided upon, the flexibility of the decompensated curve should be evaluated. Side or fulcrum bending and traction radiographs are helpful for decision making; the surgeon needs to perform an osteotomy in order to get correction of a rigid curve. In our clinical practice, our strategy would not be to revise the whole construct in the surgical management of AO. Basically, two instrumented cranial- or caudal-end vertebrae of the index procedure should be exposed. This incision also includes an extension component towards the decompensated levels. Paravertebral muscles are then dissected subperiosteally until the tip of the previous construct is seen.

Postoperative Shoulder Imbalance (PSI) and Adding-On Phenomenon 271

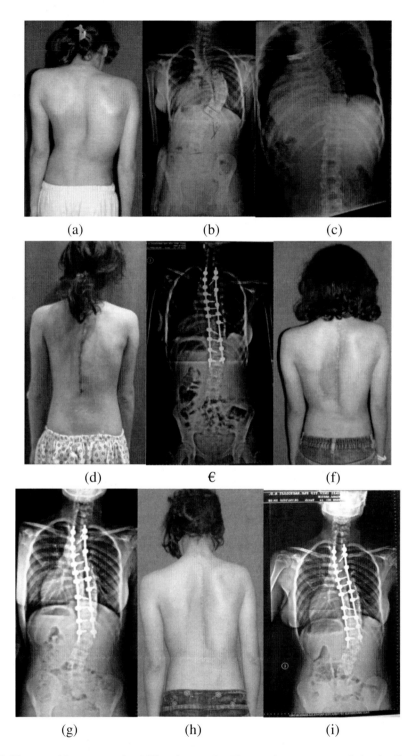

Figure 5. A 13-year-old premenarche AIS patient (a, b). Her traction x-ray revealed quite flexible lumbar curve and she considered as Lenke Type-2 (c). Postopeartive early pictures shows an acceptable correction and well-balanced spine (d, e). However, she started to deteriorate at 8 months postop. Revision operation was offered, nevertheless it was denied by the parents due to a well-balanced clinical appearance (f, g). She was remain the same at 3-year follow-up (h, ı).

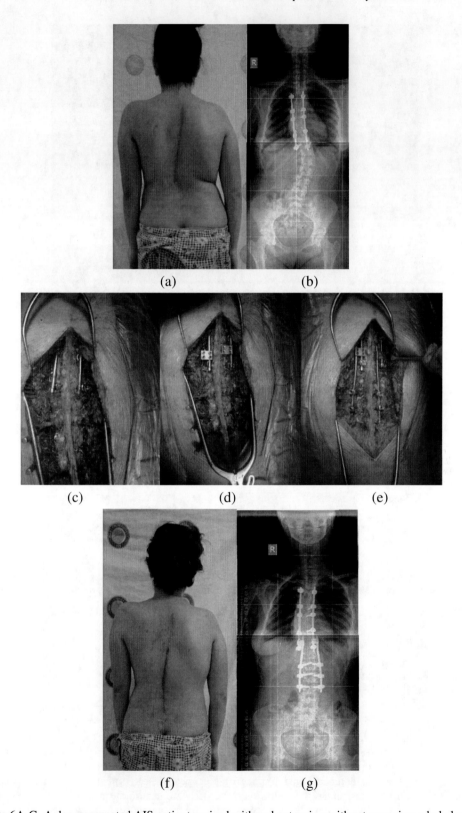

Figure 6A-G. A decompensated AIS patient revised with rod extension without exposing whole levels.

The first step is to remove the set screws of the last two levels of the instrumented portion adjacent to the decompression site and release their rods (Figure 6c). Subsequently, the distal (or proximal) ends of the rods are removed from the pedicle tulips using rod holders, and two side-to-side domino connectors are inserted into the rods (Figure 6d). The intended extension level is calculated, and new pedicle screws are inserted into the caudal or cranial adjacent vertebra (e). Desired osteotomy should be done at this stage if the curve is rigid. New extension rods are connected to the previous rods by domino connectors and placed in the recently inserted pedicle screws (Figure 6e). Desired compression, distraction or derotation maneuvers are performed in order to achieve a successful correction of the decompensated curve (Figure 6f, g).

CONCLUSION

This chapter has provided an overview of two significant factors affecting success in surgical treatment of AIS: PSI and AO.

The definition of shoulder imbalance remains controversial. Cosmetic shoulder balance is considered a major concern by patients with scoliosis, although surgeons pay more attention to the radiological shoulder balance. No consensus exists on the incidence of and risk factors for PSI; additional studies are required.

Although the clinical significance of AO is unclear, decompensation of coronal balance produces unfavorable radiological and clinical outcomes that may require revision surgery. Extension of the primary curve, disc wedging, and/or degenerative changes may necessitate the need to extend the fusion distally.

The radiological and clinical parameters mentioned throughout this chapter will help deformity surgeons to identify the onset of AO. Even better, they should assist in the meticulous preoperative planning and surgical technique that is mandatory to achieve a balanced spine and prevent AO in high-risk patients with AIS. And finally, we review some of the treatment options that are available if it nonetheless occurs.

REFERENCES

[1] Liu, Z., Hu, Z. S., Qiu, Y., Zhang, Z., Zhao, Z. H., Han, X. & Zhu, Z. Z. (2017). "Role of clavicle chest cage angle difference in predicting post- operative shoulder balance in Lenke 5C adolescent idiopathic scoliosis patients after selective posterior fusion." *Orthop Surg*, *9*(1), 86–90.

[2] Senkoylu, A., Luk, K. D., Wong, Y. W. & Cheung, K. M. (2014). "Prognosis of spontaneous thoracic curve correction after the selective anterior fusion of thoracolumbar/lumbar (Lenke 5C) curves in idiopathic scoliosis." *Spine J*, *14*, 1117-24.

[3] Akel, I., Pekmezci, M., Hayran, M., et al. (2008). "Evaluation of shoulder balance in the normal adolescent population and its correlation with radiological parameters." *Eur Spine J*, *17*, 348–354.

[4] Bago, J., Carrera, L., March, B., et al. (1996). "Four radiological measures to estimate shoulder balance in scoliosis." *J Pediatr Orthop B*, 5(1), 31–34.

[5] Qiu, X. S., Ma, W. W., Li, W. G., et al. (2009). "Discrepancy between radiographic shoulder balance and cosmetic shoulder balance in adolescent idiopathic scoliosis patients with double thoracic curve." *Eur Spine J*, 18, 45–5.

[6] Kwan, M. K., Wong, K. A., Lee, C. K. & Chan, C. Y. W. (2016). "Is neck tilt and shoulder imbalance the same phenomenon? A prospective analysis of 89 adolescent idiopathic scoliosis patients (Lenke type 1 and 2)." *Eur Spine J*, 25(2), 401-8.

[7] Kuklo, T. R., Lenke, L. G., Graham, E. J., et al. (2002). "Correlation of radiographic, clinical, and patient assessment of shoulder balance following fusion versus nonfusion of the proximal thoracic curve in adolescent idiopathic scoliosis." *Spine*, 27, 2013–2020.

[8] Smyrnis, P. N., Sekouris, N. & Papadopulos, G. (2009). "Surgical assessment of the proximal thoracic curve in adolescent idiopathic scoliosis." *Eur Spine J*, 18, 522–530.

[9] Zhang, S., Zhang, L., Feng, X. & Yang, H. (2018). "Incidence and risk factors for postoperative shoulder imbalance in scoliosis: a systematic review and meta-analysis." *Eur Spine J*, 27(2), 358-369.

[10] Lee, C. S., Hwang, C. J., Lim, E. J., Lee, D. H. & Cho, J. H. (2016). "A Retrospective study to reveal factors associated with postoperative shoulder imbalance in patients with adolescent idiopathic scoliosis with double thoracic curve." *J Neurosurg Pediatr*, 25(6), 744–752.

[11] Min, K., Hahn, F. & Ziebarth, K. (2007). "Short anterior correction of the thoracolumbar/lumbar curve in King 1 idiopathic scoliosis: the behaviour of the instrumented and non-instrumented curves and the trunk balance." *Eur Spine J*, 16(1), 65–72.

[12] Cao, K., Watanabe, K., Hosogane, N., Toyama, Y., Yonezawa, I., Machida, M., Yagi, M., Kaneko, S., Kawakami, N., Tsuji, T. & Matsumoto, M. (2014). "Association of postoperative shoulder balance with adding-on in Lenke Type II adolescent idiopathic scoliosis." *Spine*, 39(12), E705–E712.

[13] Yazsay, B., Bastrom, T. P., Newton, P. O. & Harms Study Group. (2013). "Should Shoulder Balance Determine Proximal Fusion Levels in Patients With Lenke 5 Curves?" *Spine Deform*, 1(6), 447-451.

[14] Lenke, L. G., Bridwell, K. H., O'Brien, M. F., Baldus, C. & Blanke, K. (1994). "Recognition and treatment of the proximal thoracic curve in adolescent idiopathic scoliosis treated with Cotrel-Dubousset instrumentation." *Spine*, 19, 1589-97.

[15] Suk, S. I., Kim, W. J. & Lee, C. S., et al. (2000). "Indications of proximal thoracic curve fusion in thoracic adolescent idiopathic scoliosis: recognition and treatment of double thoracic curve pattern in adolescent idiopathic scoliosis treated with segmental instrumentation." *Spine*, 25, 2342-9.

[16] Kuklo, T. R., Lenke, L. G., Won, D. S., et al. (2001). "Spontaneous proximal thoracic curve correction after isolated fusion of the main thoracic curve in adolescent idiopathic scoliosis." *Spine*, 26, 1966-75.

[17] Elfiky, T. A., Samartzis, D., Cheung, W. Y., Wong, Y. W., Luk, K. D. & Cheung, K. M. (2011). "The proximal thoracic curve in adolescent idiopathic scoliosis: surgical strategy and management outcomes." *Global Spine J*, *1*, 27-36.

[18] Menon, K. V., Pillay, H. M., Anbuselvam, M., Tahasildar, N. & Renjit Kumar, J. (2015). "Post-operative shoulder imbalance in adolescent idiopathic scoliosis: a study of clinical photographs." *Scoliosis*, *10*, 31.

[19] Luhmann, S. J., Sucato, D. J., Johnston, C. E., Richards, B. S. & Karol, L. A. (2016). "Radiographic Assessment of Shoulder Position in 619 Idiopathic Scoliosis Patients: Can T1 Tilt Be Used as an Intraoperative Proxy to Determine Postoperative Shoulder Balance?" *J Pediatr Orthop*, *36*(7), 691-4.

[20] Amir, D., Yaszay, B., Bartley, C. E., Bastrom, T. P. & Newton, P. O. (2016). "Does Leveling the Upper Thoracic Spine Have Any Impact on Postoperative Clinical Shoulder Balance in Lenke 1 and 2 Patients?" *Spine (Phila Pa 1976)*, *41*(14), 1122-7.

[21] Ono, T., Bastrom, T. P., Newton, P. O. (2012). "Defining 2 components of shoulder imbalance: clavicle tilt and trapezial prominence." *Spine (Phila Pa 1976)*, *37*(24), E1511-6.

[22] Schlechter, J., Newton, P., Upasani, V., et al. (2009). "*Risk Factors for Distal Adding-on Identified: What to Watch Out For.*" Paper presented at the annual meeting for the American Association of Orthopaedic Surgeons., Las Vegas., Nevada., February 25-28.

[23] Sponseller, P. D., Betz, R., Newton, P. O., et al. (2009). "Differences in curve behavior after fusion in adolescent idiopathic scoliosis patients with open triradiate cartilages." *Spine*, *34*, 827 – 31.

[24] Parisini, P., Di Silvestre, M., Lolli, F., et al. (2009). "Selective thoracic surgery in the Lenke type 1A: King III and King IV type curves." *Eur Spine J*, *18* (suppl 1), 82 – 8.

[25] Lehman, Jr. R. A., Lenke, L. G., Keeler, K. A., et al. (2008). "Operative treatment of ado-lescent idiopathic scoliosis with posterior pedicle screw-only constructs: minimum three-year follow-up of one hundred fourteen cases." *Spine*, *33*(14), 1598–604.

[26] Matsumoto, M., Watanabe, K., Hosogane, N., et al. (2013). "Postoperative distal adding-onand related factors in Lenke type 1A curve." *Spine*, *38*, 737–44.

[27] Suk, S. I., Lee, S. M., Chung, E. R., et al. 2005. "Selective thoracic fusion with segmental pedicle screw fixation in the treatment of thoracic idiopathic scoliosis: more than 5-year follow-up." *Spine*, *30*(14), 1602–9.

[28] Wang, Y., Hansen, E. S., Hoy, K., et al. (2011). "Distal adding-on phenomenon in Lenke 1A scoliosis: risk factor identification and treatment strategy comparison." *Spine*, *36*(14), 1113–22.

[29] Wang, Y., Bunger, C. E., Zhang, Y., et al. (2013). Distal adding-on in Lenke 1A scoliosis: how to more effectively determine the onset of distal adding-on. *Spine*, *38*(6), 490–5.

[30] Lenke, L. G., Betz, R. R., Harms, J., et al. (2013). "Adolescent idiopathic scoliosis: a new classification to determine extent of spinal arthrodesis." *J Bone Joint Surg Am*, *83-A*, 1169 – 81.

[31] King, H. A., Moe, J. H., Bradford, D. S., et al. (1983). The selection of fusion levels in thoracic idiopathic scoliosis. *J Bone Joint Surg Am*, *65*, 1302 –13.

[32] Knapp, D. R., Jr. Price, C. T., Jones, E. T., et al. (1992). "Choosing fusion levels in progressive thoracic idiopathic scoliosis." *Spine (Phila Pa 1976)*, *17*, 1159 – 65.

[33] Newton, P. O., Faro, F. D., Lenke, L. G., et al. (2003). "Factors involved in the decision to perform a selective versus nonselective fusion of Lenke 1B and 1C (King-Moe II) curves in adolescent idiopathic scoliosis." *Spine (Phila Pa 1976)*, *28*, S217 – 23.

[34] Ni, H. J., Su, J. C., Lu, Y. H., Zhu, X. D., He, S. S., Wu, D. J., et al. (2011). "Using side-bending radiographsto determine the distal fusion level in patients with single thoracic idiopathicscoliosis undergoing posterior correction with pedicle screws." *J Spinal Disord Tech*, *24*, 437–43.

[35] Lakhal, W., Loret, J. E., de Bodman, C., Fournier, J., Bergerault, F. & de Courtivron, B. Bonnard. (2014). "The progression of lumbar curves in adolescent Lenke 1 scoliosis and the distal adding-on phenomenon." *Orthop Traumatol Surg Res*, *100*(4 Suppl), S249-54.

[36] Yang, C., Li, Y., Yang, M., Zhao, Y., Zhu, X., Li, M. & Liu, G. (2016). "Adding-on Phenomenon after Surgery in Lenke Type 1, 2 Adolescent Idiopathic Scoliosis: Is it Predictable?" *Spine (Phila Pa 1976)*, *41*(8), 698-704.

[37] Cho, R. H., Yaszay, B., Bartley, C. E., et al. (2012). "Which Lenke 1A curves are at the greatest risk for adding-on. . . and why?" *Spine*, *37*(16), 1384–90.

[38] Miyanji, F., Pawelek, J. B., Van, Valin S. E., et al. (2008). "Is the lumbar modifier useful in surgical decision making?: defining two distinct Lenke 1A curve patterns." *Spine (Phila Pa 1976)*, *33*, 2545–51.

[39] Xu, W., Chen, C., Li, Y., Yang, C., Li, M., Li, Z. & Zhu, X. (2017). "Distal adding-on phenomenon in adolescent idiopathic scoliosis patients with thoracolumbar vertebra fusion: A case-control study." *Medicine (Baltimore).*, *96*(38), e8099.

[40] Cao, K., Watanabe, K., Kawakami, N., et al. (2014). "Selection of lower instrumented vertebra in treating Lenke type 2A adolescent idiopathic scoliosis." *Spine (Phila Pa 1976)*, *39*, E253–61.

[41] Murphy, J. S., Upasani, V. V., Yaszay, B., Bastrom, T. P., Bartley, C. E., Samdani, A., Lenke, L. G. & Newton, P. O. (2017). "Predictors of Distal Adding-On in Thoracic Major Curves with AR Lumbar Modifiers." *Spine (Phila Pa 1976)*, *15*, 42(4), E211-E218.

[42] Shigematsu, H., Cheung, J. P., Bruzzone, M., Matsumori, H., Mak, K. C., Samartzis, D. & Luk, K. D. (2017). "Preventing Fusion Mass Shift Avoids Postoperative Distal Curve Adding-on in Adolescent Idiopathic Scoliosis." *Clin Orthop Relat Res*, *475*(5), 1448-1460.

In: Scoliosis: Diagnosis, Classification and Management Options ISBN: 978-1-53614-464-2
Editors: F. Canavese, A. Andreacchio and H. Xu © 2018 Nova Science Publishers, Inc.

Chapter 19

HOW TO CONTROL SHOULDER BALANCE AND PREVENT IMBALANCE IN PATIENTS WITH AIS UNDERGOING SURGERY

Jun Jiang, MD and Zezhang Zhu[*], MD*

Spine Surgery Department,
Drum Tower Hospital of Nanjing University Medical School,
Nanjing, China

ABSTRACT

Restoring a leveled shoulder is the one of the main goals of surgical corrections for adolescent idiopathic scoliosis (AIS) patients. Accurate evaluation of preoperative shoulder height is an essential prerequisite for selecting upper-instrumented vertebra in AIS patients. Several radiographic parameters have been developed to describe the height difference between the left shoulder and right shoulder and to choose the optimal level of fixation.

The choice of spinal fusion level plays a key role in the successful correction of AIS patients. Postoperative residual shoulder imbalance is an important factor contributing to the patients' non-satisfactions with the operation, which is thought to be caused by the improper surgical strategy making. However, to date, how to control the shoulder balance of AIS patients during the operation remains unclear.

Maintaining postoperative shoulder balance in AIS patients is a complex process. In the author's opinion, to prevent postoperative shoulder imbalance, we should comprehensively analyze 3 important factors: a) preoperative shoulder height, b) flexibility of the proximal thoracic curve and c) correction rates of the proximal thoracic curve and the main thoracic curve, in order to make a reasonable surgical plan and to meet patients' expectations.

Keywords: shoulder imbalance, adolescent idiopathic scoliosis, surgery, upper instrumented level, shoulder, elevation

---

[*] Corresponding Author Email: zhuzezhang@126.com.

PART 1: HOW TO CONTROL SHOULDER BALANCE

Restoring a leveled shoulder is the one of the main goals of surgical corrections for AIS patients, especially in patients with a thoracic curve (Lenke type 1 or 2) [1-2]. Postoperative residual shoulder imbalance is an important factor contributing to patient non-satisfaction with the operation, which is thought to be caused by improper surgical strategy-making. However, to date, how to control the shoulder balance of AIS patients during the operation remains unclear. Previous studies concerning this issue have often emphasized the influence of the upper instrumented vertebra (UIV) on postoperative shoulder height [3-4]. They thought that the preoperative left-elevated shoulder indicated full fusion of the proximal thoracic (PT) curve (proximally fused to T2 or above) since sole correction of the right main thoracic (MT) curve will further elevate the left shoulder. In contrast, a right-elevated shoulder often indicates partial fusion (T3 level) or non-fusion of the PT curve (T4 or below). Some other investigators have focused their studies on evaluations of the flexibility of the PT curve in AIS patients. They have insisted that a rigid PT curve (Lenke type 2 curve or double thoracic curve) should be fused during the operation since it has a low ability to accommodate the correction gained from the MT curve, which often leads to decompensation of the PT curve and a residual left higher shoulder after surgery [5-6]. In clinical practice, sometimes these rules do not work. In fact, the maintenance of postoperative shoulder balance in AIS patients in a complex process. In the author's opinion, to prevent postoperative shoulder imbalance, we should comprehensively analyze 3 important factors (preoperative shoulder height, flexibility of PT curve and correction rates of the PT curve and the MT curve) to develop a reasonable surgical plan.

Radiographic Evaluation of Preoperative Shoulder Height

Accurate evaluation of preoperative shoulder height is an essential prerequisite for selecting UIV in AIS patients. Until now, several radiographic parameters have been developed to describe the height difference between the left shoulder and right shoulder, which are listed as follows [4]:

1. Radiographic shoulder height (RSH): the difference in the soft tissue shadow directly superior to the acromioclavicular joint (Fig. 1). The value is considered positive if the left is higher and negative if the right is higher. RSH is the most widely used parameter for evaluating shoulder height in AIS patients. The postoperative shoulder height is often graded as significant imbalance (RSH >3 cm), moderate imbalance (RSH: 2–3 cm), minimal imbalance (RSH: 1–2 cm), or balanced (RSH <1 cm side-to-side difference).
2. Clavicle angle (CA): the angle subtended by a horizontal line and the tangential line connecting the highest two points of each clavicle (Fig. 2). The value is positive if the left clavicle is higher and negative if the right clavicle is higher.
3. Coracoid height difference (CHD): the height difference between the right and left horizontal line traced in the superior edge of each coracoid process (Fig. 3). The value is positive if the left coracoid is higher and negative if the right coracoid is higher.
4. T1 tilt: the angle between the horizontal line and the line through the upper endplate of T1 (Fig. 4). The value is positive if the left anterior corner of T1 is higher than the right anterior corner of T1.

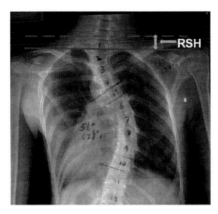

Figure 1. Illustration of the measurement of RSH (radiographic shoulder height).

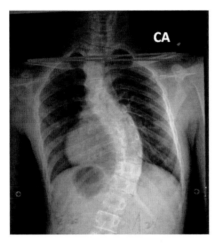

Figure 2. Illustration of the measurement of CA (clavicle angle).

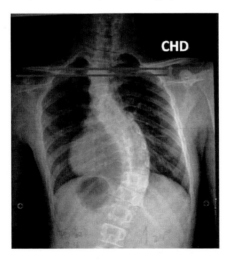

Figure 3. Illustration of the measurement of coracoid height difference (CHD).

T1 tilt describes the profile of the PT curve rather than the shoulder height. The PT curve is divided into 2 kinds based on the directionality of the T1 tilt. A positive T1 tilt is indicative of a complete PT curve with a true apex (Figure 5a), while a leveled T1 or negative T1 tilt is indicative of a fractional PT curve (Figure 5b) [6]. In 1983, King first defined a complete PT curve as a type V curve, which is characterized by a positive T1 tilt, an elevated left shoulder or a first rib and stiffness of the PT curve [7]. This type is also categorized as a type 2 curve in Lenke's classification [8]. The previous view was that the left shoulder was often elevated in AIS patients with a King type V or Lenke type 2 curve due to the presence of a complete PT curve with a positive T1 tilt. However, this is not always the case in clinical practice. In fact, the preoperative shoulder height is independent of the T1 tilt. A positive T1 tilt can be combined with three different shoulder heights in AIS patients (Figure 6). In a recent study, only a small proportion of AIS patients with a positive T1 tilt had a preoperative left-elevated shoulder, and more than half of them had a preoperative right-elevated shoulder [9]. Therefore, T1 tilt is no longer a reliable radiographic parameter for the evaluation of shoulder height. This conclusion deserves special attention by spine surgeons.

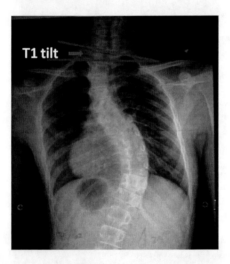

Figure 4. Illustration of the measurement of T1 tilt.

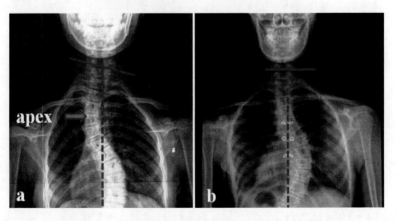

Figure 5. A complete PT curve has a positive T1 tilt and a true apical vertebra (T4) (a), and a fractional PT curve has a neutral or negative T1 tilt without true apical vertebra (b).

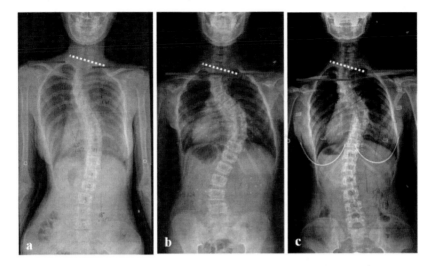

Figure 6. A positive T1 tilt combined with 3 different directionalities of shoulder tilting: left-elevated shoulder (a); leveled shoulder (b) and right-elevated shoulder (c).

Flexibility of the PT Curve

It has been widely accepted that the selection of UIV in AIS patients depends on both the flexibility of the PT curve and the directionality of the preoperative shoulder height. An unfused rigid PT curve has low spontaneous correction ability in the case of sole correction of the MT curve. Hence, accurate evaluation of the flexibility is essential for surgical decision-making. In the past experience of surgeons, a complete PT curve (with positive T1 tilt) is often rigid, while a fractional PT curve (with negative T1 tilt or leveled T1) is often flexible. This phenomenon is true in most cases. However, a complete curve can sometimes also be flexible (Fig. 7). Therefore, side-bending X-ray films of the PT curve are indispensable for AIS patients.

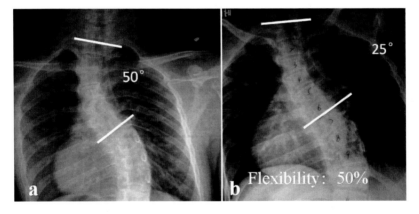

Figure 7. A complete PT curve (a) is not rigid with a flexibility of 50% (b).

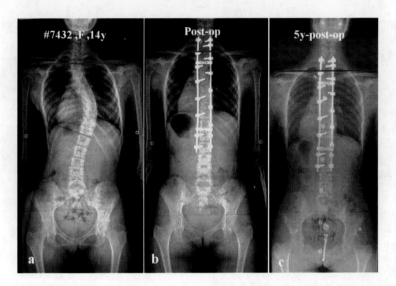

Figure 8. A 14-year-old female AIS patient with a Lenke type 2 curve (rigid PT curve) and preoperative higher left shoulder (a). This patient underwent full fusion of the PT curve (proximally fused to T1) and gained satisfactory shoulder balance after surgery (b). The leveled shoulder was well maintained at the 5-year follow-up (c).

Correction Rate of the PT Curve and MT Curve

To maintain a leveled shoulder, spinal surgeons should cautiously decide whether the PT curve should or should not be fused. In theory, correction of the PT curve can bring down the left shoulder, while correction of the MT curve can elevate the left shoulder. The spontaneous correction of an unfused PT curve is closely related to the amount of correction obtained from the MT curve in the AIS patient. With the introduction of more powerful instrumentation, such as a pedicle screw that further increases the MT correction, the risk of PT curve decompensation substantially increases. It has been widely recognized that overcorrection of the MT curve beyond the flexibility of the PT curve is a risk factor for the residual left-elevated shoulder after surgery [2]. Previous studies have also recommended fusion of the rigid PT curve in AIS patients [8]. However, an increasing number of researchers currently believe that a rigid PT curve in AIS does not always necessarily imply the inclusion of the PT curve in the fusion range. Partial or non-fusion of the PT curve has been advocated if AIS patients have a preoperative right-elevated shoulder since correction of the MT curve will elevate the left shoulder, which helps to restore the shoulder balance in patients with a right-elevated shoulder. In the current recommendation from Lenke's team, the authors suggest that in patients with flexible PT curve (Lenke type 1), the UIV is T2 if the left shoulder is higher, T3 or T4 if the shoulders are leveled and T4 or T5 if the right shoulder is higher. In patients with a rigid PT curve (Lenke type 2), the UIV is T2 if the left shoulder is higher, T2 or T3 if the shoulders are leveled and T3 if the right shoulder is higher [10].

Surgical Decision-Making

In the author's opinion, to restore shoulder balance in AIS patients, there is no rule that can be applicable in any case. The spinal surgeons should be well aware of the associations between the change in shoulder height and the 3 important factors mentioned above and comprehensively analyze these important factors when developing a surgical plan. There is no doubt that a preoperative right-elevated shoulder with a flexible PT curve may indicate proximal fusion to the T4 level or below. In contrast, a preoperative left-elevated or leveled shoulder with a rigid PT curve often indicates proximal fusion to the T2 level (Figures 8 and 9). In our experience, patients with right-elevated shoulder and a rigid PT curve can also undergo partial (T3) or non-fusion of the PT curve (T4 or below) if the MT curve is not over-corrected (Figure 10). Sometimes, if the MT curve is properly corrected, patients with a leveled shoulder and rigid PT curve can also gain shoulder balance with the PT curve left untreated (Figure 11). If the PT curve is fused in patients with a higher left shoulder, compression force should be applied on the convex side to increase the PT correction so that the left shoulder can be brought down. In addition, over-correction of the MT curve should be avoided in AIS patients, even if the PT curve is also corrected. We noticed that the influence of the MT curve on shoulder height is significantly larger than that of the PT curve. If the MT curve is over-corrected in AIS patients with a higher left shoulder, the patient may still have a residual left-elevated shoulder after surgery despite fusion of the PT curve because the decline of the left shoulder resulting from PT curve correction cannot compensate for the elevation of the left shoulder resulting from MT curve correction (Figures 12 and 13).

The Behavior of Shoulder Height during Follow-Up

An interesting association between the shoulder balance and the behavior of the unfused lumbar spine in AIS has recently been a subject of interest. In AIS patients who underwent selective thoracic fusion (lumbar spine not fused), inadequate selection of the lower instrumented vertebra (LIV) often led to complications distal to the fusion area, such as adding-on (characterized by progressive deviation of the lumbar spine or wedging of the intervertebral disc below LIV). Such complications often lead to unsatisfactory radiographic and clinical outcomes with an increased risk of re-operation in AIS patients. However, the development of adding-on can improve the postoperative shoulder imbalance in Lenke type 2 AIS patients during the follow-up period (Figure 14). Since the MT curve is on the right side, distal adding-on can make the MT curve shift further to the right side and elevate the right shoulder. Therefore, it is not difficult to understand that the residual left-elevated shoulder can be compensated by the progression of adding-on during the follow-up period. In other words, the residual shoulder imbalance is a risk factor for distal adding-on in AIS patients with selective thoracic curve fusion.

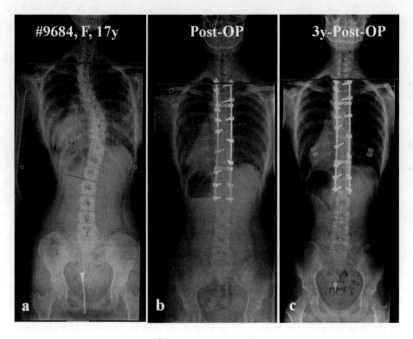

Figure 9. A 17-year-old female AIS patient with a Lenke type 2 curve (rigid PT curve) and preoperative leveled shoulder (a). This patient underwent full fusion of the PT curve (proximally fused to T2), and a leveled shoulder was obtained after surgery (b). The shoulder balance was well maintained at the 3-year follow-up (c).

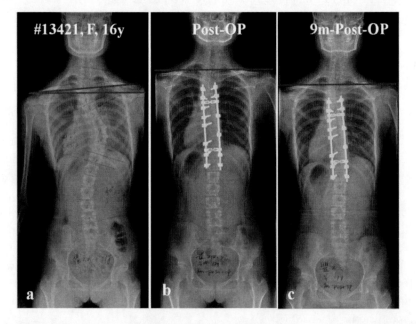

Figure 10. A 16-year-old female AIS patient with a Lenke type 2 curve and preoperative right higher shoulder (RSH: -13 mm) (a). This patient gained shoulder balance (RSH: 2 mm) with PT not fused (proximally fused to T5) (b). The shoulder balance was well maintained (RSH: 2 mm) at the 9-month follow-up (c).

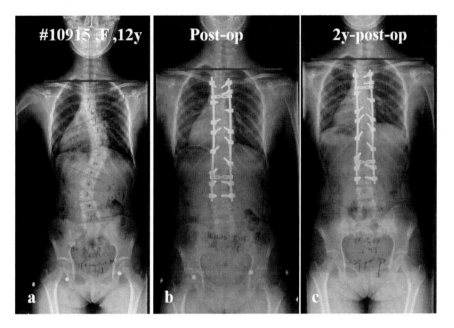

Figure 11. A 12-year-old female AIS patient with a Lenke type 2 curve and preoperative leveled shoulder (RSH: 0 mm) (a). This patient gained shoulder balance (RSH: 5 mm) with the PT curve left untreated (proximally fused to T4) (b). The shoulder balance was well maintained (RSH: 7 mm) at the 2-year follow-up (c).

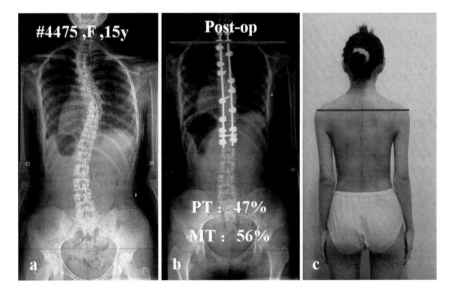

Figure 12. A 15-year-old female patient with a Lenke type 2 curve and preoperative RSH of 7.5 mm (a). This patient underwent full fusion of the PT curve (proximally fused to T1) with a PT curve correction rate of 47% and MT curve correction rate of only 56% (b). This patient had a leveled shoulder (RSH: 5 mm) after surgery due to proper correction of the MT curve (c).

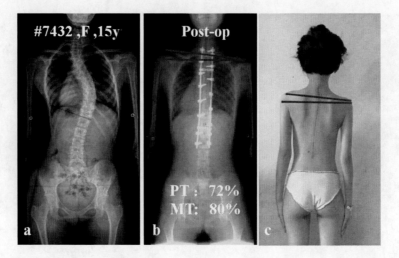

Figure 13. A 15-year-old female patient with a Lenke type 2 curve and preoperative RSH of -3 mm (a). This patient underwent full fusion of the PT curve (proximally fused to T1) with a PT curve correction rate of 72% and MT curve correction rate of 80% (b). Although the PT curve was well corrected, this patient still had a residual left-elevated shoulder (RSH: 18 mm) after surgery due to over-correction of the MT curve (c).

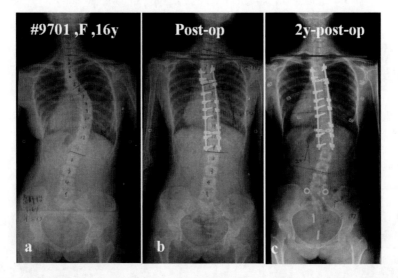

Figure 14. A 16-year-old female patient with a Lenke type 2 curve and preoperative RSH of -6 mm (a). This patient underwent thoracic fusion with distal fusion at L1 and had a residual higher left shoulder after surgery (RSH: 11.7 mm) (b). This patient had improved shoulder balance (RSH decreased to 5 mm) with the development of distal adding-on at the 2-year follow-up.

PART 2: HOW TO PREVENT ADDING-ON IN AIS PATIENTS WHO UNDERWENT POSTERIOR SURGERY

The choice of spinal fusion level plays a key role in the successful correction of AIS patients. Currently, selective thoracic fusion (STF) is becoming more and more popular in the surgical treatment of thoracic AIS patients with a nonstructural lumbar curve, with the purpose of conserving as much growth potential and lumbar spine mobility as possible [11-12]. Though a flexible lumbar curve can be spontaneously corrected after STF, an improper surgical plan can lead to annoying complications in the unfused lumbar region, which is often accompanied by an unsatisfactory clinical outcome and risk of re-operation [13].

In patient with a structural thoracic curve and nonstructural lumbar spine, the lumbar spine modifier (A, B and C) is developed in Lenke's classification to describe the profile of the lumbar curve based on the relationship of the center sacral vertical line (CSVL) and lumbar apical vertebra. The phenomenon of adding-on mostly occurs in thoracic AIS patient with a lumbar modifier of A. These patients have a single thoracic curve without a true lumbar curve (no true lumbar apex). The improper selection of lower instrumentation vertebra (LIV) in these patients can lead to progressive or extension of the primary thoracic curve combined with either the first vertebra below the instrumentation deviating from CSVL more than 5 mm or the angle of the first disc below the instrumentation increasing more than 5°, which is termed "adding-on" [14-15].

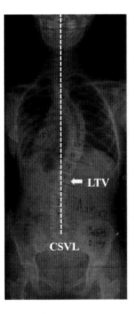

Figure 15. Illustrations of the last touching vertebra (LTV).

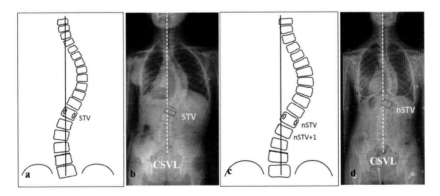

Figure 16. Illustrations of substantially touched vertebra (STV, a and b) and non-substantially touched vertebra (nSTV, c and d).

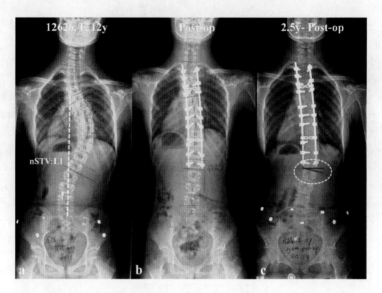

Figure 17. A 12-year-old female patient with nSTV at the L1 level (a). This patient underwent posterior corrective surgery with LIV at the level of nSTV (b). Distal adding-on was noticed in this patient at 2.5 years after surgery (c).

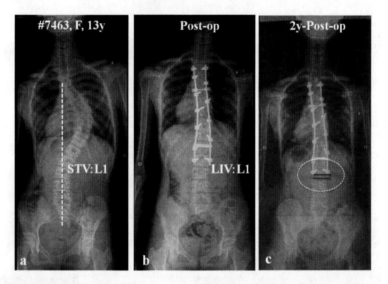

Figure 18. A 12-year-old female patient with STV at the L1 level (a). This patient underwent posterior corrective surgery with LIV at the level of STV (b). No distal adding-on was noticed in this patient at 2.5 years after surgery (c).

Until now, several risk factors associated with adding-on have been reported, including skeletal immaturity and inadequate selection of LIV, among others. However, most previous studies have focused on the relationship between the LIV and the occurrence of distal adding-on [16-17]. The inadequate selection of LIV is considered the most important risk factor for adding-on. Although many strategies of LIV selection have been suggested to prevent the development of adding-on, an increasing number of investigators recommend the last touching vertebra (LTV) as LIV [14-15]. The LTV is defined as the last cephalad vertebra touched by the CSVL, as shown in the anteroposterior X-ray film (Figure 15). However, it is difficult to accurately determine the real LTV when the CSVL slightly touches the cephalad vertebra in clinical practice. Here, the author introduces a new classification of LTV, substantially touched vertebra (STV) and non-substantially touched vertebra (nSTV), according to the position of CSVL on the vertebra [18]. The nSTV is defined as the LTV where CSVL touches the corner of the vertebra lateral to the pedicle border, while the STV is defined as the LTV where CSVL is between the pedicles or touching the pedicle (Figure 16). Distal fusion to nSTV or above is significantly associated with a high incidence of adding-on (Figure 17). The author strongly suggests selecting STV or nSTV+1 as LIV in thoracic AIS patients who have undergone posterior thoracic fusion surgery (Figures 18 and 19).

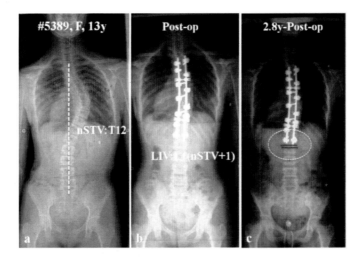

Figure 19. A 13-year-old female patient with nSTV at the T12 level (a). This patient underwent posterior corrective surgery with LIV at the level of nSTV + 1(L1) (b). No distal adding-on was observed in this patient at 2.8 years after surgery (c).

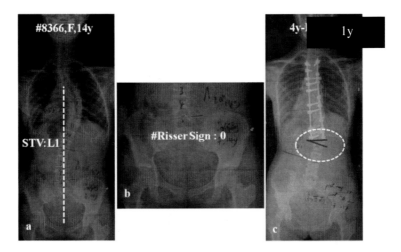

Figure 20. A 14-year-old female patient with STV at the L1 level (a). The Risser Sign was 0, indicating skeletal immaturity in this patient (b). At the 1-year-follow up, this patient still experienced distal adding-on despite distally fusion to the STV level (c).

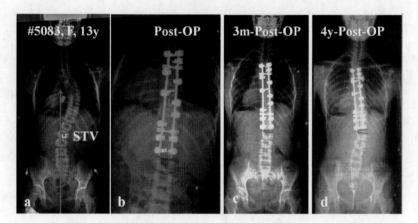

Figure 21. A 13-year-old girl with a Lenke 1A curve. L2 was STV, Risser grade was 0 (a). First erect radiograph postoperatively with fusion to L1, one level proximal to STV (b); 3-month postoperative radiograph shows adding-on, with angulation of the first disc below the instrumentation of 6.8° (c); 4-year postoperative radiograph shows adding-on progression, with an increase in the disc angulation to 12.2° (d).

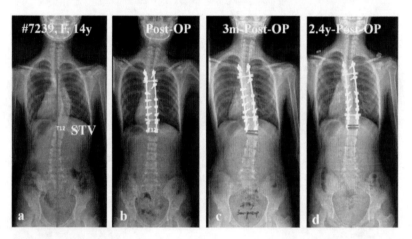

Figure 22. A 14-year-old girl with a Lenke 1A curve. T12 was STV, Risser grade was 3 (a). First erect radiograph postoperatively with fusion to T12 (b); 3-month postoperative radiograph shows adding-on, with angulation of the first disc below the instrumentation of 10.6° (c); 2.4-year postoperative radiograph shows a decrease in adding-on, with disc angulation of 2.8° (d).

In addition to the selection of LIV, some other factors related to the occurrence of adding-on merit special attention. First, Matsumoto's study has demonstrated that apical translation of the MT curve more than 25 mm immediately after surgery is a risk factor for adding-on in the follow-up period [14]. Therefore, apical translation of the MT curve should be reduced as much as possible during the correction procedure. Second, in patients with an immature skeleton, the risk of adding-on is significantly increased (Figure 20). Moreover, the authors classified distal adding-on into progressive and non-progressive adding-on [18] (Figure 21-22). In this study, among patients diagnosed with distal adding-on, the incidence of progressive and non-progressive adding-on was 39.3% and 60.7%, respectively (Figures 21-22). Skeletally immature patients with a short fusion level seemed more likely to have progressive adding-on.

If the adding-on deteriorates during the follow-up time, brace treatment or even revision surgery with LIV distally extended is indicated (Figure 23).

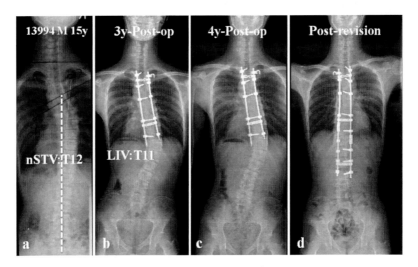

Figure 23. A 15-year-old male patient with nSTV at the T12 level (a). This patient underwent distal fusion to T11 (nSTV-1) and encountered distal adding-on at 3 years after surgery (b). The adding-on deteriorated at the 4-year follow-up (c) and received revision surgery with LIV extended to the L3 level (d).

REFERENCES

[1] Arlet, V., Ouellet, JA., Shilt, J., Shen, FH., Wood, K., Chan, D., Hicks, J., Bersusky, E., Reddi, V. (2009). Subjective evaluation of treatment outcomes of instrumentation with pedicle screws or hybrid constructs in Lenke Type 1and 2 adolescent idiopathic scoliosis: what happens when judges are blinded to the instrumentation? *Eur Spine J*, 18(XII):1927-1935.

[2] Ilharreborde, B., Even, J., Lefevre, Y., Fitoussi, F., Presedo, A., Souchet, P., Penneçot, GF., Mazda, K. (2008). How to determine the upper level of instrumentation in Lenke types 1and 2 adolescent idiopathic scoliosis: a prospective study of 132 patients. *J Pediatr Orthop*, 28(VII):733-739.

[3] Lee, CS., Hwang, C.J, Lim, EJ., Lee, DH., Cho, JH. (2016) A retrospective study to reveal factors associated with postoperative shoulder imbalance in patients with adolescent idiopathic scoliosis with double thoracic curve. *J Neurosurg Pediatr,* 25 (VI):744-752.

[4] Kuklo, TR., Lenke, LG., Graham, EJ., Won, DS., Sweet, FA., Blanke, KM., Bridwell, KH. (2002) Correlation of radiographic, clinical, and patient assessment of shoulder balance following fusion versus nonfusion of the proximal thoracic curve in adolescent idiopathic scoliosis. *Spine* (PhilaPa1976),27 (XVIII):2013-2020.

[5] Namikawa, T., Matsumura, A., Kato, M., Hayashi, K., Nakamura, H. (2015) Radiological assessment of shoulder balance following posterior spinal fusion for thoracic adolescent idiopathic scoliosis. *Scoliosis*, 10, Suppl2, S18.

[6] Lee, CK., Denis, F., Winter, RB., Lonstein, JE. (1993) Analysis of the upper thoracic curve in surgically treated idiopathic scoliosis. A new concept of the double thoracic curve pattern. *Spine* (PhilaPa1976), 18(XII):1599–1608.

[7] King, HA., Moe, JH., Bradford, DS., Winter, RB. (1983).The selection of fusion levels in thoracic idiopathic scoliosis. *J Bone Joint Surg* (Am),65(IX):1302-1313.

[8] Lenke, LG., Betz, RR., Harms, J., Bridwell, KH., Clements, DH., Lowe, TG., Blanke, K. (2001) Adolescent idiopathic scoliosis: a new classification to determine extent of spinal arthrodesis. *J Bone Joint Surg Am*, 83-A (VIII):1169-1181.

[9] Jiang, J., Qian, BP., Qiu, Y., Wang, B., Yu, Y., Zhu, ZZ. (2018)The mechanisms underlying the variety of preoperative directionalities of shoulder tilting in adolescent idiopathic scoliosis patients with double thoracic curve. *Eur Spine J*, 27(II):305-311.

[10] Rose PS, Lenke LG. (2007) Classification of Operative Adolescent Idiopathic Scoliosis: Treatment Guidelines. *Orthop Clin N Am*,38(IV):521–529.

[11] Luk, KDK., Don, AS,. Chong, CS., Wong, YW., Cheung KM. (2008) Selection of fusion levels in adolescent idiopathic scoliosis using fulcrum bending prediction: a prospective study. *Spine,* 33(xx):2192–2198

[12] Dobbs, MB., Lenke, LG., Kim, YJ., Kamath, G., Peelle, MW., Bridwell, KH. (2006) Selective posterior thoracic fusions for adolescent idiopathic scoliosis: comparison of hooks versus pedicle screws. *Spine*, 31(xx):2400–2404

[13] Fischer, CR., Kim, Y. (2011) Selective fusion for adolescent idiopathic scoliosis: a review of current operative strategy. *Eur Spine J*, 20 (VII):1048-1057.

[14] Matsumoto, M., Watanabe, K., Hosogane, N., Kawakami, N., Tsuji, T., Uno, K., Suzuki, T., Ito, M., Yanagida, H., Yamaguchi, T. (2013) Postoperative distal adding-on and related factors in Lenke type 1A curve. *Spine.* 38(IX):737–744

[15] Wang, Y., Hansen, ES., Høy, K., Wu, C., Bünger, CE. (2011) Distal adding-on phenomenon in Lenke 1A scoliosis: risk factor identification and treatment strategy comparison. *Spine.* 36(XIV):1113–22

[16] Yang, C., Li, Y., Yang, M., Zhao, Y., Zhu, X., Li, M., Liu, G.(2016) Adding-on Phenomenon After Surgery in Lenke Type 1, 2 Adolescent Idiopathic Scoliosis: Is it Predictable? *Spine (Phila Pa 1976)*,41(VIII):698-704

[17] Xu, W., Chen, C., Li, Y., Yang, C., Li, M., Li, Z., Zhu, X. (2017) Distal adding-on phenomenon in adolescent idiopathic scoliosis patients with thoracolumbar vertebra fusion: A case-control study. *Medicine (Baltimore)*, 38:e8099

[18] Qin, X., Sun, W., Xu, L., Liu, Z., Qiu, Y., Zhu, Z.(2016) Selecting the Last "Substantially" Touching Vertebra as Lowest Instrumented Vertebra in Lenke Type 1A Curve: Radiographic Outcomes With a Minimum of 2-year Follow-Up. *Spine (Phila Pa 1976)*,41(XII):E742-5

Chapter 20

POSTOPERATIVE DEEP INFECTIONS FOLLOWING SCOLIOSIS SURGERY

Qiang Jie[*], MD, Xiaowei Wang, Qingda Lu and Fei Su
*Department of Pediatric Orthopedics, Hong Hui Hospital,
Xi'an Jiao Tong University, Xi'an, Shan'xi, China*

ABSTRACT

The rate of deep surgical site infection after posterior spinal fusion with segmental spinal instrumentation in children has varied. Deep incisional surgical site infections involving deep soft tissue, and organ/space surgical site infections involving any part of the body excluding the skin incision, fascia, and muscle layers. The incidence of postoperative infection should be highly suspected when the incisional exudation, fever, and local pain are aggravated early after the spinal deformity after the internal fixation of the spinal deformity. Once the diagnosis is made, a thorough debridement, continuous drainage and drainage of the catheterization should be taken actively, with the assistance of a combined sensitive antibiotic. Treatment can effectively control infection and maximize the retention of built-in materials. For delayed infection, we first remove the implant to control infection. The two stage is based on the progress of the malformation.

Keywords: deep infection, postoperative, scoliosis, surgery

INTRODUCTION

With the improvement of the understanding of spinal deformity, the development of internal fixation technology, and the improvement of surgical techniques, surgical treatment of spinal deformity has been widely carried out and has achieved good clinical efficacy. However, due to long operation time, wide range of exfoliation, large amount of bleeding, and use of built-in materials, etc., the risk of deep incision after surgical incision greatly increase. Surgical

---

[*] Corresponding Author Email: jieqiangchina@163.com.

site infections (SSI) is one of the most serious complications of spinal deformity after internal fixation. It means longer hospital stay, higher mortality and complication rate, giving a heavy burden to the patient's physiology, psychology and economy. Therefore, how to diagnose and reasonably handle early postoperative infection of incision site, especially deep infection, has become more and more concerned by spine surgeons.

EPIDEMIOLOGY

The rate of deep surgical site infection after posterior spinal fusion with segmental spinal instrumentation in children has varied. In a review of the Scoliosis Research Society's morbidity and mortality database, they found deep surgical site infection in 321 (1.7%) of 19,360 patients. The prevalence varied by diagnosis, from 0.8% in idiopathic scoliosis to 3.8% in neuromuscular scoliosis. It was found that a 3.7% overall prevalence of surgical site infection (fifty-seven of 1543 patients) in a review of the thirty-year experience at a single institution, and the rates of surgical site infection in the four major etiologic categories of early-onset scoliosis (idiopathic, congenital, syndromic, and neuromuscular) were 0.5%, 1.4%, 3.0%, and 13.3%,respectively. It was reported that the highest prevalence of surgical site infection in patients was with myelomeningocele and those with poliomyelitis. The rates of infection in association with growth-friendly procedures have been reported to range from 5.3% to 14%.

DEFINITION

Surgical site infections (SSI) have been well described in children undergoing spinal instrumentation and arthrodesis procedures for correction of scoliosis. These infections have an adverse effect on the patients and increase health-care costs because of the frequent need for hospital readmission, surgical debridement, washout procedures, and the potential requirement for removal of spinal implants and revision surgery.

Table 1. 1992 Modifications of the CDC Definitions for Deep Surgical Site Infection

Infection occurring within 30 days after the operation if no implant is left in place or within 1 year if implant is in place and the infection appears to be related to the operation and involves deep soft tissues (e.g., fascial and muscle layers) of the incision and at least one of the following:
1. Purulent drainage from the deep incision but not from the organ/space component of the surgical site
2. A deep incision spontaneously dehisces or is deliberately opened by a surgeon when the patient has at least 1 of the following signs or symptoms: fever (>38°C), localized pain, or tenderness, unless specimens from the site are culture-negative
3. An abscess or other evidence of infection involving the deep incision is found on direct examination, during a reoperation, or by histopathologic or radiographic examination
4. Diagnosis of a deep incisional surgical site infection by a surgeon or attending physician

*Quoted from "Horan TC, Gaynes RP, Martone WJ, Jarvis WR, Emori TG. CDC definitions of nosocomial surgical site infections, 1992: a modification of CDC definitions of surgical wound infections. *Am J Infect Control*. 1992 Oct;20(5):271-4."

Surgical site infections were defined by the Centers for Disease Control and Prevention's National Healthcare Safety Network (CDC/NHSN) criteria, and were categorized as superficial incisional surgical site infections involving only the skin and subcutaneous tissue, deep incisional surgical site infections involving deep soft tissue, and organ/space surgical site infections involving any part of the body excluding the skin incision, fascia, and muscle layers. Superficial surgical site infections must occur within thirty days after surgery, but deep incisional and organ/space surgical site infections can occur within one year after surgery if an implant remains in place. A diagnosis of surgical site infection is made either clinically by a physician, with use of signs such as purulent drainage, erythema, and tenderness, or by isolating pathogens on culture from an aseptically obtained specimen from the wound.

CLASSIFICATION

The etiology of scoliosis was classified as either idiopathic or non-idiopathic scoliosis. Non-idiopathic scoliosis was divided into four categories: neuromuscular, syndromic, congenital, or other. The etiology of scoliosis is a known strong determinant of the rate of surgical site infection, with the literature demonstrating lower infection rates, ranging from 1.4% to 2.0%, in children with idiopathic scoliosis. 81.9% of the procedures performed on patients with idiopathic scoliosis were primary definitive arthrodesis, with a surgical site infection rate consistent with the literature at 1.2%. Relative to the population with idiopathic scoliosis, children with neuromuscular scoliosis have additional infection risk factors, with published rates of surgical site infection following arthrodesis ranging from 5.4% to 13.3%,Consistently, the surgical site infection rate following primary definitive arthrodesis in patients with neuromuscular scoliosis in this cohort was 13.1%. In this population with neuromuscular scoliosis, pelvic instrumentation was employed in 66.7% of primary arthrodesis and in 53.7% of all procedures. Jevsevar and Karlin found poor preoperative nutrition to be a risk factor for surgical site infection in patients with neuromuscular scoliosis. After multivariate analysis, instrumentation to the pelvis was a significant risk factor for scoliosis from all etiologies, with 13.7% of patients having complications of surgical site infection. Given these findings, there is a clear opportunity to focus efforts to improve rates of surgical site infection in the at-risk population with neuromuscular scoliosis. Patients with idiopathic scoliosis had the lowest rate of deep surgical site infection whereas those with neuromuscular or congenital scoliosis had the highest rates. The infection rates were similar between the patients with congenital scoliosis and those with neuromuscular disease. The reason for the higher-than-expected deep surgical site infection rate among the patients with congenital scoliosis is unclear.

The rates of infection in association with growth-friendly procedures have been reported to range from 5.3% to 14%. Recent studies examining infection following spinal arthrodesis have cited surgical site infection rates ranging from 3.7% to 8.5%. During the past decade, however, there has been an increasing emphasis on growing strategies (for example, rib-based and spine-based distraction and growth guidance without fusion) in preadolescent children with non-idiopathic scoliosis. In addition, there is increasing use of "growing strategies" such as vertical expandable prosthetic titanium rib, growing rods, and Shilla in children with early-onset scoliosis that allows spinal growth before definitive fusion. Many such children have complex comorbid medical conditions which increase their SSI risk. Increasingly, these repetitive procedures are being used to allow the spine of young patients with scoliosis to grow before definitive spinal arthrodesis. Following implantation, multiple lengthening procedures repeatedly expose the child to the risk of infection. To our knowledge, no previous study has established the rates of infection following these growing construct techniques. The greater number of complications associated with growing constructs is well established, with more recent studies examining the use of Vertical Expandable Prosthetic Titanium Rib (VEPTR) devices. Given the differences in operative time and exposure, growing construct lengthening procedures had the lowest overall rate (3.3%) of surgical site infection, followed by insertion (8.4%) and revision procedures (10.3%) for growing constructs.

Previous single-center studies have demonstrated that the prevalence of gram-negative pathogens in surgical site infections has ranged from 30% to 53%. Similarly, Mackenzie et al. found that 46.5% (thirty-three of seventy-one) of surgical site infections contained one or more gram-negative organisms. Nearly all (thirty-two) of these thirty-three infections were in patients with non-idiopathic scoliosis and many were due to enteric pathogens, suggesting potential wound contamination with feces or urine, complications more likely in patients with non-idiopathic scoliosis. Furthermore, detection of anaerobic flora and polymicrobial surgical site infections support this probable explanation. Sponseller et al. found that 60% of surgical site infections in patients with neuromuscular scoliosis were associated with the growth of gram-negative pathogens on culture, and 52% of surgical site infections were polymicrobial19. Our study had similar findings as 52.5% (thirty-two of sixty-one) of surgical site infections in patients with non-idiopathic scoliosis were associated with gram-negative pathogens, and more than one pathogen grew on culture in 53.5% (thirty-eight of seventy-one) of surgical site infections in patients with either idiopathic or non-idiopathic scoliosis.

The infection of the scoliosis is divided into acute postoperative infection and late infections. The acute postoperative infection is a well-recognized complication of instrumented spinal arthrodesis. Delayed infection after elective posterior or combined anterior and posterior spinal instrumentation and arthrodesis is characterized by an interval of normal postoperative recovery followed by the onset of diffuse pain, malaise, or discomfort several months to many years after surgery. The infection is a late inflammatory reaction, with spontaneous drainage, that had occurred as a result of metal corrosion. The estimated prevalence of late infection approached 1%. The symptoms of infection were swelling and pain at the site of the incision, usually followed by spontaneous drainage. Multihook instrumentation systems include bulky hardware with an extensive surface area that create small gaps between the spine and the hardware, particularly under the crosslinks. The formation of hematoma, soft tissue reaction to increased amounts of implanted hardware, and fretting corrosion promotes a favorable environment for bacterial microorganisms. The exact mechanism of bacterial seeding has not yet been clearly defined, but two possible options are considered: hematogenous seeding and intraoperative seeding. The glycocalyx around the instrumentation adheres to bacteria. Propionibacterium acnes and Staphylococcus epidermidis are the most common skin flora. They are considered nonpathogenic in humans under normal conditions (13), although recently they have been recognized as a cause of implant-related infections. These normal skin flora bacteria may have been introduced into the wound during the operation. It is not known how pathogenic they may be in patients in whom multihook instrumentation has been implanted. The bacteria may adhere to the surface of the instrumentation and become part of the biofilm known as glycocalyx. Without exception, the arthrodesis mass around the rods and the posterior elements of the spine was composed of viable bone. There was no necrotic bone (sequestrum) or bone infiltration with pus to suggest the presence of osteomyelitis. Newer multihook spinal instrumentation systems are associated with extensive hardware. As a result, delayed deep wound infections have become an increasing, but not yet well-defined problem. The incidence of such infections varies from 1% to 7%. The duration between the date of surgery and the date of identification of surgical site infection is not well established. In a large cohort, 67% (two-thirds) of surgical site infections presented within the first month after surgery and 90% presented within the first six months after surgery.

CLINICAL MANIFESTATION

Symptom

1. Fever: Frequently more than 38.5°C, fever lasts for 3 days, body temperature does not fall, or body temperature drops again and then rises. In particular, the temperature rises rapidly after the drainage tube is removed. Incision infection should be highly suspected.
2. Pain: After the analgesia pump was discontinued 3 days after operation, the surgical site or the wound was still painful and tender. The pain in the surgical site or the postoperatively reduced radioactivity pain in the extremities reappeared or aggravated. The patients with cerebrospinal fluid infection still had headaches, stiff neck, and stiffness, meningeal irritation positive
3. Local swelling
4. Skin incision
5. Increased incision skin temperature
6. Tenderness or percussive pain
7. Purulent exudation, et al.

LABORATORY EXAMINATION

1. Increased C-reactive protein (CRP) and increased erythrocyte sedimentation rate (ESR): ESR usually exceeds 2 standard deviations of the mean value, while CRP will appear to rise for the second time or remain at a high level during the 2 to 3 days after the peak is reached, and CRP is diagnosed and reacted to SSI after spinal surgery. The therapeutic effects are all more sensitive than ESR
2. Increased white blood cell count: Increased proportion of white blood cells and neutrophils.
3. The combination of the three can provide more accurate assessment and monitoring for the diagnosis of spinal infection and treatment.
4. Pathological examination: Histopathological examination of deep incision confirmed the presence of infection.

IMAGING EXAMINATION

The posterior spinal internal fixation was mostly paravertebral soft tissue infection and did not involve bone tissue. Therefore, imaging examination was performed. The investigation is not meaningful, but only when MRI is suspected

- *X-ray:* The role of X-ray in diagnosis is not very clear. There was no obvious positive performance in the early X-ray. After 4 weeks, the intervertebral space was narrowed, blurred, the bone density of the vertebral body was reduced, and the surrounding soft tissue was thickened.
- *CT:* The main manifestation of CT examination was worm-like destruction of the affected vertebral body. The pathological changes such as epidural abscess and psoas muscle abscess could be found earlier.
- *MRI:* MRI manifestations of intervertebral disc thickening, long T1 low signal, and high T2 signal in adjacent vertebrae. The sensitivity of magnetic resonance in the diagnosis of spinal infections, especially early infections, specificity and accuracy are better than X-ray and CT.
- *Ultrasonography:* B-ultrasound is an economical, safe, and effective examination method. It is found that paravertebral and psoas major muscles have irregular echogenic areas as indications for surgical treatment.
- *PET/CT:* In recent years, with the rise of 18 fluoro-deoxyglucose positron emission tomography (PET)/CT technology, it has gradually been applied to the diagnosis of post-spinal infections with specificity and sensitivity to MRI. More preferably, it can provide assistance for cases in which MRI cannot diagnose or diagnose difficult cases, but its disadvantage is that it is expensive and restricts clinical use.

DIAGNOSIS

The CDC has published definitions for different types of SSIs. A superficial incisional SSI involves only the skin or subcutaneous tissues and occurs within 30 days after the procedure. Additional criteria include purulent drainage, positive cultures from fluid or tissue obtained sterilely from the superficial incision, pain or tenderness, localized swelling, erythema, and warmth. A stitch abscess is not considered a superficial SSI. A deep incisional SSI involves the fascia and muscle layers. It occurs within 30 days after the procedure if no implant is placed, or within 1 year if an implant is placed and the infection appears to be related to the procedure. Additional criteria include purulent drainage, deep wound dehiscence, fever, pain or tenderness, and presence of an abscess or other evidence of infection diagnosed by direct examination, radiographs, or cultures. Deep SSI after spinal deformity surgery can be further classified into acute and delayed infection. The definition of a delayed SSI after spinal fusion is controversial and has been described as greater than 1 month, 2 months, 3 months, 6 months, and 1 year after the initial procedure.

The diagnosis of deep infection after spinal surgery is mainly combined with clinical symptoms, laboratory indicators, imaging and so on. A deep incisional SSI involves the fascia and muscle layers. It occurs within 30 days after the procedure if no implant is placed, or within

1 year if an implant is placed and the infection appears to be related to the procedure. At least one of the following can make a clinical diagnosis. 1) Drain or puncture pus from the deep incision instead of from the incision site or lacune. 2) Natural incisions or incisions opened by surgeons, with purulent secretions or with fever >38°C, local pain or tenderness. 3) Re-exploration, histopathology, or imaging examinations revealed evidence of deep incision abscesses or other infections. 4) Deep wound infection diagnosed by clinicians.

TREATMENT FOR INFECTION OF SCOLIOSIS

Prevent

Antibiotic

S. aureus was most frequently seen in culture positive surgical site infections. Inappropriate choice of antibiotic may result in increased SSI rates, include: incorrect dose given, incorrect timing of first dose and subsequent doses. Some studies suggested that SSI rates were increased in patients receiving clindamycin versus cefazolin or vancomycin. The Milestone et al. showed that administration of antibiotics within 1 hour of incision was an independent risk factor for SSIs. And appropriate antibiotic prophylaxis, defined as the appropriate dose of cefazolin (20 mg/kg/dose, maximum dose 2000 mg) administered within 30 minutes prior to incision with intraoperative redosing (if relevant) was provided to 23% of patients with SSIs compared to 58% of patients without SSIs. Some studies showed that all patients should receive perioperative intravenous cefazolin (or appropriate coverage in setting of allergy) for insertion or lengthening procedures. Despite the lack of significant high-quality evidence available in the literature, many surgeons have used the intrasite vancomycin powder in surgical wounds, and it continues to provide protection from infection without apparent significant risk of side effects. We suggest that an appropriate use of cefazolin for decreasing rate of SSI may be a good choice, and the use of intrasite vancomycin powder in surgical wounds depend on the situation you meet, we don't make a recommendation.

Intraoperative Irrigation

A number of intraoperative irrigation regimens, aimed at reducing postoperative SSI, for example: antibiotic irrigation, saline irrigation, povidone-iodine irrigation and so on. Some studies have shown that wound irrigation with a povidone-iodine preparation significantly reduces the total SSI rate by approximately 20 percentage points compared with a saline/gentamicin preparation alone. However, in procedures where bony fusion is necessary, surgeons have historically been cautious about the use of povidone-iodine in wound irrigation owing to its toxic effect on fibroblasts and osteoblasts, and the theoretical increased risk of developing pseudarthrosis.

Other Manners

Patients should have a chlorhexidine skin wash the night before surgical procedure. Operating room access should be limited during scoliosis surgery whenever practical. Soft tissue handling and incision planning is important in preventing postoperative infections for surgical procedures. Vancomycin powder should be used in the bone graft and/or the surgical site for insertion procedures. Hyperbaric oxygen (HBO) is a safe and potentially useful supplement to prevent postoperative deep infections in complex spine deformity in high risk neuromuscular patients and so on.

Treatment

Antibiotic

Conservative management with antibiotic therapy alone is not recommended, considering the high risk of failure, presence of extensive instrumentation, and possible consequences of delay, including increasing severity of infection, clinically significant sepsis, and osteomyelitis. Patients with deep SSI were primarily treated with parenteral antibiotics often followed by a short course of oral antibiotics. Initial antibiotic therapy would include broad-spectrum gram-positive and gram-negative coverage that would be modified based on culture results. Most authors suggest patients received a 4-6weeks of intravenous therapy followed in the majority of the cases with a short course of oral therapy.

Irrigation and Debridement

It is an important treatment to deal with SSI. When a deep wound infection is diagnosed, the routine treatment for deep infections included aggressive debridement of the wound and soft tissues, retention of all stable hardware, or primary replacement of instrumentation if fixation failure had occurred. An aggressive approach to deep wound infection emphasizing early irrigation and debridement allowed preservation of instrumentation and successful fusion. Some studies show that deep surgical site infections can be treated with single aggressive surgical debridement in most cases. Even if the infection cannot be completely cleared unless the instrumentation is removed, we recommend debridement without instrumentation removal in the early infections followed by suppressive antibiotics until adequate fusion is obtained.

Treatment of Acute Deep SSIs

The antibiotics administered based on the intraoperative cultures. Acute deep SSIs following spinal deformity surgery can be treated with aggressive irrigation and debridement, retention of instrumentation, and long-term parenteral and oral antibiotics. Implant removal is avoided during the acute postoperative period secondary to concern for deformity progression. Duration of antibiotic treatment varies, but parenteral antibiotics should be continued for a minimum of 4 to 6 weeks. Subsequent treatment with oral antibiotics may be necessary for 2 to 6 months. Some authors recommend primary wound closure over drains after debridement. Others have reported success.

Some authors recommend primary wound closure over drains after debridement. Others have reported success with use of the vacuum-assisted closure VAC) system. The VAC promotes formation of granulation tissue, debrides necrotic tissue, and acts as a sterile dressing. Canavese et al. described application of a VAC sponge at the time of initial surgical debridement in 14 patients who developed an acute deep SSI after spinal fusion. Twelve of the wounds healed by secondary intention with the VAC. Removal of instrumentation was not necessary in any of the patients and there were no recurrent infections. Van Rhee et al.

published similar findings in 6 patients who developed an acute deep SSI after PSF. All patients in both studies received long-term parenteral and oral antibiotics.

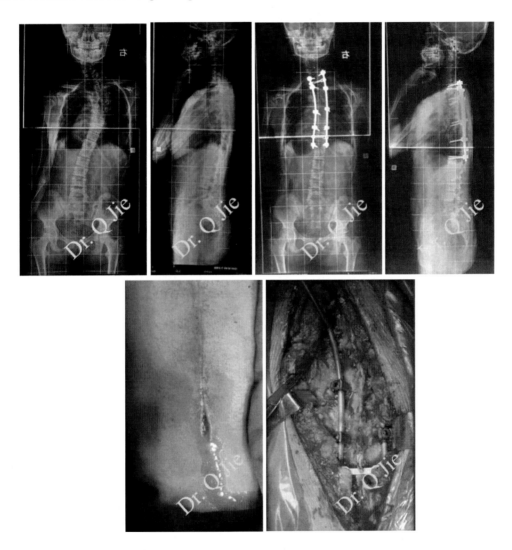

Figure 1. CASE 1: A 12 years old girl with CS, 5 days post-operation demonstrated an exudation of incision.

Management of Delayed Deep SSIs

We define the delayed SSI after spinal fusion as 3 months, and other definition of a delayed SSI after spinal fusion is controversial. The optimal treatment of deep SSI following spinal surgery remains controversial. There is a debate in previous studies as to whether infected surgical wounds should be closed primarily at the time of initial irrigation and debridement/removal of instrumentation or whether closure should be performed in a delayed, staged fashion Most authors agree that implant removal is necessary for the effective treatment of delayed deep SSIs after spinal deformity surgery. After all instrumentation is removed, the wound can be closed primarily over drains and a short course of parenteral and oral antibiotics is sufficient. And Albert F et al. have different suggestion, they recommend the routine treatment for deep infections included aggressive debridement of the wound and soft tissues, retention of all stable hardware, and primary replacement of instrumentation if fixation failure had occurred. Primary wound closure over multiple drains was performed. With this method 76.0% of deep SSI could be treated with a single surgical debridement. Further debridements were performed if clinical evidence of uncontrolled infection continued.

Both Clark and Shufflebarger, and Richards and Emara reported that deep SSIs after spinal fusion are soft tissue infections and not osteomyelitis. These authors recommended 2 to 5 days of parenteral antibiotics, followed by 7 to 14 days of oral antibiotics. Several authors have reported success with this treatment protocol. Ho et al. retrospectively examined 53 patients who developed a deep SSI after PSF for scoliosis. All patients underwent debridement, primary closure over drains, and antibiotics. Instrumentation was initially retained in 97% of acute SSIs and 59% of delayed SSIs. The authors found that retention of instrumentation was a significant predictor of further surgery. Of the 43 patients who retained their instrumentation after initial irrigation and debridement, 47% developed recurrent infection and had a second irrigation and debridement, and 12% required a third operation. Ho et al.'s results suggest that perhaps removal of instrumentation should be considered in acute deep SSIs as well. Implant removal prior to bony fusion can lead to progression of deformity. Cahill et al. retrospectively reviewed 57 patients who developed a SSI after scoliosis surgery. Instrumentation was removed in 51% of patients. Forty-four percent of these patients developed greater than 10° of curve progression. The patients who underwent implant removal within 1 year of the initial surgery had an average of 30° of progression, compared with 20° for those who underwent removal greater than 1 year postoperatively. Twenty-three percent of the patients in Hedequist et al.'s series underwent revision surgery for curve progression. Ho et al. had limited follow-up on their patients who had implants removed, but 60% had greater than 10° of deformity progression in at least one plane. Not all pseudarthroses are evident at the time of instrumentation removal and not all pseudarthroses result in progressive deformity. However, patients and families should be counseled about the possibility of curve progression, especially if implants are removed less than 1 year postoperatively. They should be advised that future revision surgery may be necessary once the infection has cleared.

Hedequist et al. retrospectively reviewed 26 patients who developed a delayed SSI after spinal fusion. They found that patients who retained their instrumentation always returned with recurrent infection and required further debridements until the implants were removed. In most cases, no repeat surgeries were necessary after instrumentation removal. Occasionally, patients with significant comorbidities underwent placement of a VAC at the initial debridement to promote formation of granulation tissue. These patients required one additional procedure for VAC removal and wound closure. The number of hospitalizations, number of hospital days, number of procedures, and cost of hospitalization correlated with the number of debridements before instrumentation removal. Average hospital charges if implants were removed during the first procedure were $81,828, compared to $101,590 if implants were removed within 3 procedures and $674,292 if implants were removed after 4 or more procedures.

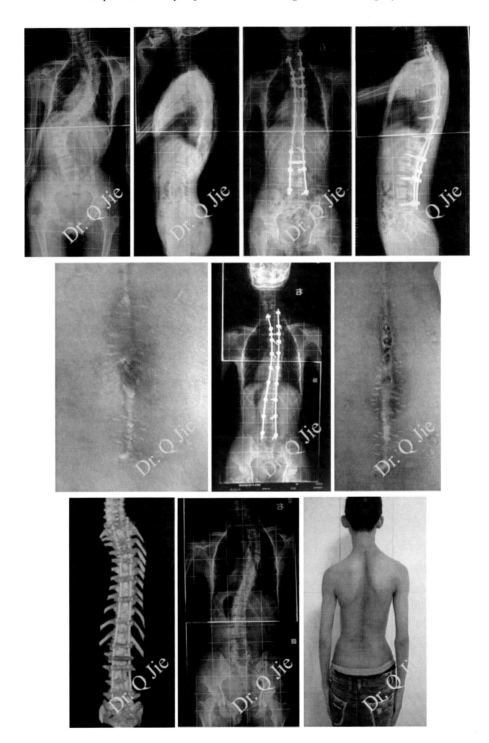

Figure 2. CASE 2: A 14-years boy with a neuromuscular scoliosis was performed a posterior fusion from T1-L5. One year post-operation demonstrated a sinus in the incision. With twice debridement, there was still a recurrence of SSI. And after the implant removed, there is no recurrence of SSI.

Controversy

Metal Type and SSI

Clinical evidence regarding the role of metal composition in pediatric spine surgery has been controversial. Di Silvestre et al. reported on 15 patients with adolescent idiopathic scoliosis (AIS) and SSI following posterior spine fusion and found that stainless steel instrumentation increases the risk of late infection (>12 months after surgery). Marks et al. reported on 28 patients with AIS and SSI following spine fusion and found no difference in risk of infection and type of metal implants. Margaret L et al. reported on 874 patients at three large children's hospitals for any etiology of scoliosis and found no relationship between implant metal type and risk of infection among pediatric patients who have undergone spine surgery.

Remove Implants

Some authors believe that delayed infection can successfully be treated with a single surgical procedure consisting of irrigation and debridement and removal of instrumentation, followed by a course of culture-guided antibiotic therapy. This progression does not, however, seem to effect patients' reported outcomes. Most author agree that delay infections required treatment with implant removal, or it would be easy recurrence. Curve progression may occur after instrumentation removal.

REFERENCES

[1] Mackenzie WG, Matsumoto H, Williams BA, Corona J, Lee C, Cody SR, Covington L, Saiman L, Flynn JM, Skaggs DL, Roye DP Jr, Vitale MG(2013). Surgical Site Infection Following Spinal Instrumentation for Scoliosis: A Multicenter Analysis of Rates, Risk Factors, and Pathogens. *J Bone Joint Surg Am*, 95(9): 800-806, S1-2.

[2] Kabirian N, Akbarnia BA, Pawelek JB, Alam M, Mundis GM Jr, Acacio R, Thompson GH, Marks DS, Gardner A, Sponseller PD, Skaggs DL(2014). Deep Surgical Site Infection Following 2344 Growing-Rod Procedures for Early-Onset Scoliosis: Risk Factors and Clinical Consequences. *J Bone Joint Surg Am*, 96(15):e128.

[3] Brandon A, Sherrod, Arynchyna, Anastasia A., Johnston, James M., Rozzelle, Curtis J., Blount, Jeffrey P., Oakes, W. Jerry and Rocque, Brandon G. (2017). Risk factors for surgical site infection following nonshunt pediatric neurosurgery: a review of 9296 procedures from a national database and comparison with a single-center experience. *J Neurosurg Pediatr*, 19(4): 407–420.

[4] Subramanyam, Rajeev, Schaffzin, Joshua, Cudilo, Elizabeth M., Rao, Marepalli B., Varughese, Anna M. (2015). Systematic review of risk factors for surgical site infection in pediatric scoliosis surgery, *Spine J*, 15(6):1422-1431.

[5] Salsgiver E, Crotty J, LaRussa SJ, Bainton NM, Matsumoto H, Demmer RT, Thumm B, Vitale MG, Saiman L (2017). Surgical Site Infections following Spine Surgery for Non-idiopathic Scoliosis. *J Pediatr Orthop*, 37(8):e476-e483.

[6] Myung KS, Glassman DM, Tolo VT, Skaggs DL (2014). Simple steps to minimize spine infections in adolescent idiopathic scoliosis. *J Pediatr Orthop*, 34(1):29-33.

[7] Menger RP, Kalakoti P, Pugely AJ, Nanda A, Sin A (2017). Adolescent idiopathic scoliosis: risk factors for complications and the effect of hospital volume on outcomes. *Neurosurg Focus*, 43(4):E3.

[8] Pourtaheri S, Miller F, Dabney K, Shah SA, Dubowy S, Holmes L (2015). Deep Wound Infections After Pediatric Scoliosis Surgery. *Spine Deform*, 3(6): 533-540.

[9] Warner SJ, Uppstrom TJ, Miller AO, O'Brien ST, Salvatore CM, Widmann RF, Perlman SL(2017). Epidemiology of Deep Surgical Site Infections After Pediatric Spinal Fusion Surgery. *Spine* (Phila Pa 1976), 42(3): E163-E168.

[10] Farley FA, Li Y, Gilsdorf JR, VanderHave KL, Hensinger RN, Speers M, Childers D, Caird MS(2014). Postoperative spine and VEPTR infections in children: a case-control study. *J Pediatr Orthop*, 34(1):14-21.

[11] Marks MC, Newton PO, Bastrom TP, Betz RR, Sponseller PD, Lonner B, Shah SA, Samdani A, Petcharaporn M, Shufflebarger H, Asghar J; Harms Study Group(2013). Surgical Site Infection in Adolescent Idiopathic Scoliosis Surgery. *Spine Deform*, 1(5):352-358.

[12] Maesani M, Doit C, Lorrot M, Vitoux C, Hilly J, Michelet D, Vidal C, Julien-Marsollier F, Ilharreborde B, Mazda K, Bonacorsi S, Dahmani S(2016). Surgical Site Infections in Pediatric Spine Surgery: Comparative Microbiology of Patients with Idiopathic and Nonidiopathic Etiologies of Spine Deformity. *Pediatr Infect Dis J,* 35(1):66-70.

[13] Rihn JA, Lee JY, Ward WT (2008). Infection after the surgical treatment of adolescent idiopathic scoliosis: evaluation of the diagnosis, treatment, and impact on clinical outcomes. *Spine* (Phila Pa 1976), 33(3):289-294.

[14] Richards BR, Emara KM (2001). Delayed infections after posterior TSRH spinal instrumentation for idiopathic scoliosis: revisited. *Spine* (Phila Pa 1976), 26(18): 1990-1996.

[15] Soultanis K, Mantelos G, Pagiatakis A, Soucacos PN (2003). Late infection in patients with scoliosis treated with spinal instrumentation. *Clin Orthop Relat Res*, (411): 116-123.

[16] Abdullah KG, Attiah MA, Olsen AS, Richardson A, Lucas TH (2015). Reducing surgical site infections following craniotomy: examination of the use of topical vancomycin. *J Neurosurg*, 123:1600-1604.

[17] Edwards JR, Peterson KD, Mu Y (2008). National Healthcare Safety Network (NHSN) report: data summary for 2006 through 2008, issued December 2009. *Am J Infect Control,* 37 (10): 783-805.

[18] Tsiodras S, Falagas ME (2006). Clinical assessment and medical treatment of spine infections. *Clin Orthop Relat Res*, 444:38-50.

[19] Yang X, Xu H, Li M, Gu S, Fang X, Wang J, Ni J, Wu D(2010). Clinical and radiographic outcomes of the treatment of adolescent idiopathic scoliosis with segmental pedicle screws and combined local autograft and allograft bone for spinal fusion: a retrospective case series. *BMC Musculoskelet Disord*, 11:159.

[20] Gemmel F, Rijk PC, Collins JM, Parlevliet T, Stumpe KD, Palestro CJ(2010). Expanding role of 18F-fluoro-D-deoxyglucose PET and PET/CT in spinal infections. *Eur Spine J*, 19(4):540-551.

[21] Van Rhee MA, de Klerk LW, Verhaar JA. Vacuum-assisted wound closure of deep infections after instrumented spinal fusion in six children with neuromuscular scoliosis. *Spine J*. 2007;7:596–600.

[22] Canavese F, Gupta S, Krajbich JI, et al. Vacuum-assisted closure for deep infection after spinal instrumentation for scoliosis. *J Bone Joint Surg Br.* 2008;90:377–81.
[23] Hedequist D, Haugen A, Hresko T, et al.: Failure of attempted implant retention in spinal deformity delayed surgical site infections. *Spine* 2009, 34:60–64. This retrospective review demonstrated that implant removal is required for effective treatment of delayed surgical site infection after pediatric spinal deformity surgery. The number of hospitalizations, number of hospital days, number of operations, and cost of hospitalization correlated with the number of debridements performed before implant removal. Patients should be counseled that curve progression can occur and may require revision surgery after clearance of the infection.

In: Scoliosis: Diagnosis, Classification and Management Options ISBN: 978-1-53614-464-2
Editors: F. Canavese, A. Andreacchio and H. Xu © 2018 Nova Science Publishers, Inc.

Chapter 21

NEUROMONITORING SIGNAL DECREMENT: WHAT TO DO

Qianyu Zhuang* and Shujie Wang
Department of Orthopaedics, Peking Union Medical College Hospital,
Wangfujing, Beijing, China

ABSTRACT

Within the past 2 decades, the management of spinal deformities has changed significantly. Neurologic complications of spine deformity surgery are perhaps the most feared risk of these procedures. Intraoperative neuromonitoring (IONM) has become an essential component for decreasing the incidence of spinal cord injury during spine deformity surgery. It provides a safety measure for patients and surgeons by providing real-time assessment of neurological function. Generally, IONM alerts can be recused frequently by taking appropriate timely interventions during surgery. Therefore, our objective in this section is to summarize some strategies associated with IONM alerts in spine deformity correction surgeries.

Keywords: spinal deformities, intraoperative neuromonitoring (IONM), somatosensory evoked potentials (SSEPs), transcranial motor evoked potentials (TcMEPs); Intraoperative intervention strategy

INTRODUCTION

Within the past 2 decades, the management of spinal deformities has changed significantly. The advent and widespread use of pedicle screw fixation, in combination with advancements in posterior and 3-column osteotomy techniques, has permitted more aggressive deformity correction. Unfortunately, neurologic complications have been associated with increased complexity, large corrections, staged procedures, and significant blood loss. Although

---

* Corresponding Author Email: zhuangqianyu@126.com.

relatively infrequent, iatrogenic neurologic deficit can be a devastating complication. Intraoperative neuromonitoring (IONM) was developed in an effort to mitigate the risks to the sensitive neural elements during spine surgery.

IONM has become an essential component for decreasing the incidence of spinal cord injury during spine deformity surgery, including spinal cord deficits, cauda equine deficits and nerve root deficits. Several techniques are generally combined by the neurophysiologist to increase the sensitivity of intraoperative monitoring. Different monitoring alerts are then presented, illustrating the different responses to monitoring changes during spinal deformity surgery depending on the time of the alert during the surgery, the lesion level determined by the IONM, etc. A veteran IONM team who know the surgical maneuvers very well can timely and accurately find an impending monitoring loss.

Neurologic complications of spine deformity surgery are perhaps the most feared risk of these procedures. Neurologic complications may occur through a variety of mechanisms, including direct trauma to the spinal cord, ischemia, and stretch during deformity correction. Currently, transcranial motor evoked potentials (TcMEPs), somatosensory evoked potentials (SSEP), descending neurogenic-evoked potentials (DNEP), spontaneous electromyography (sEMG), and triggered EMG (tEMG) can detect these neurologic changes in a timely manner, allowing for intervention and reversal of neurologic deficits before they become permanent. The primary goal of IONM is to identify an impending neurologic deficit as early as possible and to facilitate interventions to minimize the risk of a lasting neurologic injury. The objective in this section is to summarize some strategies associated with IONM alerts in spine deformity correction surgeries.

SIGNAL DECREMENT, WHAT TO DO

During spinal deformity surgery, prompt evaluation and management of factors contributing to signal loss must occur in order to avoid permanent neurologic deficits. Although the use of multiple interventions such as the removal of spinal implants, set screws, and traction may be necessary, surgeons may first want to consider the influence from anesthetic factors. In 2014, Vitale et al. published an intraoperative checklist to provide a systematic approach for management when IONM change is encountered. Increasing cord perfusion by raising MAP has also been shown to restore IONM signals (Yang et al. 2017, Laratta et al. 2018, Vitale et al. 2014, Wang, Tian, et al. 2017, Wang and Tian 2016, Wang, Yang, et al. 2016, Zhuang et al. 2014).

MONITORING TECHNIQUES

Somatosensory Evoked Potentials (SSEPs)

Somatosensory evoked potentials (SSEPs) assess the functional integrity of the spinal cord sensory pathways leading from the peripheral nerve, through the dorsal column and to the sensory cortex. From a technical point of view, the posterior tibial nerves are stimulated (duration of stimulus, 0.2 ms; frequency, ~3 Hz; intensity, ~25 mA). Peripheral recordings are made at the level of internal popliteal sciatic nerves. A cortical recording is made in Cz, in regard of the primary somatosensory cortex of both lower limbs. SSEP are the result of averaging. The acquisition time is on the order of 1 min. An increase in latencies greater than 10% and a decrease in amplitudes greater than 50% constitute warning signals. SSEPs are altered by the surgical act due to a mechanical factor or secondarily by ischemia. SSEP alterations can also be related to systemic hypotension, hematocrit decrease, hypothermia, anesthesia (volatile agents such as isoflurane, halothane, nitrous oxide attenuate SSEP and should not be used if monitoring is employed) (Gavaret et al. 2013).

Studies by Hu et al. have shown that time–frequency analysis can provide both temporal and spectral information on the SEP waveform, which allows computation of parameters in the combined time and frequency domain. The time–frequency analysis of SSEP waveforms reveals stable and easily identifiable characteristics. Peak power is recommended as a more reliable monitoring parameter than amplitude, while peak time monitoring was not superior to latency measurement. Applying time–frequency analysis to SEP can improve the reliability of intraoperative spinal cord monitoring (Hu et al. 2003, Wang, Li, et al. 2017, Hu, Liu, and Luk 2011, Hu et al. 2002).

Transcranial Motor Evoked Potentials (TcMEPs)

TcMEPs are common elicited using subcutaneous needle electrodes by stimulation of constant voltage (from 250 to 500V) and multiple trains of 6–7 pulses, with duration of 200-400 μs for each pulse (Axon Systems Inc., Hauppauge, NY). The inter-stimulus interval was 2.5-4.0 ms for each stimulation trains. The filter bandpass was 30 to 1000 Hz and the time base were 100-ms window. The stimulation strength for preoperative spinal deficits (PPSDs) would be much stronger than normal neurological patient. The two pairs of stimulation electrodes were inserted subcutaneously into motor cortex regions C3–C4. Recording Muscles: in order to obtain optimal TcMEPs waveform in the limps of PPSDs, we recorded it at the muscles with higher strength (quadriceps, tibialis anterior, flexor hallucis longus, gastrocnemius, biceps femoris, abductor hallucis, etc.). However, the patient with lower extremity motor weakness of 0-1/5 strength for specific muscle groups often cannot be recorded reliable MEP baselines even if the maximum TcMEPs stimulation strength are used, for instance, there is no TcMEPs in our 11 paralyses and 6 incomplete paraplegia patients (Wang, Tian, et al. 2015, Wang, Yang, et al. 2016, Zhuang et al. 2014).

In addition, Zhuang et al. have explored the warning criteria of TcMEPs which included 3 main items: a more than 80% amplitude loss; synchronously and logically associated with high-risk surgical maneuver (pedicle screw insertion, osteotomy, correction, etc.); systemic and anesthetic factors being ruled out. Only when the data meet all above three criteria, it will be defined as a formal alert and then reported to the surgeon. The exact time and the surgical procedure when the signal decreased will be recorded and reported, too (Zhuang et al. 2014).

Descending Neurogenic-Evoked Potentials (DNEP)

Descending neurogenic-evoked potentials (DNEP) were used during any procedure involving the thoracic spine. All DNEP responses were recorded bilaterally from the sciatic nerve at the popliteal fossa. Stimulation was applied until a repeatable response could be obtained with minimum intensity. Muscle relaxation was required to prevent stimulation-induced movement of paraspinous musculature as well as limit muscle artifact in the response. Warning criteria for DNEPs were defined as an 80% decrease in amplitude and/or 10% increase in latency of the signal compared with baseline values.

Spontaneous Electromyography (sEMG) and Triggered EMG (tEMG)

Spontaneous electromyography (sEMG) may be a potential tool for detecting the early neurologic injury. And the sEMG combined with MEP in bilateral muscles was also used to explore early mechanical spinal cord injury. Calancie et al. first described the use of electrical stimulation of pedicle screws for evaluation of placement in an animal model. Since that time, tEMGs have been shown to be an effective tool for detecting pedicle breaches (Calancie et al. 1992).

There are numerous neuromonitoring tests in the surgeon's armamentarium to assist in performing safe spinal deformity surgery, with promising results previously discussed. Each neuromonitoring modality has potential benefits and drawbacks, but the use of multimodal neuromonitoring can be quite successful at alerting the surgeon to potential neurologic injury and guiding prompt intraoperative correction. A frequently used combination involves monitoring both SSEPs and MEPs. Somatosensory Evoked Potentials (SSEPs) should be used in all spine deformity cases. Transcranial Motor Evoked Potentials (TcMEPs) and/or Descending Neurogenic Evoked Potentials (DNEPs) should be used in all spine deformity cases. Vitale et al. recently published a consensus based best practice guideline for positive neuromonitoring warning signs in pediatric deformity. (Figure 1) the SSEP criteria for surgeon notification are an intraoperative unilateral or bilateral amplitude loss of at least 60% or 10% increase in latency. The tcMEP warning criteria of amplitude loss of at least 60% in the same study showed 100% specificity and sensitivity. The tEMG has sensitivity of 94% and specificity of 90% from an animal study using pedicle screws with a threshold of 10 V (Laratta et al. 2018, Vitale et al. 2014).

ANESTHESIA AND SYSTEMIC FACTORS

Total intravenous anesthesia (TIVA) is often utilized when IONM is used during spine surgery. The use of muscle relaxants permits a more reliable recording on the SSEP signals but can easily misinterpret the TcMEP findings (Owen 1999). In order to limit such undesirable interactions, TIVA is more commonly used in major adult deformity spinal cases in conjunction with SSEP and TcMEP signals, which provides a more accurate assessment of the entire spinal cord in real time. Balanced anesthesia, such as sevoflurane or desflurane, along with propofol and remifentanyl infusion is used as the standard protocol for monitoring. For cases relying on the use of TcMEPs, TIVA with Propofol, remifentanil, and sufentanil are used to prevent any potential interactions with the IONM modalities. Halogenated inhalation agents are only used in exceptional cases when patients have reactive airway disease or difficult blood pressure control while on TIVA. Isoflurane is well recognized to affect TcMEP recordings significantly.

Likewise, desflurane has been shown to alter the amplitude of SSEPs in rats and TcMEPs at 1 MAC. At 2 MAC, TcMEPs were completely unobtainable (Lo et al. 2006). And the use of a small quantity of N$_2$O/desflurane can acquire TcMEPs successfully signal during scoliosis surgery. Generally, the TIVA from the studies of Wang et al. were recommended, a bolus dose of propofol (3 mg/kg) and fentanyl (2.5 ug/kg) combined with a short-acting muscle relaxant and inhalation agents (sevoflurane or nitrous oxide). No muscle relaxants or inhalation agents were given after induction and intubation. Subsequently, maintenance of anesthesia was Propofol (5-8 mg/kg/h) based on hemodynamic response; remifentanil (0.1 ug/kg/min); and a total dose of 5-6 ug/kg fentanyl (intermittent infusion) were used during the whole operation (Wang, Tian, et al. 2017, Wang and Tian 2016, Wang, Yang, et al. 2016, Zhuang et al. 2014, Wang, Zhuang, et al. 2015, Wang, Tian, et al. 2015, Wang, Tian, et al. 2016, Wang, Zhang, et al. 2016).

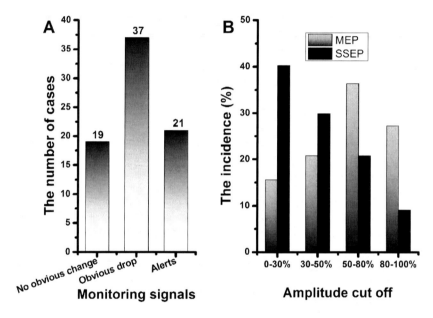

Figure 1. Final checklist for the response to intraoperative neuromonitoring changes in patients with a stable spine. (Vitale, et al. (2014). "Best Practices in Intraoperative Neuromonitoring in Spine Deformity Surgery: Development of an Intraoperative Checklist to Optimize Response." Spine Deform 2(5): 333-339.).

Return of IONM Signals by an Increase of MAP Alone

TcMEPs provide direct information on the corticospinal tract and indirect information on the status of the spinothalamic tract which correlates with the vascular supply of the anterior spinal artery. SSEP's provide information of the dorsal columns. Previous studies have defined spinal cord compromise as a decrease in amplitude of 50% to 80% or an increase in latency of >10% from baseline of TcMEP or SSEP. Increasing cord perfusion by raising Mean Arterial Pressure (MAP) has also been shown to restore IONM signals in other series. The findings of Yang et al. suggest raising MAPs above 85 mmHg should be considered the first step in response to IONM signal decrement, as this alone was successful in 20% of patients without sacrificing deformity correction. Concurrently, 60% of patients from their study had a return of IONM signals after an increase of blood pressure in conjunction with other interventions. Pediatric spine centers where the anesthesiologists are familiar with spinal deformity and cognizant of the need to keep the blood pressure elevated while the correction is being performed. Thus, the number of times blood pressure alone is a factor may be even higher at institutions where the operative team is less familiar with the procedure (Yang et al. 2017).

Intraoperative Blood Loss

On the other hand, intraoperative blood loss is also an important and potential high-risk factor for IONM loss. Because the intraoperative evoked potential or electroencephalogram can detect the pathophysiological state occurring in acute ischemia in which neurons are nonfunctional but still alive and salvageable by reperfusion, there is time to reverse the processes and prevent further irreversible ischemic neural damage. In addition, lumbosacral and cervical enlargements have 40% greater flow than the thoracic cord containing less gray matter. The thoracic cord ischemia has more influence on rapid muscle TcMEPs deterioration than cervical or lumbar segments, which is also an important reason for monitoring loss during severe scoliosis correction surgeries (Wang, Yang, et al. 2016).

Temperature

Low temperatures increase latencies of evoked potential and higher temperatures reduce them. The effect can be generalized according to body temperature or localized to a limb cooled by exposure or intravenous infusion, or to a spinal cord segment exposed to air or cool irrigation. Deep hypothermia obliterates muscle MEPs and SSEPs (Macdonald et al. 2013). In addition, there is a relationship between complete spinal cord injury and body surface temperature. This finding can be applied to aid the MEP monitoring as an ancillary measurement. Body surface temperature change may aid in maximizing the benefits of MEP by overcoming the limitations, such as the inability to differentiate between simple concussion and severe irreversible neurological damage (Yang et al. 2015).

A critical neurophysiologic alert triggered a sequence of interventional steps based on a predetermined algorithm. Regardless of whether the change was related to a particular surgical action, the anesthesiologist was always directed to raise the mean arterial blood pressure to at least 80 mm Hg to promote better spinal cord perfusion. In addition, the body temperature and blood loss should also be our consideration when the IONM alerts. If, after temporary cessation of the surgery and institution of hemodynamic management, the response amplitude failed to show signs of recovery over the course of 10 min, corrective forces were considered to reverse (Pastorelli et al. 2011).

PROPER SURGICAL RESPONDING STRATEGIES

According to Barry et al., the reasons for a signal change or loss were ranked according to frequency of occurrence (Table 1). Identifying the source or reason for a significant change or loss of IONM signals largely determined intervention strategy. True-positive reversals were not always achieved with single interventions. Although IONM signals degraded 406 times, intervention was required 441 times (Table 2). Intervention was not always successful (Raynor et al. 2013).

An adapted response to a IONM alert during scoliosis correction surgery is necessary: (1) release the correction and pursue the instrumentation or distraction if the potentials normalize rapidly, (2) reduce the correction to a level ensuring that the potentials normalize, (3) remove the material if normal values do not return, (4) leave the material in place in under correction so that instability that may compromise neurological recuperation is not induced (Gavaret et al. 2013).

Table 1. Causes of data degradation

	Instances	Patients in True-Positive Population	% of Total Population	Permanent Nerve Root Deficit	Permanent Cord Deficit
Screw placement	123	117	0.99		
Blood pressure	48	46	0.39		2
Patient positioning	39	37	0.32		
Wound retractor pressure	38	36	0.31		
Correction	32	30	0.26	1	1
Unknown	24	23	0.19	1	4
Shoulder taping	23	22	0.19		
Rod placement	13	12	0.11		
Halo-femoral traction	12	11	0.10		
Bony compression	12	11	0.10		
Traction weight	11	10	0.09		
Cage placement	7	7	0.06	1	
Spinal subluxation	7	7	0.06		2
Other	6	6	0.05		2
Osteotomy closure	3	3	0.02		
Tumor	3	3	0.02	1	
Cerebral ischemia	2	2	0.02		
Hook placement	1	1	0.01		
Segmental cross clamping	1	1	0.01		
Body temperature	1	1	0.01		
	406	386	3.28	4	11

(Significant Change or Loss of Intraoperative Monitoring Data: A 25-Year Experience in 12,375 Spinal Surgeries. Raynor, Barry; Bright, Joseph; Lenke, Lawrence; Rahman, Ra; Bridwell, Keith; Riew, K; Buchowski, Jacob; MD, MS; Luhmann, Scott; Padberg, Anne. Spine. 38(2):E101-E108, January 15, 2013).

IONM alert triggered identification procedures during 3-Column Osteotomies including (1) rule out IONM systematic and anesthetic factors; (2) verification of no residual bony or annulus structures around the resected area (corrective space), for the risk of impingement on the spinal cord, especially on the concave side of the vertebral canal; (3) if there was unstable spinal column, due to inadequate pedicle screw anchors connected to the temporary rod, or mismatched rod shape; (4) palpation and inspection on the tension of the spinal cord circumferentially, ensuring the tension on the concave side does not exceed the initial state, ensuring no excessive kinking of the dural sac near the convex side; (5) observe the excessive opposite displacement between two aspects of resected area (Wang, Xie, et al. 2017).

The surgery of posterior vertebral column resection (PVCR) has been a procedure known to be a high risk for neurologic complications. The surgical procedure of abrupt subluxation, laminar impingement, or cord buckling can all lead to spinal cord deficits. Because of the PVCR acutely destabilizes and separates vertebral columns, according to current data (Figure 2), the IONM often drops suddenly during the procedure of PVCR completion. Fortunately, most IONM loss may be reversible and will recover with placing the bilateral rod accordingly. In addition, according to Wang et al. there are at least 30 cases presenting IONM recovery after implanting the unilateral or bilateral temporary rod in this study.

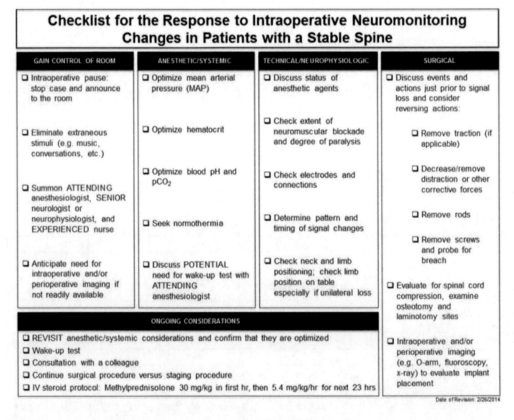

Figure 2. The number of intraoperative monitoring (IONM) changes after vertebral column resection completion. There are 19 cases showing no obvious monitoring change, 37 cases showing obvious IONM degenerations, and 21 cases showing significant IOM loss with alerts. (Wang S, Yang Y, Zhang J, Tian Y, Shen J, Wang S. Frequent neuromonitoring loss during the completion of vertebral column resections in severe spinal deformity surgery. Spine J. 2016).

Table 2. Intervention techniques

		Interventions	% of True-Positive Patients	% of Total Population
Instrumentation adjustment				
Redirect pedicle screw		75	17.0	0.61
Remove pedicle screw		58	13.2	0.47
Release correction		35	7.9	0.28
Remove all instrumentation		13	2.9	0.11
Recontour rods		6	1.4	0.05
Exchange fixation point		5	1.1	0.04
Realign spinal subluxation		4	0.9	0.03
Remove cage		3	0.7	0.02
	Total	199	45.1	1.61
Positioning adjustment				
Reposition patient		38	8.6	0.31
Release shoulder tape		26	5.9	0.21
Reduce traction weight		25	5.7	0.20
	Total	89	20.2	0.72
In situ adjustment				
Reposition retractors		39	8.8	0.32
Further decompression		29	6.6	0.23
Remove cross clamps		1	0.2	0.01
	Total	69	15.6	0.56
Systemic				
Raise blood pressure		52	11.8	0.42
Raise temperature		1	0.2	0.01
	Total	53	12.0	0.43
Other				
No intervention		17	3.9	0.14
Other		5	1.1	0.04
Abort		8	1.8	0.06
Unknown		1	0.2	0.01
	Total	31	7.0	0.25
	Grand Total	441.0	100.0	3.56

(Significant Change or Loss of Intraoperative Monitoring Data: A 25-Year Experience in 12,375 Spinal Surgeries. Raynor, Barry; Bright, Joseph; Lenke, Lawrence; Rahman, Ra; Bridwell, Keith; Riew, K; Buchowski, Jacob; MD, MS; Luhmann, Scott; Padberg, Anne. Spine. 38(2):E101-E108, January 15, 2013).

The approach aiming at the acute IONM loss during intraoperative PVCR reconstruction is fairly systematic. The first step is to make sure that the mean arterial blood pressure is greater than 80 mm Hg meanwhile excluding anesthetic factors. Generally, the IONM loss during this surgical point is sudden and we do not have sufficient time to perform a wake-up test. So, it is necessary to place bilateral rod immediately to further stabilize the spinal column. Moreover, the methylprednisolone is probably useful for patients with preoperative spinal deficits. Once the signals return promptly after these maneuvers, the surgeons can continue to perform the following surgical procedures (Wang, Yang, et al. 2016).

The Stagnara Wake-Up Test

The Stagnara wake-up test was used selectively. A lack of any usable monitoring data necessitated its use as the sole indicator of neurological status in a small number of patients. It was also used to confirm motor function after a loss or significant change in monitoring signals in some of the study population. A wake-up test was considered positive if the patient was unable to move any or all extremities sensitive to surgical variables. A negative wake-up test meant that the patient demonstrated movement in upper and/or lower extremities consistent with preoperative neurological status (Raynor et al. 2013).

CONCLUSION

Intraoperative neuromonitoring is best performed with a team approach: Surgeon, anesthesiologist, and qualified neuromonitoring personnel should all be involved in the identification and communication of neuromonitoring changes. The varied surgical population has provided an extensive array of reasons for loss or significant change of IOM data. Different spinal surgical procedures have unique and varying types of neurological risk. Determining the actual cause is critical in reducing any postoperative neurological deficit. And the approach aiming at IONM loss during intraoperative scoliosis correction surgery is fairly systematic. Once the IONM signals return promptly after the interventions, the surgeons can continue to perform the following deformity correction procedures. The ultimate goal was to confirm the utility of intraoperative neurological monitoring with appropriate intraoperative interventions to reduce postoperative neurological deficits and optimize patient outcomes.

REFERENCES

Calancie, B., Lebwohl, N., Madsen, P. and Klose, K. J. 1992. "Intraoperative evoked EMG monitoring in an animal model. A new technique for evaluating pedicle screw placement." *Spine (Phila Pa 1976)* 17 (10):1229-35.

Gavaret, M., Jouve, J. L., Pereon, Y., Accadbled, F., Andre-Obadia, N., Azabou, E., Blondel, B., Bollini, G., Delecrin, J., Farcy, J. P., Fournet-Fayard, J., Garin, C., Henry, P., Manel, V., Mutschler, V., Perrin, G., Sales de Gauzy, J. and Sfcr French Society of Spine Surgery. 2013.

Hu, Y., Liu, H. and Luk, K. D. 2011. "Time-frequency analysis of somatosensory evoked potentials for intraoperative spinal cord monitoring." *J Clin Neurophysiol* 28 (5):504-11. doi: 10.1097/WNP.0b013e318231c15c.

Hu, Y., Luk, K. D., Lu, W. W. and Leong, J. C. 2002. "Comparison of time-frequency analysis techniques in intraoperative somatosensory evoked potential (SEP) monitoring." *Comput Biol Med* 32 (1):13-23.

Hu, Y., Luk, K. D., Lu, W. W. and Leong, J. C. 2003. "Application of time-frequency analysis to somatosensory evoked potential for intraoperative spinal cord monitoring." *J Neurol Neurosurg Psychiatry* 74 (1):82-7.

"Intraoperative neurophysiologic monitoring in spine surgery. Developments and state of the art in France in 2011." *Orthop Traumatol Surg Res* 99 (6 Suppl):S319-27. doi: 10.1016/j.otsr.2013.07.005.

Laratta, J. L., Ha, A., Shillingford, J. N., Makhni, M. C., Lombardi, J. M., Thuet, E., Lehman, R. A. and Lenke, L. G. 2018. "Neuromonitoring in Spinal Deformity Surgery: A Multimodality Approach." *Global Spine J* 8(1):68-77. doi: 10.1177/2192568217706970.

Lo, Y. L., Dan, Y. F., Tan, Y. E., Nurjannah, S., Tan, S. B., Tan, C. T. and Raman, S. 2006. "Intraoperative motor-evoked potential monitoring in scoliosis surgery: comparison of desflurane/nitrous oxide with propofol total intravenous anesthetic regimens." *J Neurosurg Anesthesiol* 18 (3):211-4. doi: 10.1097/01.ana.0000211007.94269.50.

Macdonald, D. B., Skinner, S., Shils, J., Yingling, C. and Monitoring American Society of Neurophysiological. 2013. "Intraoperative motor evoked potential monitoring - a position statement by the American Society of Neurophysiological Monitoring." *Clin Neurophysiol* 124 (12):2291-316. doi: 10.1016/j.clinph.2013.07.025.

Owen, J. H. 1999. "The application of intraoperative monitoring during surgery for spinal deformity." *Spine (Phila Pa 1976)* 24 (24):2649-62.

Pastorelli, F., Di Silvestre, M., Plasmati, R., Michelucci, R., Greggi, T., Morigi, A., Bacchin, M. R., Bonarelli, S., Cioni, A., Vommaro, F., Fini, N., Lolli, F. and Parisini, P. 2011. "The prevention of neural complications in the surgical treatment of scoliosis: the role of the neurophysiological intraoperative monitoring." *Eur Spine J* 20 Suppl 1:S105-14. doi: 10.1007/s00586-011-1756-z.

Raynor, B. L., Bright, J. D., Lenke, L. G., Rahman, R. K., Bridwell, K. H., Riew, K. D., Buchowski, J. M., Luhmann, S. J. and Padberg, A. M. 2013. "Significant change or loss of intraoperative monitoring data: a 25-year experience in 12,375 spinal surgeries." *Spine (Phila Pa 1976)* 38 (2):E101-8. doi: 10.1097/BRS.0b013e31827aafb9.

Vitale, M. G., Skaggs, D. L., Pace, G. I., Wright, M. L., Matsumoto, H., Anderson, R. C., Brockmeyer, D. L., Dormans, J. P., Emans, J. B., Erickson, M. A., Flynn, J. M., Glotzbecker, M. P., Ibrahim, K. N., Lewis, S. J., Luhmann, S. J., Mendiratta, A., Richards, 3rd B. S., Sanders, J. O., Shah, S. A., Smith, J. T., Song, K. M., Sponseller, P. D., Sucato, D. J., Roye, D. P. and Lenke, L. G. 2014. "Best Practices in Intraoperative Neuromonitoring in Spine Deformity Surgery: Development of an Intraoperative Checklist to Optimize Response." *Spine Deform* 2 (5):333-339. doi: 10.1016/j.jspd.2014.05.003.

Wang, S., and Tian, Y. 2016. "Exploration of the Intraoperative Motor Evoked Potential." *Spine (Phila Pa 1976)* 41 (6):470-5. doi: 10.1097/BRS.0000000000001240.

Wang, S., Zhang, J., Tian, Y. and Shen, J. 2016. "Rare true-positive outcome of spinal cord monitoring in patients under age 4 years." *Spine J*. doi: 10.1016/j.spinee.2016.05.002.

Wang, S., Zhuang, Q., Zhang, J., Tian, Y., Zhao, H., Wang, Y., Zhao, Y., Li, S., Weng, X., Qiu, G. and Shen, J. 2015. "Intra-operative MEP monitoring can work well in the patients with neural axis abnormality." *Eur Spine J*. doi: 10.1007/s00586-015-4205-6.

Wang, S., Tian, Y., Wang, C., Lu, X., Zhuang, Q., Peng, H., Hu, J., Zhao, Y., Shen, J. and Weng, X. 2016. "Prognostic value of intraoperative MEP signal improvement during surgical treatment of cervical compressive myelopathy." *Eur Spine J*. doi: 10.1007/s00586-016-4477-5.

Wang, S., Tian, Y., Zhang, J., Shen, J., Zhao, Y., Zhao, H., Li, S., Yu, B. and Weng, X. 2015. "Intraoperative motor evoked potential monitoring to patients with preoperative spinal deficits: judging its feasibility and analyzing the significance of rapid signal loss." *Spine J.* doi: 10.1016/j.spinee.2015.09.028.

Wang, S., Tian, Y., Lin, X., Ren, Z., Zhao, Y., Zhai, J., Zhang, X., Zhao, Y., Dong, Y., Zhao, C. and Tian, Y. 2017. "Comparison of intraoperative neurophysiologic monitoring outcomes between cervical and thoracic spine surgery." *Eur Spine J.* doi: 10.1007/s00586-017-5194-4.

Wang, S., Yang, Y., Zhang, J., Tian, Y., Shen, J. and Wang, S. 2016. "Frequent neuromonitoring loss during the completion of vertebral column resections in severe spinal deformity surgery." *Spine J.* doi: 10.1016/j.spinee.2016.08.002.

Wang, Y. Z., Li, G. S., Luk, K. D. K. and Hu, Y. 2017. "Component analysis of somatosensory evoked potentials for identifying spinal cord injury location." *Scientific Reports* 7. doi: ARTN 235110.1038/s41598-017-02555-w.

Wang, Y., Xie, J., Zhao, Z., Li, T., Bi, N., Zhang, Y. and Shi, Z. 2017. "Proper Responding Strategies to Neuromonitoring Alerts During Correction Step in Posterior Vertebral Column Resection Patients With Severe Rigid Deformities Can Reduce Postoperative Neurologic Deficits." *Spine (Phila Pa 1976)* 42 (22):1680-1686. doi: 10.1097/BRS.0000000000002320.

Yang, J. H., Suh, S. W., Park, Y. S., Lee, J. H., Park, B. K., Ham, C. H. and Choi, J. W. 2015. "Change in body surface temperature as an ancillary measurement to motor evoked potentials." *Spinal Cord* 53 (11):827-834. doi: 10.1038/sc.2015.90.

Yang, J., Skaggs, D. L., Chan, P., Shah, S. A., Vitale, M. G., Neiss, G., N. Feinberg, and Andras, L. M. 2017. "Raising Mean Arterial Pressure Alone Restores 20% of Intraoperative Neuromonitoring Losses." *Spine (Phila Pa 1976).* doi: 10.1097/BRS.0000000000002461.

Zhuang, Q. Y., Wang, S. J., Zhang, J. G., Zhao, H., Wang, Y. P., Tian, Y., Zhao, Y., Li, S. G., Weng, X. S., Qiu, G. X. and Shen, J. X. 2014. "How to Make the Best Use of Intraoperative Motor Evoked Potential Monitoring? Experience in 1162 Consecutive Spinal Deformity Surgical Procedures." *Spine* 39 (24):E1425-E1432. doi: 10.1097/Brs.0000000000000589.

Chapter 22

EVALUATION AND CONSERVATIVE MANAGEMENT OF SPINAL DEFORMITIES IN PATIENTS WITH CEREBRAL PALSY

*Michèle Kläusler and Erich Rutz**
Pediatric Orthopedic Department, University Children's Hospital Basel UKBB, Basel, Switzerland

ABSTRACT

Scoliosis is a frequent condition in patients with cerebral palsy (CP), with an incidence rate between 20 to 25%. The incidence is related to the severity of neurologic involvement and thereby correlated to the Gross Motor Function Classification System (GMFCS) level. Though the cause for scoliosis in CP patients is still not entirely clear it is thought to be due to a combination of muscle weakness, truncal imbalance and asymmetric tone in paraspinous and intercostal muscles. Risk factors for progression are spinal curves greater than 40° Cobb angle before age of 15 years, total body involvement, being bedridden and a thoracolumbar curve.

A detailed assessment and evaluation is important for the discussion of non-operative versus operative treatment. Thereby information about extent of the neuromuscular disease, anatomical factors and functional impairments should be collected.

There are several conservative treatment options for neuromuscular scoliosis. The two main options are observation and bracing, though seating modification and medication is also part of the non-operative treatment. Bracing is recommended at a very early stage of scoliosis or trunk instability, which is when the patient becomes incapable of keeping in an upright position while sitting. In these early stages patients should be provided with a short lumbar brace for functional indications. For patients with scoliosis with a Cobb angle >20° we recommend to use a double-shelled brace when in upright position.

Keywords: spinal deformity, scoliosis, children, cerebral palsy, conservative, management

---

[*] Corresponding Author Email: erich_rutz@hotmail.com.

INTRODUCTION

Incidence

The incidence rate of adolescent idiopathic scoliosis (scoliosis without an obvious reason) is 1 to 2% if we use the general definition of scoliosis (10° of lateral curvature calculated by Cobb's method on a radiograph) whereas the prevalence of scoliosis in individuals with CP is much higher [1].

The most common found incidence of scoliosis in the overall CP population lies in between 20% to 25% [2-6], although in literature you will find an incidence from 6% to almost 100%. The different study design (especially age of studied population), the type of CP, the severity of neurologic involvement and the ambulatory status can explain this wide range of results [7]. For example Balmer and MacEwen [2] studied 100 radiographs of children in an outpatient clinic and found scoliosis of more than 10° Cobb angle in 21 children, whereas studies based on institutionalized adult patients, which are likely to be more impaired in cognitive and physical function have a much higher incidence of scoliosis.

Patients with spastic CP have the highest incidence (about 70%) of scoliosis whereas those with athetoid CP have the lowest rate (from 6% to 50%) [3, 8].

A study of Koop et al. [9] showed scoliosis greater than 40° Cobb angle in adulthood in 30% of CP patients with quadriplegia, 10% of those with diplegia, and 2% of those with hemiplegia. The forming of most of these curvatures started before these individuals reached 10 years of age.

In 1981, Madigan and Wallace [3] published a survey study of 272 institutionalized cerebral palsy patients, in which they studied their screening radiographs for scoliosis. They found scoliosis greater than 10° Cobb angle in 64% of the residents with CP and were also able to demonstrate that the severity of neurologic involvement is related to the incidence of scoliosis. Furthermore, they found an inverse relationship between ambulatory status and screening radiographs. 44% of the independent ambulators, 54% of the dependent ambulators, 61% of the independent sitters, 75% of the dependent sitters and 76% of the bedridden residents showed scoliosis. All of the bedridden patients were spastic and most them spastic quadriplegic. Almost all of the dyskinetic and ataxic group could walk independently or with help.

In 2012 Persson-Bunke et al. [10] published a study with a total population of 666 children with cerebral palsy which found a statistically significant relationship between Gross Motor Function Classification (GCMFS) level [11] and development of scoliosis. They found that nearly all children with a moderate or severe clinical scoliosis or a radiograph with scoliosis with a curve of more than 20° had a GMFCS level III-V. 50% of the children with a GCMFS level IV-V developed a severe scoliosis. They could also show that children with a GCMFS level I-II had no significant risk to develop scoliosis.

Pathophysiology

At this point in time, is not entirely clear what is the cause for scoliosis in CP, but it is thought to be due to a combination of muscle weakness, truncal imbalance, and asymmetric tone in paraspinous and intracostal muscles [7]. Multiple researchers have found a relation between the direction of wind-swept deformity and trunk decompensation, the convexity of the scoliosis being on the opposite side [1]. Rutz and Brunner [12] state that in their experience scoliosis is mainly a result of inadequate gravity control, which typically leads to lateral flexion of the thorax over the relative mobile spine, therefore the lumbar curve.

However it is long known that bone growth is reduced by pressure and increased by tension. Hence, lateral bending caused by inadequate trunk control is already a risk factor for scoliosis if there is enough time given.

Madigan and Wallace [3] also found that the incidence of scoliosis was higher in the group of CP patients with hip displacement and dislocated hips. They could not find any difference between bilaterally dislocated or only one-sided dislocated hips. And they concluded that scoliosis is rather influenced by the degree of neurologic impairment than the stability of the hip.

In 2010 Loeters et al. [13] published a systematic review article, finally looking at 10 studies, which were looking at the risk factors of developing a scoliosis in children with cerebral palsy. They found no clear association between age, type, location of the scoliotic curve and the progression of scoliosis. The single weak evidence they found was the association between the severity of CP, hip dislocation and pelvic obliquity and scoliosis. This given there is still a further need for research in about this topic.

There is also some data that suggests that certain spasticity treatments, in particular selective dorsal rhizotomy (SDR) and intrathecal baclofen possibly induce a progression of scoliosis.

The most recent systematic review study by Grunt et al. in 2011 [14] about the long-term outcome and adverse effects of SDR in children with CP found 6 studies with a follow-up time of 5 to 20 years, which assessed the incidence of spinal abnormalities and/or back pain after SDR. Even though a lot of patients showed spinal abnormalities over time, there has not been any comparison to a group who did not receive SDR and for this reason it remains unclear to what extent these abnormalities are due to SDR.

The best SDR candidates are CP patients with pure spasticity and good trunk control (unusually GMFCS I and II). There is little risk for these patient to develop scoliosis. SDR should be avoided in patients with GMFCS IV and V, because these patients often suffer from a mixed type CP with dystonia predominating [7].

Secondly for the intrathecal baclofen there are a few retrospective reviews and case reports which found a faster progression of the scoliotic curve after the insertion of a baclofen pump. The recent study by Segal et al. [15] reported a six-fold increase. On the other hand Shilt et al. [16] in a study with 50 patients with CP and baclofen pump insertion and matched controls found no difference. Also in this case it is to say that CP patients who usually get a baclofen pump are more severely involved patients and because of that there is a higher risk for progressive scoliosis also without a baclofen pump.

Since a clear relationship between SDR as well as intrathecal baclofen pump and progressive scoliosis could not be found there is still a need for long-term, randomized prospective studies.

Natural History

There are several studies on the topic of the natural history of untreated scoliosis in patients with CP, which look at the risk factors for progression and its impact on overall function and health. Factors, which are related to progression are type of involvement, poor functional status and curve location [7]. Thometz and Simons [5] discovered that thoracolumbar curves, followed by lumbar curves have the fastest progression rate and thoracic curves having the slowest progression.

Saito et al. [4] found in their study of 37 institutionalized children (mean age 7.8 years at starting and follow-up time of 17.3 years) with severe spastic cerebral palsy and scoliosis that risk factors for progression of scoliosis in spastic cerebral palsy are a spinal curve of 40° Cobb angle before age 15 years; having a total body involvement, being bedridden and a thoracolumbar curve. To prevent progression to severe scoliosis these patients might benefit from an early surgical intervention. In adult individuals with cerebral palsy it is common that also after skeletal maturation there is an increase in curve size [5].

A recent retrospective study by Lee et al. (2016) [17], has found that there was no significant annual change in Cobb angle, thoracic kyphosis and lumbar lordosis angles in the GMFCS level I-II and III. But in the GMFCS level IV-V group they could show a significant annually increase of 3.4° in the scoliosis Cobb angle, apical vertebral translation increase of 5.4 mm and increase by 2.2° of the thoracic kyphosis angle.

It is known that untreated severe scoliosis has a negative effect on a patient's health and function, especially in regards to the cardiopulmonary system and the sitting balance [7]. Majd et al. in 1997 [8] published a study about the natural history of scoliosis in the institutionalized adult cerebral palsy population in which they included 46 CP patients with scoliosis, which had an average follow-up period (evaluated periodically by radiographs and a clinical examination) of 8.5 years after diagnosis. They found that the patients who had a functionally decline during the course in the beginning had an average Cobb angle of 41.1° and a final curve of 80.6° (average progression rate of 4.4° per year), compared to an initial curve of 33.9° and a final curve of 56.5° (average progression rate of 3.0° per year) in stable patients. In this case it is important to say, that this study did not include any independently ambulatory patients in the beginning. Also Saito et al. [4] who's study included patients with severe cerebral palsy also found that patients who needed more nursing time to complete various activities in their daily life had a much higher Cobb angle than the patients who did not have a an increase in need for assistance (73° vs. 34°). Compared to that Kalen et al. [18] did no find a difference in incidence of decubiti, highest functional level achieved, functional loss, oxygen saturation or pulse in patients with untreated scoliosis in 14 residents with a Cobb angle >45° compared with 42 residents with mild or no curves.

It is important to mention that sitting balance is very crucial in the daily life of a wheelchair bound patient with CP. If the curve of scoliosis is so great, that the wheelchair cannot be modified anymore the patient will rely on his upper extremities to remain in an upright position and he is not able to use his upper extremities for other task anymore [7].

CLINICAL ASSESSMENT AND EVALUATION

In the initial evaluation of any patient with spinal deformity it is necessary to identify the underlying diagnosis and to determine any functional limitations caused by the spinal deformity [19]. A discussion with the patient and parents helps to assess the key components of the neuromuscular disease. The evaluation should include details of the birth history, the perinatal period, developmental milestones, family history and the age at diagnosis. The age of onset of neuromuscular scoliosis is usually earlier than adolescent idiopathic scoliosis.

The clinical examination of the patient helps to evaluate the degree of deformity. It should be started by a careful inspection. The inspection may show a shoulder asymmetry, a rip prominence, pelvic obliquity, trunk imbalance and "wind-swept" hip deformity. It is also important to pay attention to the presence of limb-length discrepancy, funnel and pigeon breast, contractures, spasticity, hip dislocation, and any skin breakdowns.

The physical examination should be done in a lying (recumbent and procumbent) as well as in a sitting position and if possible also while standing and during ambulation [20].

In upright position it is possible to assess finger-floor-distance, measure a rip-prominence, measure with a perpendicular if the spine is balanced and define the range of movement of the spine.

In a recumbent position there is no effect of gravity (no weight-bearing of head and trunk) and in this position it is simpler to assess the level of passive correctability respectively the structural part of the deformity. By marking of the spinal processes it is possible to get a rough overview over the extension of the scoliosis. The lying position is also important for the planning process of the conservative treatment and surgical therapy. Through traction on arms and limbs in a procumbent position as well as with the help of the recurve maneuver, during which the knee of the examiner is placed in the curve apex, it is possible to obtain information about the passive (over-)correctability.

While sitting there is no influence of a possible limb-length discrepancy. The examination of movement of the lumbar region is best in a sitting position because of the fixation of the pelvis. Through traction on the head it is possible to assess the level of passive ability of erection. Brace adjustment and evaluation of seating modifications should also be done in a sitting position.

In case of a scoliosis the examiner has to distinguish between its anatomical forms (kypho- and lordoscoliosis) and its distribution (cervical, thoracic, lumbar). Also the relation between hip joint asymmetry and position of the pelvis are of interest. It is of importance to recognize habitual trunk side leaning while sitting or standing. In severely disabled patients the spine and trunk musculature can have a serious spastic activity increase. Furthermore the assessment should include a neurological examination.

A crucial part of the clinical examination is also the assessment of the functional impairment [19]. Because of the underlying cause of their disorder patients with neuromuscular scoliosis are in general more affected in their functioning compared to those patients with idiopathic scoliosis. For an unassisted ambulation these patients may need bracing or assistive devices. There can be problems with the sitting balance on a static surface as well as in a wheelchair. In severe cases the patients need both arms to keep their balance while sitting. A conversation with the patient, family, caregivers, therapists and teachers can help to gather more information about the patient's function level in daily life.

As a next step an imaging should be done to quantify and monitor the degree of deformity. Usually plain films are used to evaluate and monitor curves. If possible x-rays of the spine should be done while sitting or standing in order to allow an evaluation of the deformity with the effect of gravity compared to non-weight-bearing imaging. Functional x-rays help to evaluate the correctability and plan the treatment.

An evaluation of the complications of the neuromuscular disease is also very important in the process of evaluation. Due to the spinal deformity the patient can develop respiratory problems, because of the weakness of the intrinsic and accessory muscles. If there is a thoracic spinal deformity there might be a decreased volume of the thorax, which can cause a diminished forced vital capacity as well as a restrictive lung disease. Worst case this can progress to alveolar hypoventilation, carbon dioxide retention, pulmonary hypertension and right-sided heart failure. The reduced pulmonary function carries also an increased risk of pneumonia and recurrent respiratory infections [21]. Furthermore there is also a higher prevalence of sleep disordered breathing in patients with neuromuscular disease [22].

The data collected through this whole evaluation process is important for the discussion of non-operative versus operative treatment.

CONSERVATIVE TREATMENT

Non-operative treatment options for scoliosis in CP patient are mainly observation and bracing, but also seating modifications and medication is part of the conservative treatment. The aim is the improvement of the sitting control and the reduction or modification of the curve progression without surgical treatment [23].

In general there are two options to provide external support to the spine when there is a presence of neuromuscular scoliosis, one of them are customized seating arrangements and the other one are braces [1]. Almost all patient with a neuromuscular disease have difficulties such as poor balance control and dynamic instability of the trunk. In the beginning the patient will only present with dynamic instability of the trunk, this can be easily tested by asking the patient to put his hands up while sitting. The aim of any intervention is to retain comfortable sitting and to enable functional use of the upper extremity [12].

A study by Terjesen et al. [24] published in 2000 of 86 patients with spastic quadriplegic cerebral palsy found some evidence that braces may slow down curve progression. Though it is still not clear if spinal bracing reduces the amount of surgery indications [1]. And it is still not clear if bracing can stop progression [1, 4, 7, 24-28].

But still, spinal bracing is a well-described and established conservative treatment option for children with CP [24, 26, 27, 29-32]. There have been multiple alternative modalities investigated such as physical therapy, electrical stimulation and botulinum toxin A. Whereas there could not be shown any effectiveness for physical therapy and electrical stimulation, there is a scant evidence for benefit in using botulinum toxin A in treating scoliosis in individuals with CP [7].

The start of the bracing treatment is recommended at a very early stage, when the patient becomes incapable of keeping in an upright position while sitting (positive hands up test) [12]. In these early stages patients should be provided with a short lumbar brace for functional indications. Patients with scoliosis with a Cobb angle >20° should wear a double-shelled brace when in an upright position.

Early Treatment with Short Lumbar Brace

There is a recent published study about short-term results of early treatment with short lumbar bracing (Figure 1) in 31 children (14 boys, 17 girls; mean age 12.6 years, range 3-24 years) with a neuromuscular disease resulting in dynamic trunk instability [33]. Of the 31 included children, 21 suffered from spastic quadriplegia and the other 10 patients from other neuromuscular disorders. At the study onset the mean lumbar Cobb angle was 25.3° (range 10-48°) and the thoracic Cobb angle 9.9° (range 2-15°). After the mean follow-up time of 28.3 months (range 12-38 months) the mean lumbar Cobb angle measured 16.0° (range 0-52°), which is a significant correction ($p < 0.001$), and the mean thoracic Cobb angle was 7.1° (range 0-35°). That means the correction of the lumbar Cobb angle was on average 36.7% and the correction of the thoracic Cobb angle 39.4%. In only 3 cases there was a progression of the Cobb angles during the study period. On average there were 2.0 short braces per patient were used during the study time of 28.3 months.

We recommend this treatment for mildly affected cases, but they emphasize that close observation clinically as well radiologically is important.

Double Shelled Braces

At our department all patients with scoliosis with a Cobb angle over 20° get a double-shelled brace (Figure 2). The main problem is that patients, parents and caregivers not always accept them well. As already described by Terjesen et al. [24] a very important part of the conservative treatment with bracing the braces have to be checked for correct fitting. We recommend a tight fit at the pelvis, an adequate spacer between pelvis and ribs, and a wider fit at the thorax for breathing. It is important to have a large open window at the belly to allow eating while wearing the brace. It is important that the brace is simple to handle. An important part in the production process of the brace is taking the mold. Best way to get immediate and optimal correction so is to take it in overcorrection (bending to the convex side) of the patient. With the mold in overcorrection large contact areas in the corrective position are provided without putting on pressure locally the way form pads do. It is important to remember that soft tissue stays compressible and for this reason braces always have the tendency to be too wide at the pelvis dorsally over the glutei as well as the waist and too tight at the ribs. Though a tight fitting in addition provides a broader contact area and can better control the included segments. It is important to pay attention to the pelvis, because a wide fitting there does not allow accurate control of the lumbar spine. It is crucial that the brace is always worn when the patient is under influence of gravity and while in an upright position (while sitting and standing). After the final corrections have been made the braces always have to be checked by radiographs (at minimum an anterior-posterior view under load without and with the brace). This is fundamental to check any correction that should be at least 30%.

Figures 3 and 4 present clinical cases.

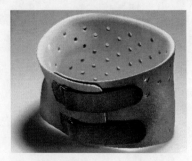

Figure 1. Short lumbar brace. (Picture with permission from Basler Orthopädie, René Ruepp AG, Basel, Switzerland).

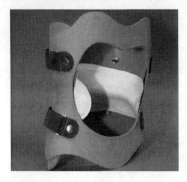

Figure 2. Double shelled brace. (Picture with permission from Basler Orthopädie, René Ruepp AG, Basel, Switzerland).

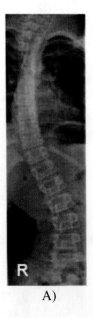
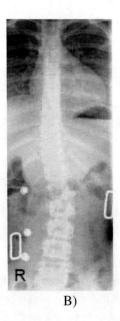

A)   B)

Figure 3. Clinical case I. Satisfactory correction of a neuromuscular scoliosis in a 12 years old girl with spastic quadriplegia. A) Without a brace; the Cobb angles were 35° (lumbar) and 25° (thoracic). B) With a short lumbar brace; the angles were 12° (lumbar) and 4° (thoracic).

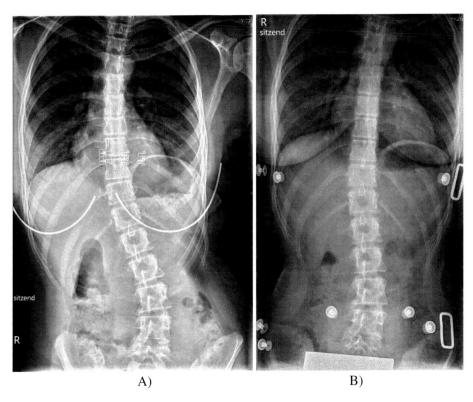

A) B)

Figure 4. Clinical case II. Satisfactory correction of a neuromuscular scoliosis in a 16 years old girl with spastic quadriplegia. A) Without a brace; the Cobb angles were 26° (lumbar) and 12° (thoracic). B) With a double shelled brace; the angles were 14° (lumbar) and 8° (thoracic).

Seating Modifications

As mentioned earlier another treatment option, especially also for patients, which cannot tolerate bracing well but also for patients with bracing, are seating modifications [7]. These modifications usually include adaptation on the patient's wheelchair with a variety of supports. There are many different seating modifications that can be used such as custom-molded seatbacks for sever spinal deformity or 2- and 3-point body support systems. The best static correction can be achieved with the 3-point force configuration [34]. Though it is important that modifications are individually determined and tailored.

CONCLUSION

In our opinion, spinal braces are a good treatment option for functional reasons in order to improve head and hand function as well as potentially preventing spinal deformities which often develop when side leaning positions are prevalent. If there is a dynamic instability of the trunk we suggest an early treatment with a short lumbar brae for functional reasons. If scoliosis (Cobb angle >20°) is present braces need to be implemented early and they need to be worn constantly to prevent progression. For these requirements we recommend short bivalve braces, which with optimal correction seem to fit best.

REFERENCES

[1] Koop SE. Scoliosis in cerebral palsy. *Developmental medicine and child neurology*. 2009;51 Suppl 4:92-8.

[2] Balmer GA, MacEwen GD. The incidence and treatment of scoliosis in cerebral palsy. *The Journal of bone and joint surgery British volume*. 1970;52(1):134-7.

[3] Madigan RR, Wallace SL. Scoliosis in the institutionalized cerebral palsy population. *Spine*. 1981;6(6):583-90.

[4] Saito N, Ebara S, Ohotsuka K, Kumeta H, Takaoka K. Natural history of scoliosis in spastic cerebral palsy. *Lancet*. 1998;351(9117):1687-92.

[5] Thometz JG, Simon SR. Progression of scoliosis after skeletal maturity in institutionalized adults who have cerebral palsy. *The Journal of bone and joint surgery American volume*. 1988;70(9):1290-6.

[6] McCarthy JJ, D'Andrea LP, Betz RR, Clements DH. Scoliosis in the child with cerebral palsy. *The Journal of the American Academy of Orthopaedic Surgeons*. 2006;14(6):367-75.

[7] Imrie MN, Yaszay B. Management of spinal deformity in cerebral palsy. *The Orthopedic clinics of North America*. 2010;41(4):531-47.

[8] Majd ME, Muldowny DS, Holt RT. Natural history of scoliosis in the institutionalized adult cerebral palsy population. *Spine*. 1997;22(13):1461-6.

[9] Koop S, Lonstein J, Winter R, Denis F, editors. *The natural history of spine deformity in cerebral palsy*. 25th Annual Meeting, Scoliosis Research Society; 1991.

[10] Persson-Bunke M, Hagglund G, Lauge-Pedersen H, Wagner P, Westbom L. Scoliosis in a total population of children with cerebral palsy. *Spine* (Phila Pa 1976). 2012;37(12):E708-13.

[11] Palisano RJ, Hanna SE, Rosenbaum PL, Russell DJ, Walter SD, Wood EP, et al. Validation of a model of gross motor function for children with cerebral palsy. *Physical therapy*. 2000;80(10):974-85.

[12] Rutz E, Brunner R. Management of spinal deformity in cerebral palsy: conservative treatment. *Journal of children's orthopaedics*. 2013;7(5):415-8.

[13] Loeters MJ, Maathuis CG, Hadders-Algra M. Risk factors for emergence and progression of scoliosis in children with severe cerebral palsy: a systematic review. *Dev Med Child Neurol*. 2010;52(7):605-11.

[14] Grunt S, Becher JG, Vermeulen RJ. Long-term outcome and adverse effects of selective dorsal rhizotomy in children with cerebral palsy: a systematic review. *Developmental medicine and child neurology*. 2011;53(6):490-8.

[15] Segal LS, Wallach DM, Kanev PM. Potential complications of posterior spine fusion and instrumentation in patients with cerebral palsy treated with intrathecal baclofen infusion. *Spine*. 2005;30(8):E219-24.

[16] Shilt JS, Lai LP, Cabrera MN, Frino J, Smith BP. The impact of intrathecal baclofen on the natural history of scoliosis in cerebral palsy. *Journal of pediatric orthopedics.* 2008;28(6):684-7.

[17] Lee SY, Chung CY, Lee KM, Kwon SS, Cho KJ, Park MS. Annual changes in radiographic indices of the spine in cerebral palsy patients. *Eur Spine J.* 2016;25(3):679-86.

[18] Kalen V, Conklin MM, Sherman FC. Untreated scoliosis in severe cerebral palsy. *Journal of pediatric orthopedics.* 1992;12(3):337-40.

[19] Allam AM, Schwabe AL. Neuromuscular scoliosis. *PM & R: the journal of injury, function, and rehabilitation.* 2013;5(11):957-63.

[20] Döderlein L. *Infantile Zerebralparese: Diagnostik, konservative und operative Therapie:* [*Infantile cerebral palsy: diagnosis, conservative and operative therapy.*] Steinkopff Verlag; 2007.

[21] Kim H, Murphy N, Kim CT, Moberg-Wolff E, Trovato M. Pediatric rehabilitation: 5. Transitioning teens with disabilities into adulthood. PM & R: *The journal of injury, function, and rehabilitation.* 2010;2(3):S31-7.

[22] Krachman SL, Criner GJ, Chatila W. Cor pulmonale and sleep-disordered breathing in patients with restrictive lung disease and neuromuscular disorders. *Seminars in respiratory and critical care medicine.* 2003;24(3):297-306.

[23] Cloake T, Gardner A. The management of scoliosis in children with cerebral palsy: a review. *J Spine Surg.* 2016;2(4):299-309.

[24] Terjesen T, Lange JE, Steen H. Treatment of scoliosis with spinal bracing in quadriplegic cerebral palsy. *Developmental medicine and child neurology.* 2000;42(7):448-54.

[25] Kotwicki T, Jozwiak M. Conservative management of neuromuscular scoliosis: personal experience and review of literature. *Disability and rehabilitation.* 2008;30(10):792-8.

[26] Winter RB, Carlson JM. Modern orthotics for spinal deformities. *Clinical orthopaedics and related research.* 1977(126):74-86.

[27] James WV. Spinal bracing in children with atonic cerebral palsy. *The Ulster medical journal.* 1975;44(1):53-5.

[28] Zadek RE. Orthopedic management of the child and multiple handicaps. *Pediatric clinics of North America.* 1973;20(1):177-85.

[29] Baumann JU. *Zeitschrift fur Orthopadie und ihre Grenzgebiete.* [*Conservative therapy of scoliosis in cerebral palsy*]. 1976;114(4):496-8.

[30] Brunner R, Gebhard F. Neurogenic spinal deformities. I. Conservative and surgical treatment of spinal deformities. *Der Orthopade.* 2002;31(1):51-7.

[31] Nuzzo RM. Dynamic bracing: elastics for patients with cerebral palsy, muscular dystrophy and myelodysplasia. *Clinical orthopaedics and related research.* 1980(148):263-73.

[32] Bunnell WP, MacEwen GD. Non-operative treatment of scoliosis in cerebral palsy: preliminary report on the use of a plastic jacket. *Developmental medicine and child neurology.* 1977;19(1):45-9.

[33] Rutz E, Brunner R. Lumbales Kurzkorsett zur Behandlung der neuromuskularen Skoliose. [Lumbar short corset for the treatment of neuromuscular scoliosis.] *Medizinisch orthopadische technik.* 2008;128(3):71.

[34] Holmes KJ, Michael SM, Thorpe SL, Solomonidis SE. Management of scoliosis with special seating for the non-ambulant spastic cerebral palsy population--a biomechanical study. *Clin Biomech* (Bristol, Avon). 2003;18(6):480-7.

In: Scoliosis: Diagnosis, Classification and Management Options   ISBN: 978-1-53614-464-2
Editors: F. Canavese, A. Andreacchio and H. Xu   © 2018 Nova Science Publishers, Inc.

Chapter 23

NEUROMUSCULAR SCOLIOSIS: SURGICAL CONSIDERATIONS AND MANAGEMENT OF COMPLICATIONS

Ismat Ghanem[1,2], Maroun Rizkallah[1],* and Federico Canavese[3]

[1]Faculty of Medicine, Saint-Joseph University,
Beirut, Lebanon
[2]Hôtel-Dieu de France University Hospital, Saint-Joseph University,
Beirut, Lebanon
[3]University Hospital Estaing, University Clermont Auvergne,
Clermont Ferrand, France

ABSTRACT

Scoliosis deformity is frequently diagnosed in Cerebral palsy (CP) patients. Its incidence and progression is related to the functional level of the patient. The direct etiology of scoliosis in CP patients is not clear, but its natural history is well documented. A little place for conservative management is reserved for bracing and sitting adjustments for patients with small curves. When surgery is indicated, preoperative assessment and multidisciplinary approach remain very important as they can help prevent major complications especially infection. Pelvic obliquity correction through fixation to the pelvis as well as adequate seating remains the most important objectives of treatment. Surgery has changed during the last 50 years especially for instrumentation, technique and approach, but randomized control studies are still needed to answer conflictual questions, as available literature could not favor any technique.

Keywords: scoliosis, cerebral palsy, surgical treatment, complication

---

* Corresponding Author Email: maroun.rizkallah@gmail.com (Rizkallah Maroun, Saint Joseph University, Faculty of Medicine, Beirut, Lebanon, Department of Orthopedic Surgery, Hôtel-Dieu de France Hospital, Saint Joseph University, Beirut, Lebanon, Alfred Naccache Street, Achrafieh, Beirut, Lebanon)

INTRODUCTION

Scoliosis is a three dimensional deformity of the spine with lateral, antero-posterior and rotational components (Gomez, Hresko, and Glotzbecker 2016). In most cases it is idiopathic (Gomez, Hresko, and Glotzbecker 2016; R Vialle, Mary, and Marty 2012). Non-idiopathic cases are often secondary to neuromuscular diseases affecting the neuro-musculo-skeletal (NMS) system (Mary, Servais, and Vialle 2018). Scoliosis incidence in the cerebral palsy population ranges from 6% to almost 100% as 20 to 25% of CP patients will at some point of their lifetime develop scoliosis (Balmer and MacEwen 1970; Madigan and Wallace, n.d.; Saito et al. 1998; Thometz and Simon 1988; J. J. McCarthy et al. 2006; R Vialle, Thévenin-Lemoine, and Mary 2013). In CP patients, scoliosis cannot be managed the same way as in adolescents with idiopathic scoliosis (J. J. McCarthy et al. 2006). Among all types of scoliosis, scoliosis in CP deformities entails the highest morbidity and mortality rates (J. J. McCarthy et al. 2006). This chapter reviews the pathophysiology, the natural history as well as medical and surgical treatments of CP scoliosis together with complications associated to the latter.

PATHOPHYSIOLOGY AND RISK FACTORS

The specific etiology of scoliosis in CP patients is not well understood but seems to be an association of muscle weakness, trunk imbalance, and asymmetric tone in the paraspinous and intercostal muscles (Mary, Servais, and Vialle 2018; Brooks and Sponseller 2016; Halawi, Lark, and Fitch 2015). Whether the development of scoliosis is due to the primary cerebral insult or to its secondary consequences is still unclear (Brooks and Sponseller 2016; R Vialle, Thévenin-Lemoine, and Mary 2013).

The incidence of scoliosis in CP depends on a variety of factors such as the type of CP, the severity of neurologic involvement, and the ambulatory status (Hägglund et al. 2018). For example, the incidence is higher in patients having spastic versus athetoid forms of CP (6% vs. 50%) (Madigan and Wallace, n.d.; Saito et al. 1998; Thometz and Simon 1988; J. J. McCarthy et al. 2006; Langerak et al. 2009). Madigan and Wallace, in their survey of institutionalized CP patients found that 64% of the 272 evaluated patients had scoliosis greater than 10 degrees on screening radiographs and that the incidence of scoliosis was directly correlated to the severity of neurologic involvement(Madigan and Wallace, n.d.). In support to this conclusion, they pointed to the reverse relationship between ambulatory status and scoliosis (44% of independent ambulators, 54% of dependent ambulators, 61% of independent sitters, and 75% of dependent sitters or bedridden residents had scoliosis) (Madigan and Wallace, n.d.). Even more, Golan and colleagues found that none of their patients with curves greater than 45 degrees were ambulating, whereas 34% of those with curves less than 45 degrees were ambulatory (Golan et al. 2007). Having a higher gross motor function level (GMFCS) is associated with a higher incidence of scoliosis (Madigan and Wallace, n.d.). Hagglund et al. found in their prospective study that the incidence of scoliosis was related to age and GMFCS level. In individuals at the lowest level of gross motor function (GMFCS V) scoliosis was seen in 10/131 before 5 years of age. At the age of 20 years, 75% of these individuals had a Cobb angle $\geq 40°$. No one in the highest level of motor function (GMFCS I) developed a Cobb angle $\geq 40°$. (Hägglund et al. 2018).

On the other hand, having a subluxated or dislocated hip is positively correlated with scoliosis as incidence of scoliosis rises to around 75% in patients with subluxated and dislocated hips (J. J. McCarthy et al. 2006). Interestingly, no difference was found between patients with unilateral or bilateral dislocated hips, underscoring the importance of severity of involvement rather than the balance of the pelvis (J. J. McCarthy et al. 2006). Similarly, history of previous hip surgery, intractable epilepsy, and female gender are predictors of severe scoliosis in children with cerebral palsy (Bertoncelli et al. 2017)

Selective dorsal rhizotomy (SDR) and intrathecal baclofen, which constitutes the treatment commonly used for CP patients, may result in progressive scoliosis (Ravindra et al. 2017). SDR is done with the intention of decreasing spasticity (Aquilina, Graham, and Wimalasundera 2015). It has been implicated by some investigators in increasing spinal deformities with the incidence of scoliosis ranging from 16% to 57% in patients with SDR (Langerak et al. 2009; Golan et al. 2007; Steinbok et al. 2005; Johnson et al., n.d.; Spiegel et al., n.d.; Turi and Kalen, n.d.; Peter et al. 1990; Peter, Hoffman, and Arens 1993; Ravindra et al. 2017). In the long term follow up of patients operated of SDR, Langerak demonstrated an incidence of 57% of scoliosis (Langerak et al. 2009). Most of the operated patients were GMFCS I or II. Those patients rarely develop scoliosis and have a good trunk control. The previously reported scoliosis cases were less than 30 degree and the scoliosis had no clinical impact. It is still unclear how SDR affects spinal deformity but it is felt that a greater attention to the integrity of the laminae would possibly prevent the development of scoliosis (Langerak et al. 2009). When SDR is indicated in patients with severe CP, it remains a safe procedure (Ravindra et al. 2017). On the other hand, no causal relationship has been proved between the use of intrathecal Baclofen and the evolution of scoliosis knowing that it is used in deeply affected patients in whom the scoliosis is often severe(Ginsburg and Lauder 2007; Sansone et al., n.d.; Segal, Wallach, and Kanev 2005; Shilt et al. 2008; Scannell and Yaszay 2015). However it seems that the use of intrathecal baclofen accelerates up to 6 times the progression of a preexisting scoliosis (Ginsburg and Lauder 2007; Sansone et al., n.d.). There are some reports that compare matched patients and demonstrate no increased incidence of scoliosis with Baclofen pump use (Shilt et al. 2008). Another recent report shows no difference in the rates of new-onset neuromuscular scoliosis for those with CP and intra thecal baclofen (ITB) pumps and those without ITB pumps; however, there was a higher rate of progression as well as an increased rate of posterior spine fusion surgery in individuals with CP who had ITB pumps compared to those who did not have ITB pumps (Walker, Novotny, and Krach 2017). Note of importance is that patients that need a Baclofen pump often have a natural history of severe progressive scoliosis (Scannell and Yaszay 2015).

NATURAL HISTORY

In opposition to risk factors and pathophysiology, spinal deformity progression in children with CP has been well described (Oda et al. 2017). As with the development of any other deformity in CP, the incidence and progression of the deformity is related to the functional level of the patient (Hägglund et al. 2018; Oda et al. 2017). Scoliosis is the most common form of spinal deformity in cerebral palsy; its incidence has been reported to be as high as 77% in some studies (Koop 2009; Thometz and Simon 1988). The results of the majority of the studies show that natural history of scoliosis is actually correlated to the severity of involvement of the CP child (Koop 2009; Thometz and Simon 1988; Oda et al. 2017). Koop found a higher incidence of scoliosis in patients with quadriplegic involvement (Koop 2009). In their study 30% of quadriplegic children developed scoliosis of greater than 40 degrees at skeletal maturity compared with only 2% in children with hemiplegia (Koop 2009). In a more recent study, Persson-Bunke and colleagues analyzed the correlation between the incidence of scoliosis and children's GMFCS level (Persson-Bunke et al. 2012). They demonstrated that only children with GMFCS level IV and V developed clinically significant scoliosis of greater than 40 degrees (Persson-Bunke et al. 2012). Severely involved children develop scoliosis at a younger age (< 15 years of age) (Lee et al. 2016). Thus, they have a higher risk for progression even after skeletal maturity (Lee et al. 2016). Thometz and Simon showed that after skeletal maturity, curves below 50 degrees progressed at a rate of 0.8 degree per year, whereas those above 50 degrees progressed at a rate of 1.4 degree per year (Thometz and Simon 1988). While curves progress in ambulatory children at a rate of 0.9 degree per year, they tend to progress at a higher rate of 2.4 degree per year in nonambulatory children (Thometz and Simon 1988).

Scoliosis in CP children often has a long C shape and frequently involves the pelvis (Vialle, Thévenin-Lemoine, and Mary 2013; Lonstein and Akbarnia 1983). This curve pattern is more frequent in quadriplegics patients (Vialle, Thévenin-Lemoine, and Mary 2013). The more functional patients are, the more idiopathic like the curves become (Porter, Michael, and Kirkwood 2007). The more severe the scoliosis, the higher functional impairment as well as affections of activities of daily living (Porter, Michael, and Kirkwood 2007; Vialle, Thévenin-Lemoine, and Mary 2013). Ultimately, scoliosis will induce a pelvic obliquity that will affect seating position (Porter, Michael, and Kirkwood 2007). Patient can develop contact pressure and ulceration related to the imbalanced position leading to pain and infections (Porter, Michael, and Kirkwood 2007). The loss of upright sitting ability may also cause a decrease in pulmonary function leading to feeding problems and exacerbating gastroesophageal reflux(R Vialle, Thévenin-Lemoine, and Mary 2013).

Majd and colleagues, in their survey of institutionalized adults with CP, found that those patients who experienced a decline in function had the greatest Cobb angle and rate of progression (80 vs 56 degrees and 4.4 vs 3.0 degrees per year respectively)(Majd, Muldowny, and Holt 1997). Saito and colleagues found that 20 of their 37 patients required increased amounts of nursing time to complete various activities of daily living (Saito et al. 1998). The average Cobb angle for those 20 patients was 73 degrees versus 34 degrees in those patients who did not require increased assistance (Saito et al. 1998). In these instances, the treatment should be centered on correcting spinal balance, relieving pain, and maintaining spinal stability in the safest way possible. The restoration of sitting ability and overall functional improvement should be achieved after treatment focusing on maintaining an upright position, so to become a "functional quadriplegic". (Shook JE 1991)

TREATMENT

The goals of treatment differ depending on the curve type and the child's level of function (Cloake and Gardner 2016). In more functional individuals, treatment focuses on prevention of curve progression and on maintaining spinal balance (Cloake and Gardner 2016). In ambulatory children, spinal curvature may be treated with the same guidelines of adolescent idiopathic scoliosis treatment (Cloake and Gardner 2016). However, these scenarios are less common. The most common case is a quadriplegic child with severe neuromuscular scoliosis and significant pelvic obliquity, resulting in pain, discomfort, and loss of seating balance.

NON OPERATIVE TREATMENT

Non-operative treatment options consist of observation and bracing, but also include seating modifications as well as medical management of co-morbidities (Cloake and Gardner 2016). CP patients present dynamic instability and poor balance control of the trunk(R Vialle, Thévenin-Lemoine, and Mary 2013). At the early stage, the patient presents with dynamic instability; the patient can correct it by himself by asking him to "hands up". As previously stated, the aim of any treatment is to maintain a comfortable sitting and to allow functional movements of the upper extremities. In fact, seating modifications in cerebral palsy patients could be divided in two groups: bracing and customized seating arrangements (Koop 2009).

Although different from adolescent idiopathic scoliosis, spinal bracing in children with CP is a well-described and established option for non-operative treatment (Terjesen, Lange, and Steen 2000; R. B. Winter and Carlson, n.d.; James 1975; Zadek 1973; Baumann 1976; Bunnell and MacEwen 1977). Braces may slow down curve progression in quadriplegic CP (Terjesen, Lange, and Steen 2000), but it is unclear if it reduces the need for surgery (Koop 2009). Spinal bracing reduces however curve size and slows down progression to severe curves during growth (Terjesen, Lange, and Steen 2000). However, no data can prove actually that bracing stops the evolution of the disease (Saito et al. 1998; Imrie and Yaszay 2010; Terjesen, Lange, and Steen 2000; Zadek 1973).

For patients that cannot tolerate braces, seating modification is a good alternative (Angsupaisal, Maathuis, and Hadders-Algra 2015). It usually involves adapting a patient's wheelchair with various supports (Angsupaisal, Maathuis, and Hadders-Algra 2015). However, it does not alter the natural history of the scoliosis (Cloake and Gardner 2016; Canavese et al. 2014). There are multiple types of seating modifications that can be used, from custom-molded seatbacks for patients with severe spinal deformity to 2- and 3-point body support systems (Angsupaisal, Maathuis, and Hadders-Algra 2015). The 3-point force configuration has been shown to achieve the best static correction of the scoliotic spine based on external measurements (K. J. Holmes et al. 2003). All seating modifications need to be personally adapted and molded to provide the best support and comfort to the patient (K. J. Holmes et al. 2003).

OPERATIVE TREATMENT

The main goals of operative treatment are to stop scoliosis progression and to restore sitting capacity, thus achieving good sagittal and frontal balance and restoring pelvic level (Cloake and Gardner 2016). Surgery is indicated when curve progresses beyond 50 degrees but even then, there are no strict guidelines (Cloake and Gardner 2016; Canavese et al. 2014). Sitting capacity and function of the upper limbs have to be considered in the surgical decision (Saito et al. 1998; Lonstein and Beck, n.d.; Thomson and Banta 2001). Overall, indications for surgery are: significant curve resulting in functional disturbance and/or cardio-respiratory compromise, progressive spinal deformity not controllable with orthosis; small curve with inevitable progression; and painful deformities (Canavese et al. 2014).

In contrast to adolescent idiopathic scoliosis, a thorough pre-operative evaluation has to be done carefully as to assess all co-morbidities associated (Cloake and Gardner 2016). Success of surgery relies on a multidisciplinary approach as well as on a good pre-operative planning (Cloake and Gardner 2016). Each case has its own management and advices for parents, caregivers and patients have to be taken into account. Ideally, the multidisciplinary team should include a scoliosis surgeon, general and neuro-pediatricians, a pediatric respiratory physician and a physiotherapist, an anesthetist and a cardiologist (Cloake and Gardner 2016).

PREOPERATIVE ASSESSMENT

Musculoskeletal Assessment

All associated clinical complaints have to be cleared and evaluated before going to surgery. Pelvic obliquity, hip dislocation, sitting ability, curve flexibility and skin conditions are major problems than can affect surgery planning or decision (Porter, Michael, and Kirkwood 2007; Oda et al. 2017).

Adduction contracture, pelvic obliquity, hip dislocation and scoliosis are closely related and each of them affects and accelerates the progression of the other (Oda et al. 2017). Pelvic obliquity and hip dislocation are frequently seen in patients with scoliosis (C. Holmes, Brock, and Morgan 2018). It is still not clear witch deformity has to be addressed first but when discussed with the caregiver, the issue has to be cleared so not to face any complication. Treating scoliosis may reduce hip subluxation and correct pelvic obliquity but it may also exacerbate hip dislocation (Persson-Bunke, Hägglund, and Lauge-Pedersen 2006; Senaran et al., n.d.; Cooperman et al., n.d.; Lonstein and Beck, n.d.; Letts et al. 1984; Pritchett 1990). Hip contracture and dislocation can secondarily deform the spine dynamically when the patient attempts to accommodate the hip deformity while sitting (Senaran et al., n.d.). For patients with both scoliosis and hip dislocation, dynamic physical examination with the patient prone with the lower limbs hanging outside the examination table helps identify the major cause of pelvic obliquity: upper cause i.e., the spine, lower cause i.e., the lower limbs and mainly the hips, or both. In cases where pelvic obliquity is predominantly caused by hip muscle imbalance or subluxation, hip surgery is usually addressed first. In the opposite case, spinal deformity should be corrected first (Canavese et al. 2014). When both the hips and the spine are equally responsible of the pelvic obliquity the authors of the current chapter prefer to address the spine first. On the other hand, it is also important to assess any hamstring or rectus femoris tightness that can affect the position of the pelvis (Flynn and Miller, n.d.). Muscular release can be done during the same procedure as to prevent any *"sacral sitting"* position post-operatively (Rang et al. 1981).

Neuromuscular Scoliosis: Surgical Considerations and Management of Complications 337

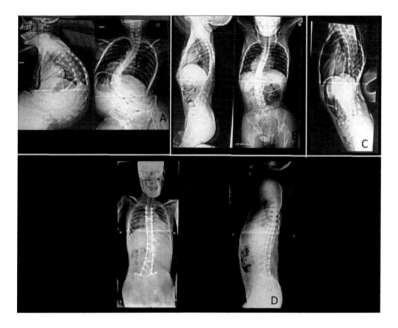

Figure 1. Case of a 14 year old male who presented with aggravating neuromuscular scoliosis and kyphosis. A: Pre-operative AP and lateral D1-S1 x-rays. B: Traction AP and lateral D1-S1 x-rays. C: Lateral spine x-rays over sandbag. D: Post-operative AP and lateral D1-S1 x-rays.

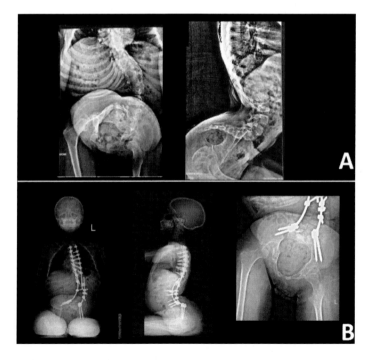

Figure 2. Case of a 16 year old girl who presented with aggravating neuromuscular scoliosis and kyphosis. A: Pre-operative AP and lateral lumbosacral x-rays. B: Post-operative AP and lateral D1-S1 x-rays and AP pelvis x-ray. This is an example of an insufficiently corrected pelvis obliquity in the post-operative course.

Curve pattern, reducibility, ability to sit and to voluntarily correct the position have to be evaluated (Cloake and Gardner 2016). Patient function has also to be evaluated to prevent any deterioration following surgery (Cloake and Gardner 2016). An optimal 3D balance must be restored and postoperative sitting ischiatic pressure distribution must be symmetrical after surgery as it reflects the good correction of pelvic obliquity. Any insufficient correction of 3D imbalance and pelvic obliquity is more deleterious to the patient than the preoperative situation (Figure 2). In fact T2-S1 fusion prevents the patient from adapting to his pelvic obliquity by moving his trunk. Finally, an overall check of the skin has to be done and any sore or maceration have to be treated pre-operatively (Cloake and Gardner 2016).

Pulmonary Assessment

Even though it is hard to evaluate pulmonary function in CP patients, it is important to eliminate a subclinical aspiration. Frequent pneumonia, coughing while eating and sputtering are signs of aspiration and require medical optimization before proceeding to surgery for scoliosis. Moreover, pulmonary function may be affected by scoliosis or oropharyngeal dysfunction. Respiratory evaluation has to be done to prevent postoperative complications and longer mechanical ventilation following surgery (S. Winter 1994; Borkhuu et al., n.d.).

Sleep disordered breathing with or without nocturnal hypercapnic hypoventilation is a common complication of respiratory muscle weakness in children and adolescents with neuromuscular disorders and cerebral palsy (Mellies et al. 2003). Nocturnal hypercapnic hypoventilation is a sign of respiratory muscle fatigue and poor prognosis (Canavese et al. 2014). It is recommended to perform a polysomnographic evaluation searching for sleep-disordered breathing in patients with neuromuscular compromise and spinal deformity (Canavese et al. 2014). Children with neuromuscular scoliosis are at risk for sleep-disordered breathing when inspiratory vital capacity is less than 60% during daytime hours (Mellies et al. 2003). Moreover, these patients are at risk of hypercapnic hypoventilation during night-time if inspiratory vital capacity is less than 40% and PaCO2 is higher than 40 mmHg (Mellies et al. 2003). The use of pre-operative non-invasive ventilation (NIV) training to strengthen respiratory muscles has shown promises in improving outcomes in patients with neuromuscular disease following spinal surgery (Khirani et al. 2014). NIV has been gaining popularity in the management of respiratory disease in pediatric patients with CP and represents a safe and effective option to help mitigate against and manage respiratory complications (Young et al. 2007).

Gastro-Intestinal Assessment

As previously discussed, gastroesophageal reflux disease (GERD) has to be treated before scoliosis surgery (Rang et al. 1981). GERD increases the risk of pneumonia as an independent risk factor. It also increases the risk of postoperative surgical site infection (Cloake and Gardner 2016). Malnutrition has also to be addressed as weight for chronologic age below the fifth percentile is associated with an increased postoperative complication score (Lipton et al. 1999). Feeding tube or gastrostomy may be needed to accelerate rehabilitation of the nutritional status to prevent complications (García-Contreras et al. 2014).

Preoperative laboratory tests have to include albumin and lymphocyte count because it has been proved that in CP patients, serum albumin less than 35 g/L and total blood lymphocyte count less than 1.5 g/L are associated with an increased infection rate, a longer length of intubation, and a longer hospital stay (S. Winter 1994).

Neurological Assessment

It is well known that a great majority of CP patients are under medication for seizure control. Care must be taken to make sure that patients are well stabilized and seizures well controlled. Added to that, valproic acid can induce bleeding especially if a bleeding test is abnormal. So it is preferable to stop valproic acid at least one month before surgery. These medications can also alter Vitamin D and calcium metabolism and thus induce osteopenia (S. L. Winter et al. 1996; Allen and Ferguson 1982). On the other hand, if a Baclofen pump is positioned, care must be taken to secure it or to stop it during the surgery to prevent any breaking during spinal deformity correction.

IMAGING STUDIES

AP and lateral X-rays have to be done to analyze the curve pattern and magnitude. An AP of the pelvis may also be needed for a better analysis of pelvic obliquity and hips (Mary, Servais, and Vialle 2018). Since flexibility of the curve could not be assessed via voluntary bending radiographs, a variety of special films can be taken to assess the flexibility of the spinal deformity, including fulcrum bending, push-pull, and traction films(R Vialle, Thévenin-Lemoine, and Mary 2013). In general, for this patient population, traction radiographs are preferred (Mary, Servais, and Vialle 2018).

SURGERY PLANNING

Surgery planning includes the choice of fusion levels, surgical correction technique, bone grafting and neuromonitoring if any.

Extent of Fusion Levels

Most surgeons agree on the level of the proximal level of fusion. Since most of severely involved CP patients have poor neck and trunk control, it is always recommended to start instrumentation as proximal as possible at the thoracic spine, generally T2, in order to prevent proximal junctional kyphosis and possible subsequent pullout of proximal anchors (Piazzolla et al. 2011).

There does not seem to be any consensus regarding distal instrumentation level and whether to include the pelvis or not (Canavese et al. 2014). Most surgeons recommend including the pelvis in the fusion especially in patients having major pelvic obliquity (Allen and Ferguson 1982; Maloney, Rinsky, and Gamble, n.d.; Neustadt, Shufflebarger, and Cammisa, n.d.; Modi et al. 2010). Modi et al. showed that patients having more than 15 degrees of pelvic obliquity who were not fused to the pelvis had an initial correction of the pelvis balance but then lost this correction progressively (Modi et al. 2010). Other publications showed good results with fusion to L5 and sparing of the pelvis. McCall and Hayes have suggested that sparing the pelvis and maintaining a mobile L5/S1 segment ameliorates wheel chair seating (McCall and Hayes 2005). To do that, they used a pedicle screw at L5 and found that it is was safe and strong enough (McCall and Hayes 2005). It is felt however, that independently from the ambulatory status, patients having pelvic obliquity should be fused to the pelvis (McCall and Hayes 2005). Instrumentation and fusion should be extended to the pelvis in non-ambulatory patients with pelvic obliquity (Canavese et al. 2014). Although some authors believe that instrumented fusion may stop at L5 or above when patient are still ambulatory and show minimal or no sign of pelvic obliquity (Canavese et al. 2014), we prefer to include the pelvis any time there is anterior trunk imbalance even in GMFCS III or IV. In fact, our experience shows that in this patient category, any attempt to avoid instrumenting to the pelvis was associated with a distal junctional kyphosis that required secondary extension to the pelvis at a later stage. Small amounts of pelvic obliquity (less than 10 to 15 degrees) are compatible with comfortable seating. On the other hand, larger fixed obliquities are not compatible with comfortable seating, and must be corrected by operative means or, if not fixed, by wheelchair modifications (Neustadt, Shufflebarger, and Cammisa, n.d.).

Instrumentation

Historically, spinal instrumentation begun with the Harrington rod in the early 1960s. This was followed by the segmental fixation concept pioneered by Resina and Alves from Portugal in 1963 who introduced segmental wiring for the treatment of scoliotic curves (Resina and Alves 1977). The stainless steel wires are passed through a hole at the base of the spinous processes (one wire per vertebra) and twisted around to two straight rods placed on either side of the spine (Resina and Alves 1977). This technique allows translation of the spine and correction of the deformity (mostly on the frontal plane) by using an even distribution of corrective forces (Canavese et al. 2014). At that time, it was revolutionary but included a high risk of pseudarthrosis, three months of bed rest and a low level of correction (Sullivan and Conner, n.d.; Bonnett, Brown, and Grow 1976). In 1976, Luque developed his instrumentation including rods and sub-laminar wires that has quickly won the ground and was qualified by surgeons as the best technique in CP patients (Luque 1982). It was then modified to extend to the pelvis by the Galveston technique in 1982(Allen and Ferguson, n.d.). Bell then modified the double rod technique and proposed a unit-rod (U-rod), which was fixed to the pelvis (Bell, Moseley, and Koreska 1989). Luque's technique and its modifications did show amelioration in curve correction and were associated with less pseudarthrosis. In the 1980s, Cotrel and Dubousset introduced a new concept in scoliosis correction using segmental hook fixation, proved at that time to be the most effective corrective method (Yazici, Asher, and Hardacker 2000); it was later gradually replaced by segmental pedicle screw fixation which showed to insure more solid constructs.

Pedicle screws are now widely used in CP scoliosis (Modi, Suh, Song, et al. 2008; Modi, Suh, Fernandez, et al. 2008; Modi, Suh, et al. 2009; Modi, Hong, et al. 2009; Watanabe et al. 2008). Mody et al. (Modi, Suh, Fernandez, et al. 2008) reported safe and effective use of pedicle screws in patients with CP. Pedicle screws in the pelvis, iliac bone or sacrum are more effective and more reliable to correct pelvic obliquity than Galveston or unit rod (Sponseller et al. 2009). Does this justify the cost of the screw instrumentation? The question cannot be answered yet but a study is going on actually comparing the different surgical instrumentations and technique and may give an answer to this question.

There are currently no studies directly comparing the current methods of spinal instrumentation in the CP population. Second generation techniques as well as pedicle screw instrumentation have all been shown to provide effective correction of deformity in terms of Cobb angle correction and reduction in pelvic obliquity (Cloake and Gardner 2016).

In order to better prepare the surgical procedure, several questions should be answered

IS PREOPERATIVE TRACTION STILL INDICATED?

Traditionally, traction was used pre-operatively so to improve trunk balance without neurologic risk and to improve pulmonary capacity in severe and stiff curves. Pre-operative traction can be of different types; halo-gravity being the less invasive, allowing mobility with low traction forces (Rinella et al. 2005). Traction is also used in staged surgery to improve the results of anterior release.

New trends use asymmetric intra-operative traction technique to improve alignment. Following Lenke's experience (Huang and Lenke 2001), Takeshika performed an asymmetric intraoperative halo-femoral traction on 20 patients. They had a better pelvic obliquity correction without an increase in complications (Takeshita et al. 2006). Vialle et al. had also similar result with asymmetric intraoperative traction, with better correction of Cobb angle and pelvic obliquity (Vialle, Delecourt, and Morin 2006). Also, Jackson et al. recently showed that intraoperative traction may be a viable alternative to an anterior release in severe CP scoliosis (major curves ≥ 100 degrees) which was associated to increased operative times (Jackson et al. 2018).

IS ANTERIOR APPROACH STILL NEEDED?

Anterior approach is classically used for curves between 75 and 100 degrees that are stiff and do not correct to less than 50 degrees on bending radiographs (Swank, Cohen, and Brown 1989). With the advent of pedicle screw instrumentation, the use of anterior release is somehow less needed as much correction can be achieved by posterior approach. Few studies evaluated only CP patients: Sush et al. published a study on severe and stiff neuromuscular scoliosis that was operated only by posterior approach associating pedicle screws and osteotomies (Suh et al. 2009). They had a 59.4% correction of Cobb angle and a 46.1% correction of pelvic obliquity (Suh et al. 2009). Watanabe and al published a report including 44 patients having a neuromuscular scoliosis; they showed that curves between 100 and 159 degree can be operated safely by posterior approach only (Watanabe et al. 2008).

Anterior approach was also classically used for young patients with open triradiate cartilage to prevent crankshaft (Westerlund et al. 2001). But actual studies are proving that isolated posterior approach can be safely performed in very young patients without any crankshaft risk as pedicle screw insertion passes the anterior vertebral physis and creates an epiphysiodesis effect (Smucker and Miller, n.d.; Westerlund et al. 2001).

IS BONE GRAFT NEEDED IN NEUROMUSCULAR SCOLIOSIS?

Allografts are not commonly used in children, even in adolescent idiopathic scoliosis. Previous studies have shown that in neuromuscular scoliosis both allograft and autograft should be used to prevent pseudarthrosis in osteopenic patients (R. E. McCarthy et al. 1986; Yazici and Asher 1997). However, allograft use is associated with an increased risk of surgical site infection (Borkhuu et al. 2008). Nerveless more recent studies have proved that adding allograft that have been mixed with gentamycin lowered the incidence of deep wound infection in CP patients (Borkhuu et al. 2008).

IS NEUROMONITORING IMPORTANT IN CP PATIENTS?

CP patients have an underlying neurologic background that makes neuromonitoring technically more demanding and less reliable (Mo et al. 2017). It remains recommended like in adolescent idiopathic scoliosis (DiCindio et al. 2003; Langeloo et al. 2001). Transcranial electric motor evoked potentials (TceMEPs) and somatosensory evoked potentials (SSEPs) can be used; they both can detect and prevent neurologic complications in CP patients (Mo et al. 2017).

SURGICAL COMPLICATIONS OF SCOLIOSIS SURGERY

Spine surgery in CP patients is still burdened with an average complication rate of 8–33%, including increased hospital stay, death (around 1%), deep infections, and revision surgery. This is often due to the presence of multiple comorbidities. High risk of complication is associated with non-ambulatory status and greater angle of scoliosis curve (Lipton et al. 1999). The complication rates increased with time and more and more complications are reported in recent literature (Cloake and Gardner 2016). This can be explained by the improvement in complication recording but also by the fact that more severe patients are now being operated (Cloake and Gardner 2016). The most frequent complication used to be infection; surgical site infection in particular as its incidence is 4 – 10%, about threefold higher than that associated to idiopathic scoliosis surgery. However, in a recent meta-analysis of complications following surgery for neuromuscular scoliosis, pulmonary complications were found to be most common (22.7%), followed by implant-related complications (12.5%) and infections (10.9%) (Sharma et al. 2013)

Bleeding is another complication of scoliosis surgery in CP. Significant bleeding averaging around 700–2,000 ml has been reported, but bleeding can reach up to 5,500 ml, particularly for vertebral column resections, equivalent to 260% of the total blood volume of the patient (Hasler 2013). On the other hand, the risk of respiratory/pulmonary complications ranges from 26.9 to

57.1%, with the most reported complications being pneumonia, pneumothorax, or atelectasis (Legg et al. 2014).

Proximal kyphosis is another encountered complication. Instrumentation up to T2/T3 as well as smooth correction of hyperkyphosis and a local hook clamp (pedicle hook and transverse process hook) for smooth transition between fused and unfused areas support the prevention of junctional kyphosis. Furthermore, increased thoracic kyphosis results in a slight, but statistically significant, increased risk of death. Pseudarthrosis is more frequent in CP patient than in adolescents with idiopathic scoliosis and was classically associated with the use of Luque Galveston technique (Sharma et al. 2013). With the recent use of pedicle screws, the incidence of this complication decreased dramatically (Piazzolla et al. 2011). Nonetheless, the risk of a hardware-related complication ranges from 7.5 to 43.8%. Prominent hardware, screw failure, or wire breakage/failure/pullout are most often reported. Finally, due to these complications, reoperation risk ranges from 19.5 to 32.5% in the available medical literature (Legg et al. 2014).

All in all, early post-operative complications include inadequate correction, skin breakdown, surgical site infection, cardio-respiratory, neurologic and nutritional issues, prolonged ileus, constipation, fluid overload, bleeding and death. Late post-operative complications include chronic infections, non-union, coccyx and/or ischiatic pain, crankshaft phenomenon, implant related issues, such as dislodgment and/or loss of correction (Canavese et al. 2014).

Strategies to reduce complication rates in CP patients undergoing spinal fusion are under investigation (Cloake and Gardner 2016). Use of vancomycin powder may reduce the rate of wound infection in spinal surgery (Cloake and Gardner 2016). In a large retrospective review, the overall infection rate was reported to be less than 1% when using vancomycin powder (Cloake and Gardner 2016). Recent best practice guidelines advocate the use of intra-wound vancomycin in high-risk patients such as those with CP (Vitale et al. 2013).

CONCLUSION

Neuromuscular scoliosis is a common manifestation in children with CP. Without timely therapeutic intervention, scoliotic curves will continue to progress and cause impairment in function and increased risk of poor health. Management options range from external bracing for minor curves to surgical instrumentation for larger curves. As CP is a multi-system disease, careful consideration must be given to the preoperative optimization and to the postoperative management of the child. A multi-disciplinary approach involving pediatric specialists will allow for this.

There have been major advances in the management of scoliosis in neuromuscular scoliosis patients, but many challenges remain. Further multicenter studies and randomized clinical trials are needed, particularly in the areas of preoperative assessment, surgical techniques, neuromonitoring and infection prevention.

The state of knowledge regarding neuromuscular scoliosis is a dynamic process and current literature review is mandatory. The somewhat large bibliography for this subject reflects the many opinions and findings currently presented.

REFERENCES

Allen, B. L. & Ferguson, R. L. n.d. "The Galveston Technique for L Rod Instrumentation of the Scoliotic Spine." *Spine*, 7 (3), 276–84. http://www.ncbi.nlm.nih.gov/pubmed/7112242.

Allen, B. L. & Ferguson, R. L. (1982). "L-Rod Instrumentation for Scoliosis in Cerebral Palsy." *Journal of Pediatric Orthopedics*, 2 (1), 87–96. http://www.ncbi.nlm.nih.gov/pubmed/7076839.

Angsupaisal, Mattana., Carel, G. B. Maathuis. & Mijna, Hadders-Algra. (2015). "Adaptive Seating Systems in Children with Severe Cerebral Palsy across International Classification of Functioning, Disability and Health for Children and Youth Version Domains: A Systematic Review." *Developmental Medicine & Child Neurology*, 57 (10), 919–30. doi:10.1111/dmcn.12762.

Aquilina, Kristian., David, Graham. & Neil, Wimalasundera. (2015). "Selective Dorsal Rhizotomy: An Old Treatment Re-Emerging." *Archives of Disease in Childhood*, 100 (8), 798–802. doi:10.1136/archdischild-2014-306874.

Balmer, G A. & MacEwen, G. D. (1970). "The Incidence and Treatment of Scoliosis in Cerebral Palsy." *The Journal of Bone and Joint Surgery. British*, Volume 52 (1), 134–37. http://www.ncbi.nlm.nih.gov/pubmed/5436198

Baumann, J U. 1976. *Zeitschrift Fur Orthopadie Und Ihre Grenzgebiete. [Conservative Therapy of Scoliosis in Cerebral Palsy.]* 114 (4): 496–98. http://www.ncbi.nlm.nih.gov/pubmed/1007417.

Bell, D. F., Moseley, C. F. & Koreska, J. (1989). "Unit Rod Segmental Spinal Instrumentation in the Management of Patients with Progressive Neuromuscular Spinal Deformity." *Spine*, 14 (12), 1301–7. http://www.ncbi.nlm.nih.gov/pubmed/2617359.

Bertoncelli, Carlo M., Federico, Solla., Peter, R Loughenbury., Athanasios, I Tsirikos., Domenico, Bertoncelli. & Virginie, Rampal. (2017). "Risk Factors for Developing Scoliosis in Cerebral Palsy: A Cross-Sectional Descriptive Study." *Journal of Child Neurology*, 32 (7), 657–62. doi:10.1177/0883073817701047.

Bonnett, C., Brown, J. C. & Grow, T. (1976). "Thoracolumbar Scoliosis in Cerebral Palsy. Results of Surgical Treatment." *The Journal of Bone and Joint Surgery. American*, Volume 58 (3), 328–36. http://www.ncbi.nlm.nih.gov/pubmed/1262364.

Borkhuu, Battugs., Andrzej, Borowski., Suken, A. Shah., Aaron, G. Littleton., Kirk, W. Dabney. & Freeman, Miller. (2008). "Antibiotic-Loaded Allograft Decreases the Rate of Acute Deep Wound Infection After Spinal Fusion in Cerebral Palsy." *Spine*, 33 (21), 2300–2304. doi:10.1097/BRS.0b013e31818786ff.

Borkhuu, Battugs., Durga, Nagaraju., Freeman, Miller., Mohamed, Hassan Moamed Ali., David, Pressel., Judith, Adelizzi-Delany., Margy, Miccolis., Kirk, Dabney. & Larry, Holmes. n.d. "Prevalence and Risk Factors in Postoperative Pancreatitis after Spine Fusion in Patients with Cerebral Palsy." *Journal of Pediatric Orthopedics*, 29 (3), 256–62. doi:10.1097/BPO.0b013e31819bcf0a.

Brooks, Jaysson T. & Paul, D Sponseller. (2016). "What's New in the Management of Neuromuscular Scoliosis." *Journal of Pediatric Orthopedics*, 36 (6), 627–33. doi:10.1097/BPO.0000000000000497.

Bunnell, W. P. & MacEwen, G. D. (1977). "Non-Operative Treatment of Scoliosis in Cerebral Palsy: Preliminary Report on the Use of a Plastic Jacket." *Developmental Medicine and Child Neurology*, *19* (1), 45–49. http://www.ncbi.nlm.nih.gov/pubmed/ 844664.

Canavese, Federico., Marie, Rousset., Benoit, Le Gledic., Antoine, Samba. & Alain, Dimeglio. (2014). "Surgical Advances in the Treatment of Neuromuscular Scoliosis." *World Journal of Orthopedics*, *5* (2), 124–33. doi:10.5312/wjo.v5.i2.124.

Cloake, Thomas. & Adrian, Gardner. (2016). "The Management of Scoliosis in Children with Cerebral Palsy: A Review." *Journal of Spine Surgery*, *2* (4), 299–309. doi:10.21037/jss.2016.09.05.

Cooperman, D. R., Bartucci, E., Dietrick, E. & Millar, E. A. n.d. "Hip Dislocation in Spastic Cerebral Palsy: Long-Term Consequences." *Journal of Pediatric Orthopedics*, *7* (3), 268–76. http://www.ncbi.nlm.nih.gov/pubmed/3584441.

DiCindio, Sabina., Mary, Theroux., Suken, Shah., Freeman, Miller., Kirk, Dabney., Robert, P Brislin. & Daniel, Schwartz. (2003). "Multimodality Monitoring of Transcranial Electric Motor and Somatosensory-Evoked Potentials during Surgical Correction of Spinal Deformity in Patients with Cerebral Palsy and Other Neuromuscular Disorders." *Spine*, *28* (16), 1851-5-6. doi:10.1097/01.BRS.0000083202.62956.A8.

Flynn, John M. & Freeman, Miller. n.d. "Management of Hip Disorders in Patients with Cerebral Palsy." *The Journal of the American Academy of Orthopaedic Surgeons*, *10* (3), 198–209. http://www.ncbi.nlm.nih.gov/pubmed/12041941.

García-Contreras, Andrea A., Edgar, M Vásquez-Garibay., Enrique, Romero-Velarde., Ana Isabel, Ibarra-Gutiérrez., Rogelio, Troyo-Sanromán. & Imelda, E Sandoval-Montes. (2014). "Intensive Nutritional Support Improves the Nutritional Status and Body Composition in Severely Malnourished Children with Cerebral Palsy." *Nutricion Hospitalaria*, *29* (4), 838–43. doi:10.3305/nh.2014.29.4.7247.

Ginsburg, Glen M. & Anthony, J Lauder. (2007). "Progression of Scoliosis in Patients with Spastic Quadriplegia after the Insertion of an Intrathecal Baclofen Pump." *Spine*, *32* (24), 2745–50. doi:10.1097/BRS.0b013e31815a5219.

Golan, Jeff Dror., Jeffery, Alan Hall., Gus, O'Gorman., Chantal, Poulin., Thierry, Ezer Benaroch., Marie-Andrée, Cantin. & Jean-Pierre, Farmer. (2007). "Spinal Deformities Following Selective Dorsal Rhizotomy." *Journal of Neurosurgery*, *106* (6 Suppl), 441–49. doi:10.3171/ped.2007.106.6.441.

Gomez, Jaime A., Timothy Hresko, M. & Michael, P Glotzbecker. (2016). "Nonsurgical Management of Adolescent Idiopathic Scoliosis." *The Journal of the American Academy of Orthopaedic Surgeons*, *24* (8), 555–64. doi:10.5435/JAAOS-D-14-00416.

Hägglund, Gunnar., Katina, Pettersson., Tomasz, Czuba., Måns, Persson-Bunke. & Elisabet, Rodby-Bousquet. (2018). "Incidence of Scoliosis in Cerebral Palsy." *Acta Orthopaedica*, March, 1–5. doi:10.1080/17453674.2018.1450091.

Halawi, Mohamad J., Robert, K Lark. & Robert, D Fitch. (2015). "Neuromuscular Scoliosis: Current Concepts." *Orthopedics*, *38* (6), e452-6. doi:10.3928/01477447-20150603-50.

Hasler, Carol C. (2013). "Operative Treatment for Spinal Deformities in Cerebral Palsy." *Journal of Children's Orthopaedics*, *7* (5), 419–23. doi:10.1007/s11832-013-0517-4.

Holmes, Carlee., Kim, Brock. & Prue, Morgan. (2018). "Postural Asymmetry in Non-Ambulant Adults with Cerebral Palsy: A Scoping Review." *Disability and Rehabilitation*, January, 1–10. doi:10.1080/09638288.2017.1422037.

Holmes, K. J., Michael, S. M., Thorpe, S. L. & Solomonidis, S. E. (2003). "Management of Scoliosis with Special Seating for the Non-Ambulant Spastic Cerebral Palsy Population-- a Biomechanical Study." *Clinical Biomechanics (Bristol, Avon)*, *18* (6), 480–87. http://www.ncbi.nlm.nih.gov/pubmed/12828895.

Huang, M. J. & Lenke, L. G. (2001). "Scoliosis and Severe Pelvic Obliquity in a Patient with Cerebral Palsy: Surgical Treatment Utilizing Halo-Femoral Traction." *Spine*, *26* (19), 2168–70. http://www.ncbi.nlm.nih.gov/pubmed/11698899.

Imrie, Meghan N. & Burt, Yaszay. (2010). "Management of Spinal Deformity in Cerebral Palsy." *The Orthopedic Clinics of North America*, *41* (4), 531–47. doi:10.1016/j.ocl.2010.06.008.

Jackson, Taylor J., Burt, Yaszay., Joshua, M Pahys., Anuj, Singla., Firoz, Miyanji., Suken, A Shah., Paul, D Sponseller., et al. (2018). "Intraoperative Traction May Be a Viable Alternative to Anterior Surgery in Cerebral Palsy Scoliosis ≥100 Degrees." *Journal of Pediatric Orthopedics*, March. doi:10.1097/BPO.0000000000001151.

James, W. V. (1975). "Spinal Bracing in Children with Atonic Cerebral Palsy." *The Ulster Medical Journal*, *44* (1), 53–55. http://www.ncbi.nlm.nih.gov/pubmed/1124561.

Johnson, Michael B., Liav, Goldstein., Susan, Sienko Thomas., Joseph, Piatt., Michael, Aiona. & Michael, Sussman. n.d. "Spinal Deformity after Selective Dorsal Rhizotomy in Ambulatory Patients with Cerebral Palsy." *Journal of Pediatric Orthopedics*, *24* (5), 529–36. http://www.ncbi.nlm.nih.gov/pubmed/15308903.

Khirani, Sonia., Chiara, Bersanini., Guillaume, Aubertin., Manon, Bachy., Raphaël, Vialle. & Brigitte, Fauroux. (2014). "Non-Invasive Positive Pressure Ventilation to Facilitate the Post-Operative Respiratory Outcome of Spine Surgery in Neuromuscular Children." *European Spine Journal*, *23* (S4), 406–11. doi:10.1007/s00586-014-3335-6.

Koop, Steven E. (2009). "Scoliosis in Cerebral Palsy." *Developmental Medicine and Child Neurology*, *51*, Suppl 4, (October), 92–98. doi:10.1111/j.1469-8749.2009.03461.x.

Langeloo, D. D., Journée, H. L., Polak, B. & de Kleuver, M. (2001). "A New Application of TCE-MEP: Spinal Cord Monitoring in Patients with Severe Neuromuscular Weakness Undergoing Corrective Spine Surgery." *Journal of Spinal Disorders*, *14* (5), 445–48. http://www.ncbi.nlm.nih.gov/pubmed/11586146.

Langerak, Nelleke G., Christopher, L Vaughan., Edward, B Hoffman., Anthony, A Figaji., Graham Fieggen, A. & Jonathan, C Peter. (2009). "Incidence of Spinal Abnormalities in Patients with Spastic Diplegia 17 to 26 Years after Selective Dorsal Rhizotomy." *Child's Nervous System: ChNS: Official Journal of the International Society for Pediatric Neurosurgery*, *25* (12), 1593–1603. doi:10.1007/s00381-009-0993-5.

Lee, Seung Yeol., Chin, Youb, Chung., Kyoung, Min Lee., Soon-Sun, Kwon., Kyu-Jung, Cho. & Moon, Seok Park. (2016). "Annual Changes in Radiographic Indices of the Spine in Cerebral Palsy Patients." *European Spine Journal: Official Publication of the European Spine Society, the European Spinal Deformity Society, and the European Section of the Cervical Spine Research Society*, *25* (3), 679–86. doi:10.1007/s00586-014-3746-4.

Legg, Julian., Evan, Davies., Annie, L Raich., Joseph, R Dettori. & Ned, Sherry. (2014). "Surgical Correction of Scoliosis in Children with Spastic Quadriplegia: Benefits, Adverse Effects, and Patient Selection." *Evidence-Based Spine-Care Journal*, *5* (1), 38–51. doi:10.1055/s-0034-1370898.

Letts, M., Shapiro, L., Mulder, K. & Klassen, O. (1984). "The Windblown Hip Syndrome in Total Body Cerebral Palsy." *Journal of Pediatric Orthopedics*, 4 (1), 55–62. http://www.ncbi.nlm.nih.gov/pubmed/6693570.

Lipton, G. E., Miller, F., Dabney, K. W., Altiok, H. & Bachrach, S. J. (1999). "Factors Predicting Postoperative Complications Following Spinal Fusions in Children with Cerebral Palsy." *Journal of Spinal Disorders*, 12 (3), 197–205. http://www.ncbi.nlm.nih.gov/pubmed/ 10382772.

Lonstein, J. E. & Akbarnia, A. (1983). "Operative Treatment of Spinal Deformities in Patients with Cerebral Palsy or Mental Retardation. An Analysis of One Hundred and Seven Cases." *The Journal of Bone and Joint Surgery. American*, Volume 65 (1), 43–55. http://www.ncbi.nlm.nih.gov/pubmed/6848534.

Lonstein, J. E. & Beck, K. n.d. "Hip Dislocation and Subluxation in Cerebral Palsy." *Journal of Pediatric Orthopedics*, 6 (5), 521–26. http://www.ncbi.nlm.nih.gov/pubmed/3760161.

Luque, E R. (1982). "Segmental Spinal Instrumentation for Correction of Scoliosis." *Clinical Orthopaedics and Related Research*, no. 163, (March), 192–98. http://www.ncbi.nlm.nih.gov/pubmed/7067252.

Madigan, R. R. & Wallace, S. L. n.d. "Scoliosis in the Institutionalized Cerebral Palsy Population." *Spine*, 6 (6), 583–90. http://www.ncbi.nlm.nih.gov/pubmed/7336281.

Majd, M. E., Muldowny, D. S. & Holt, R. T. (1997). "Natural History of Scoliosis in the Institutionalized Adult Cerebral Palsy Population." *Spine*, 22 (13), 1461–66. http://www.ncbi.nlm.nih.gov/pubmed/9231964.

Maloney, W. J., Rinsky, L. A. & Gamble, J. G. n.d. "Simultaneous Correction of Pelvic Obliquity, Frontal Plane, and Sagittal Plane Deformities in Neuromuscular Scoliosis Using a Unit Rod with Segmental Sublaminar Wires: A Preliminary Report." *Journal of Pediatric Orthopedics*, 10 (6), 742–49. http://www.ncbi.nlm.nih.gov/pubmed/2250058.

Mary, P., Servais, L. & Vialle, R. (2018). "Neuromuscular Diseases: Diagnosis and Management." *Orthopaedics & Traumatology, Surgery & Research : OTSR*, 104 (1S), S89–95. doi:10.1016/j.otsr.2017.04.019.

McCall, Richard E. & Beth, Hayes. (2005). "Long-Term Outcome in Neuromuscular Scoliosis Fused Only to Lumbar 5." *Spine*, 30 (18), 2056–60. http://www.ncbi.nlm.nih.gov/pubmed/16166895.

McCarthy, James J., Linda, P D'Andrea., Randal, R Betz. & David, H Clements. (2006). "Scoliosis in the Child with Cerebral Palsy." *The Journal of the American Academy of Orthopaedic Surgeons*, 14 (6), 367–75. http://www.ncbi.nlm.nih.gov/pubmed/16757676.

McCarthy, R. E., Peek, R. D., Morrissy, R. T. & Hough, A. J. (1986). "Allograft Bone in Spinal Fusion for Paralytic Scoliosis." *The Journal of Bone and Joint Surgery. American*, Volume 68 (3), 370–75. http://www.ncbi.nlm.nih.gov/pubmed/3512570.

Mellies, Uwe., Regine, Ragette., Christian, Schwake., Holger, Boehm., Thomas, Voit. & Helmut, Teschler. (2003). "Daytime Predictors of Sleep Disordered Breathing in Children and Adolescents with Neuromuscular Disorders." *Neuromuscular Disorders: NMD*, 13 (2), 123–28. http://www.ncbi.nlm.nih.gov/pubmed/12565909.

Mo, Andrew Z., Anthony, O Asemota., Arun, Venkatesan., Eva, K Ritzl., Dolores, B Njoku. & Paul, D Sponseller. (2017). "Why No Signals? Cerebral Anatomy Predicts Success of Intraoperative Neuromonitoring During Correction of Scoliosis Secondary to Cerebral Palsy." *Journal of Pediatric Orthopedics*, 37 (8), e451–58. doi:10.1097/BPO.0000000000000707.

Modi, Hitesh N., Jae-Young, Hong., Satyen, S Mehta., Srinivasalu, S., Seung-Woo, Suh., Ju-Won, Yi., Jae-Hyuk, Yang. & Hae-Ryong, Song. (2009). "Surgical Correction and Fusion Using Posterior-Only Pedicle Screw Construct for Neuropathic Scoliosis in Patients with Cerebral Palsy: A Three-Year Follow-up Study." *Spine*, 34 (11), 1167–75. doi:10.1097/BRS.0b013e31819c38b7.

Modi, Hitesh N, Seung-Woo Suh, Hae-Ryong Song, Harry M Fernandez, and Jae-Hyuk Yang. 2008. "Treatment of Neuromuscular Scoliosis with Posterior-Only Pedicle Screw Fixation." *Journal of Orthopaedic Surgery and Research* 3 (June): 23. doi:10.1186/1749-799X-3-23.

Modi, Hitesh N, Seung-Woo Suh, Jae-Hyuk Yang, Jae Woo Cho, Jae-Young Hong, Surya Udai Singh, and Sudeep Jain. 2009. "Surgical Complications in Neuromuscular Scoliosis Operated with Posterior- Only Approach Using Pedicle Screw Fixation." *Scoliosis* 4 (May): 11. doi:10.1186/1748-7161-4-11.

Modi, Hitesh N., Seung, Woo Suh., Harry, Fernandez., Jae, Hyuk Yang. & Hae-Ryong, Song. (2008). "Accuracy and Safety of Pedicle Screw Placement in Neuromuscular Scoliosis with Free-Hand Technique." *European Spine Journal : Official Publication of the European Spine Society, the European Spinal Deformity Society, and the European Section of the Cervical Spine Research Society*, 17 (12), 1686–96. doi:10.1007/s00586-008-0795-6.

Modi, Hitesh N., Seung, Woo Suh., Hae-Ryong, Song., Jae, Hyuk Yang. & Nirmal, Jajodia. (2010). "Evaluation of Pelvic Fixation in Neuromuscular Scoliosis: A Retrospective Study in 55 Patients." *International Orthopaedics*, 34 (1), 89–96. doi:10.1007/s00264-008-0703-z.

Neustadt, J. B., Shufflebarger, H. L. & Cammisa, F. P. n.d. "Spinal Fusions to the Pelvis Augmented by Cotrel-Dubousset Instrumentation for Neuromuscular Scoliosis." *Journal of Pediatric Orthopedics*, 12 (4), 465–69. http://www.ncbi.nlm.nih.gov/pubmed/1613088.

Oda, Yoshiaki., Tomoyuki, Takigawa., Yoshihisa, Sugimoto., Masato, Tanaka., Hirofumi, Akazawa. & Toshifumi, Ozaki. (2017). "Scoliosis in Patients with Severe Cerebral Palsy: Three Different Courses in Adolescents." *Acta Medica Okayama*, 71 (2), 119–26. doi:10.18926/AMO/54980.

Persson-Bunke, Måns., Gunnar, Hägglund. & Henrik, Lauge-Pedersen. (2006). "Windswept Hip Deformity in Children with Cerebral Palsy." *Journal of Pediatric Orthopedics. Part B*, 15 (5), 335–38. http://www.ncbi.nlm.nih.gov/pubmed/16891960.

Persson-Bunke, Måns., Gunnar, Hägglund., Henrik, Lauge-Pedersen., Philippe, Wagner. & Lena, Westbom. (2012). "Scoliosis in a Total Population of Children with Cerebral Palsy." *Spine*, 37 (12), E708-13. doi:10.1097/BRS.0b013e318246a962.

Peter, J. C., Hoffman, E. B. & Arens, L. J. (1993). "Spondylolysis and Spondylolisthesis after Five-Level Lumbosacral Laminectomy for Selective Posterior Rhizotomy in Cerebral Palsy." *Child's Nervous System : ChNS : Official Journal of the International Society for Pediatric Neurosurgery* 9 (5): 285-7-8. http://www.ncbi.nlm.nih.gov/pubmed/8252520.

Peter, J. C., Hoffman, E. B., Arens, L. J. & Peacock, W. J. (1990.) "Incidence of Spinal Deformity in Children after Multiple Level Laminectomy for Selective Posterior Rhizotomy." *Child's Nervous System : ChNS : Official Journal of the International Society for Pediatric Neurosurgery*, 6 (1), 30–32. http://www.ncbi.nlm.nih.gov/pubmed/ 2311112.

Piazzolla, Andrea., Solarino, G., De Giorgi, S., Mori, C. M., Moretti, L. & De Giorgi, G. (2011). "Cotrel-Dubousset Instrumentation in Neuromuscular Scoliosis." *European Spine*

Journal: Official Publication of the European Spine Society, the European Spinal Deformity Society, and the European Section of the Cervical Spine Research Society, 20, Suppl 1 (May), S75-84. doi:10.1007/s00586-011-1758-x.

Porter, David., Shona, Michael. & Craig, Kirkwood. (2007). "Patterns of Postural Deformity in Non-Ambulant People with Cerebral Palsy: What Is the Relationship between the Direction of Scoliosis, Direction of Pelvic Obliquity, Direction of Windswept Hip Deformity and Side of Hip Dislocation?" *Clinical Rehabilitation*, 21 (12), 1087–96. doi:10.1177/0269215507080121.

Pritchett, J. W. (1990). "Treated and Untreated Unstable Hips in Severe Cerebral Palsy." *Developmental Medicine and Child Neurology*, 32 (1), 3–6. http://www.ncbi.nlm.nih.gov/pubmed/2105251.

Rang, M., Douglas, G., Bennet, G. C. & Koreska, J. (1981). "Seating for Children with Cerebral Palsy." *Journal of Pediatric Orthopedics*, 1 (3), 279–87. http://www.ncbi.nlm.nih.gov/pubmed/7334107.

Ravindra, Vijay M., Michael, T Christensen., Kaine, Onwuzulike., John, T Smith., Kyle, Halvorson., Douglas, L Brockmeyer., Marion, L Walker. & Robert, J Bollo. (2017). "Risk Factors for Progressive Neuromuscular Scoliosis Requiring Posterior Spinal Fusion after Selective Dorsal Rhizotomy." *Journal of Neurosurgery. Pediatrics*, 20 (5), 456–63. doi:10.3171/2017.5.PEDS16630.

Resina, J. & Alves, A. F. (1977). "A Technique of Correction and Internal Fixation for Scoliosis." *The Journal of Bone and Joint Surgery. British*, Volume 59 (2), 159–65. http://www.ncbi.nlm.nih.gov/pubmed/873976.

Rinella, Anthony., Lawrence, Lenke., Camden, Whitaker., Yongjung, Kim., Soo-sung, Park., Michael, Peelle., Charles, Edwards., Charles, Edwards. & Keith, Bridwell. (2005). "Perioperative Halo-Gravity Traction in the Treatment of Severe Scoliosis and Kyphosis." *Spine*, 30 (4), 475–82. http://www.ncbi.nlm.nih.gov/pubmed/15706347.

Saito, N., Ebara, S., Ohotsuka, K., Kumeta, H. & Takaoka, K. (1998). "Natural History of Scoliosis in Spastic Cerebral Palsy." *Lancet (London, England)*, 351 (9117), 1687–92. doi:10.1016/S0140-6736(98)01302-6.

Sansone, Jason M., David, Mann., Kenneth, Noonan.., Deborah, Mcleish., Michael, Ward. & Bermans, J Iskandar. n.d. "Rapid Progression of Scoliosis Following Insertion of Intrathecal Baclofen Pump." *Journal of Pediatric Orthopedics*, 26 (1), 125–28. doi:10.1097/01.bpo.0000191555.11326.bd.

Scannell, Brian. & Burt, Yaszay. (2015). "Scoliosis, Spinal Fusion, and Intrathecal Baclofen Pump Implantation." *Physical Medicine and Rehabilitation Clinics of North America*, 26 (1), 79–88. doi:10.1016/j.pmr.2014.09.003.

Segal, Lee S., David, M Wallach. & Paul, M Kanev. (2005). "Potential Complications of Posterior Spine Fusion and Instrumentation in Patients with Cerebral Palsy Treated with Intrathecal Baclofen Infusion." *Spine*, 30 (8), E219-24. http://www.ncbi.nlm.nih.gov/pubmed/15834321.

Senaran, Hakan., Suken, A Shah., Joseph, J Glutting., Kirk, W Dabney. & Freeman, Miller. n.d. "The Associated Effects of Untreated Unilateral Hip Dislocation in Cerebral Palsy Scoliosis." *Journal of Pediatric Orthopedics*, 26 (6), 769–72. doi:10.1097/01.bpo.0000242426.60995.29.

Sharma, Shallu., Chunsen, Wu., Thomas, Andersen., Yu, Wang., Ebbe, Stender Hansen. & Cody, Eric Bünger. (2013). "Prevalence of Complications in Neuromuscular Scoliosis

Surgery: A Literature Meta-Analysis from the Past 15 Years." *European Spine Journal: Official Publication of the European Spine Society, the European Spinal Deformity Society, and the European Section of the Cervical Spine Research Society*, 22 (6), 1230–49. doi:10.1007/s00586-012-2542-2.

Shilt, Jeffrey S., Lawrence, P Lai., Michael, N Cabrera., John, Frino. & Beth, P Smith. (2008). "The Impact of Intrathecal Baclofen on the Natural History of Scoliosis in Cerebral Palsy." *Journal of Pediatric Orthopedics*, 28 (6), 684–87. doi:10.1097/ BPO.0b013e3 18183d591.

Shook, J. E. & Lubicky, J. (1991). "Paralytic Spinal Deformity. Scoliosis." In *The Textbook of Spinal Surgery*. 1st Edition, 279–322.

Smucker, J. D. & Miller, F. n.d. "Crankshaft Effect after Posterior Spinal Fusion and Unit Rod Instrumentation in Children with Cerebral Palsy." *Journal of Pediatric Orthopedics*, 21 (1), 108–12. http://www.ncbi.nlm.nih.gov/pubmed/11176363.

Spiegel, David A., Randall, T Loder., Katie, A Alley., Sarah, Rowley., Sarah, Gutknecht., Deborah, L Smith-Wright. & Mary, Elizabeth Dunn. n.d. "Spinal Deformity Following Selective Dorsal Rhizotomy." *Journal of Pediatric Orthopedics*, 24 (1), 30–36. http://www.ncbi.nlm.nih.gov/pubmed/14676531.

Sponseller, Paul D., Suken, A Shah., Mark, F Abel., Daniel, Sucato., Peter, O Newton., Harry, Shufflebarger., Lawrence, G Lenke., et al. (2009). "Scoliosis Surgery in Cerebral Palsy: Differences between Unit Rod and Custom Rods." *Spine*, 34 (8), 840–44. doi:10.1097/BRS.0b013e31819487b7.

Steinbok, Paul., Tufan, Hicdonmez., Bonita, Sawatzky., Richard, Beauchamp. & Diane, Wickenheiser. (2005). "Spinal Deformities after Selective Dorsal Rhizotomy for Spastic Cerebral Palsy." In *Journal of Neurosurgery*, 102, 363–73. doi:10.3171/ped.2005.102.4.0363.

Suh, Seung Woo., Hitesh, N Modi., Jaehyuk, Yang., Hae-Ryong, Song. & Ki-Mo, Jang. (2009). "Posterior Multilevel Vertebral Osteotomy for Correction of Severe and Rigid Neuromuscular Scoliosis: A Preliminary Study." *Spine*, 34 (12), 1315–20. doi:10.1097/ BRS.0b013e3181a028bc.

Sullivan, J. A. & Conner, S. B. n.d. "Comparison of Harrington Instrumentation and Segmental Spinal Instrumentation in the Management of Neuromuscular Spinal Deformity." *Spine*, 7 (3), 299–304. http://www.ncbi.nlm.nih.gov/pubmed/7112244.

Swank, S. M., Cohen, D. S. & Brown, J. C. (1989). "Spine Fusion in Cerebral Palsy with L-Rod Segmental Spinal Instrumentation. A Comparison of Single and Two-Stage Combined Approach with Zielke Instrumentation." *Spine*, 14 (7), 750–59. http://www.ncbi.nlm.nih.gov/pubmed/2772727.

Takeshita, Katsushi., Lawrence, G Lenke., Keith, H Bridwell., Yongjung, J Kim., Brenda, Sides. & Marsha, Hensley. (2006). "Analysis of Patients with Nonambulatory Neuromuscular Scoliosis Surgically Treated to the Pelvis with Intraoperative Halo-Femoral Traction." *Spine*, 31 (20), 2381–85. doi:10.1097/01.brs.0000238964.73390.b6.

Terjesen, T., Lange, J. E. & Steen, H. (2000). "Treatment of Scoliosis with Spinal Bracing in Quadriplegic Cerebral Palsy." *Developmental Medicine and Child Neurology*, 42 (7), 448–54. http://www.ncbi.nlm.nih.gov/pubmed/10972416.

Thometz, J. G. & Simon, S. R. (1988). "Progression of Scoliosis after Skeletal Maturity in Institutionalized Adults Who Have Cerebral Palsy." *The Journal of Bone and Joint Surgery. American*, Volume 70 (9), 1290–96. http://www.ncbi.nlm.nih.gov/pubmed/3182881.

Thomson, J. D. & Banta, J. V. (2001). "Scoliosis in Cerebral Palsy: An Overview and Recent Results." *Journal of Pediatric Orthopedics. Part B*, *10* (1), 6–9. http://www.ncbi.nlm.nih.gov/pubmed/11269813.

Turi, M. & Kalen, V. n.d. "The Risk of Spinal Deformity after Selective Dorsal Rhizotomy." *Journal of Pediatric Orthopedics*, *20* (1), 104–7. http://www.ncbi.nlm.nih.gov/pubmed/10641698.

Vialle, R., Mary, P. & Marty, C. (2012). "*Diagnostique, Physiopathologie et Analyse de La Déformation*," [Diagnosis, Physiopathology and Deformation Analysis,] no. 88299.

Vialle, Raphaël., Christophe, Delecourt. & Christian, Morin. (2006). "Surgical Treatment of Scoliosis with Pelvic Obliquity in Cerebral Palsy: The Influence of Intraoperative Traction." *Spine*, *31* (13), 1461–66. doi:10.1097/01.brs.0000219874.46680.87.

Vialle, R., Thévenin-Lemoine, C. & Mary, P. (2013). "Neuromuscular Scoliosis." *Orthopaedics & Traumatology, Surgery & Research : OTSR*, *99* (1 Suppl), S124-39. doi:10.1016/j.otsr.2012.11.002.

Vitale, Michael G., Matthew, D. Riedel., Michael, P. Glotzbecker., Hiroko, Matsumoto., David, P. Roye., Behrooz, A. Akbarnia., Richard, C. E. Anderson., et al. (2013). "Building Consensus." *Journal of Pediatric Orthopaedics*, *33* (5), 471–78. doi:10.1097/BPO.0b013e3182840de2.

Walker, Kevin R., Susan, A Novotny. & Linda, E Krach. (2017). "Does Intrathecal Baclofen Therapy Increase Prevalence And/or Progression of Neuromuscular Scoliosis?" *Spine Deformity*, *5* (6), 424–29. doi:10.1016/j.jspd.2017.03.006.

Watanabe, Kei., Lawrence, G Lenke., Keith, H Bridwell., Yongjung, J Kim., Kota, Watanabe., Young-Woo, Kim., Youngbae, B Kim., Marsha, Hensley. & Georgia, Stobbs. (2008). "Comparison of Radiographic Outcomes for the Treatment of Scoliotic Curves Greater than 100 Degrees: Wires versus Hooks versus Screws." *Spine*, *33* (10), 1084–92. doi:10.1097/BRS.0b013e31816f5f3a.

Westerlund, L. E., Gill, S. S., Jarosz, T. S., Abel, M. F. & Blanco, J. S. (2001). "Posterior-Only Unit Rod Instrumentation and Fusion for Neuromuscular Scoliosis." *Spine*, *26* (18), 1984–89. http://www.ncbi.nlm.nih.gov/pubmed/11547196.

Winter, R. B. & Carlson, J. M. n.d. "Modern Orthotics for Spinal Deformities." *Clinical Orthopaedics and Related Research*, no. *126*, 74–86. http://www.ncbi.nlm.nih.gov/pubmed/598143.

Winter, S. (1994). "Preoperative Assessment of the Child with Neuromuscular Scoliosis." *The Orthopedic Clinics of North America*, *25* (2), 239–45. http://www.ncbi.nlm.nih.gov/pubmed/8159398.

Winter, S. L., Kriel, R. L., Novacheck, T. F., Luxenberg, M. G., Leutgeb, V. J. & Erickson, P. A. (1996). "Perioperative Blood Loss: The Effect of Valproate." *Pediatric Neurology*, *15* (1), 19–22. http://www.ncbi.nlm.nih.gov/pubmed/8858695.

Yazici, M. & Asher, M. A. (1997). "Freeze-Dried Allograft for Posterior Spinal Fusion in Patients with Neuromuscular Spinal Deformities." *Spine*, *22* (13), 1467–71. http://www.ncbi.nlm.nih.gov/pubmed/9231965.

Yazici, M., Asher, M. A. & Hardacker, J. W. (2000). "The Safety and Efficacy of Isola-Galveston Instrumentation and Arthrodesis in the Treatment of Neuromuscular Spinal Deformities." *The Journal of Bone and Joint Surgery. American*, Volume *82* (4), 524–43. http://www.ncbi.nlm.nih.gov/pubmed/10761943.

Young, H. K., Lowe, A., Fitzgerald, D. A., Seton, C., Waters, K. A., Kenny, E., Hynan, L. S., Iannaccone, S. T., North, K. N. & Ryan, M. M. (2007). "Outcome of Noninvasive Ventilation in Children with Neuromuscular Disease." *Neurology*, *68* (3), 198–201. doi:10.1212/01.wnl.0000251299.54608.13.

Zadek, R E. 1973. "Orthopedic Management of the Child and Multiple Handicaps." *Pediatric Clinics of North America*, *20* (1), 177–85. http://www.ncbi.nlm.nih.gov/pubmed/4268517.

Chapter 24

RADIOGRAPHIC ASSESSMENT AND FOLLOW-UP OF PATIENTS WITH SCOLIOSIS

Mohsen Karami[*], *MD*
Department of Orthopaedic Surgery,
Shahid Beheshti University of Medical Sciences, Tehran, Iran

ABSTRACT

Radiologic assessment of scoliosis is an inevitable part of patient evaluation. It includes standing x-rays, MRI, and/or CT scans. Upright x-rays are essential for measuring scoliotic curves and planning further treatment modalities. A thorough knowledge of these measurements is the first step in clinical assessment and decision making for every scoliosis patient.

Keywords: scoliosis, radiologic assessment, MRI, CT scan

INTRODUCTION

In spite of modern radiologic imaging, traditional radiologic assessment of a new scoliosis diagnosis and its follow-up are essential. Provided that a patient has a positive clinical screen test for scoliosis, upright radiologic films are the next step in diagnosis and for treatment planning.

It is vital to know the standard films for diagnosis and measurements on these films. The measurements may affect a patient's treatment planning and his/her subsequent decision-making.

Emerging technologies have also had implications on diagnosis and treatment options. Magnetic Resonance Imaging (MRI) and Computed Tomography (CT) scans are useful imaging technologies that may help physicians and change treatment strategies. Low dose radiation technology is becoming the gold standard for scoliosis diagnosis and its follow-up.

---

[*] Corresponding Author Email: mkarami@sbmu.ac.ir.

IMAGING TECHNIQUES

Radiographs

A patient referred to a spine clinic for scoliosis evaluation should receive plain standing radiography including Postero Anterior (PA) and Lateral (LA) films (Figure 1). Patient position during x-ray exposure may significantly affect the measurement. Long cassette film of 36 by 14 inches, formerly the standard for a traditional upright film, has been replaced by digital radiology in the form of picture archiving and communication systems (PACS) and for an emerging technology, EOS™ machine.

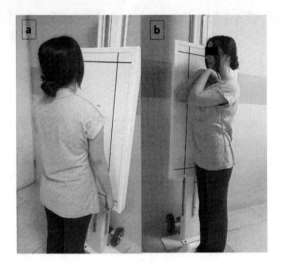

Figure 1a and b, common positioning during x-ray acquisition of upright posteroanterior and lateral films.

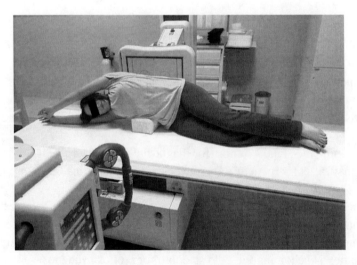

Figure 2. Patient position in fulcrum lateral bending x-ray, the fulcrum is inserted on the convex side of the curve.

In reading an upright PA film, it is important to view the entirety of the spine, evaluate each vertebra for congenital anomalies and existing curves, examine for missing/fractured/adhesed ribs, look for heart and lung anomalies (dextro-cardia), assess the pelvis bone (Risser sign and triradiate cartilage closure and pelvic tilt) and check for coronal balance (shoulders and clavicles tilting and shift of the whole spine to one side). In the standing lateral x-ray, vertebral profile (congenital anomalies, vertebral destruction or its sequela), existing sagittal curves, sagittal profile of the spine, and pelvis parameters should be noted.

Other useful films, when surgical decision making is necessary, include bilateral supine bending films (to verify each curve correction to opposite side and curve flexibility) and traction films (to verify flexibility of very severe curves, especially neuromuscular ones). Fulcrum bending radiograph in curve flexibility assessment of patients with adolescent idiopathic scoliosis (AIS) determines true thoracic curve flexibility and how to choose between a high or low-density construct for AIS surgery [1, 2] (Figure 2). For upper thoracic and thoracolumbar/lumbar curves, the traditional supine bending method is acceptable [3]. Fulcrum hyperextension LA radiograph is also useful in measuring flexibility of kyphotic curvature.

Patient Positioning and X-Ray Exposure Consideration

To obtain standing LA x-ray, a patient's position has a negative impact on their sagittal profile. Standing with the hands supported while flexing the shoulders 30 degrees during lateral x-ray acquisition results in sagittal parameter measurements comparable with a functional standing position with arms at the side. This is the most effective method to move the arms anterior to the vertebral column with the least effect on overall sagittal balance [4] (Figure 3).

To obtain traction films, a Cotrel table is the most reliable method to put traction on both a patient's pelvis and chin, allowing simultaneous capture of the x-ray. If a Cotrel table is not accessible, the patient traction can be achieved through simultaneous manual traction on the patient's leg and chin in the opposite direction. Adolescent female patients should always be asked about their last menstrual period and the possibility of pregnancy. For patient protection, PA film is superior to antero-posterior positioning to reduce x-ray exposure to the breasts.

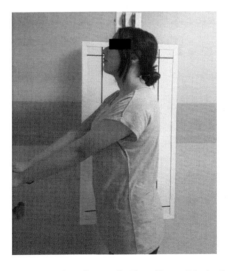

Figure 3. Patient position in upright lateral radiograph. Standing with the hands supported while flexing the shoulders 30 degrees.

The patient should stand as upright as possible with the knees completely straight and the bare feet together (Figure 1). If lower limb length inequality is suspected, the patient should place an appropriate lift under the short limb. If the patient is unable to stand, an unsupported sitting position can be used instead.

Radiographic follow-up is an inseparable part of scoliosis management that imposes further radiation risks to the patient. Scoliosis follow-up routinely needs only a PA upright x-ray, and the evaluation periods can range from four months to one or even five years. For example, a four-month follow-up x-ray is acceptable for an 11-year-old premenstrual girl and a one year follow-up period is acceptable for a 13-year-old girl who has experienced her menstrual period eighteen months ago. The routine interval is typically four to six months for a growing child.

Measurement of Coronal Parameters

Three distinct curves can be marked on a PA upright x-ray for any patient who presents with scoliosis. Each defined curve has an upper and a lower end vertebra, an apex vertebra or disk, and an angle which can be measured according to Cobb method [5] (Figure 4). Each tilted vertebra starting from the end vertebra gradually goes to a horizontal position in the apex of the curve. The most tilted vertebra at both ends of the curve is defined as the upper and lower end vertebra. The superior endplate of the upper end vertebra and the inferior endplate of the lower end vertebra are marked to measure the angle between them, known as the Cobb angle of that curve. To be measured conveniently using a goniometer, it is better to draw perpendicular lines to the endplate lines, with the inferior angle at the intersection point of that perpendicular line being equal to the Cobb angle (Figure 4). The angle can be directly measured using PACS software as well as other commercially available applications. Computer-based measurements are reliable when used for Cobb angles [6]. If a second curve is present below or above the primary curve, next or behind the original curve's lower or upper end vertebra becomes the cephalic or caudal end vertebra for the second curve, and the same line along its inferior or superior surface can be used.

There can be significant inter-observer variability when measuring Cobb curves. To combat this, a second set of vertebrae can be measured. The highest measured angle shows the correct selection of the end vertebra. The radiographic measurements of the Cobb angle and vertebral rotation (VR) should be precise, because these measurements will have significant influence on treatment decision planning. The inter-observer and intra-observer reliabilities of the Cobb method has been reported .94-.99 [6], but the mean error of most studies are less than 5 degrees [6-9].

Other coronal parameters that are measurable on a PA film are: T1, clavicles, and pelvic tilt angles regarding to horizontal line. Coronal shift or list is the distance between the center of the C7 body to the center sacral vertical line (CSVL) (Figure 5). Coronal imbalance has been defined as a shift of more than 1-2cm [10]. Another useful parameter to assess trunk balance is thoracic apical vertebral translation, which is the distance measured between the midpoint of the apical thoracic vertebra and CSVL [11-12].

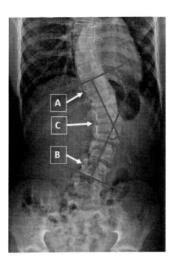

Figure 4. Cobb angle measurement, Upper end vertebra (A), lower end vertebra (B), the apex (C) and the lines which were drawn to measure Cobb angle.

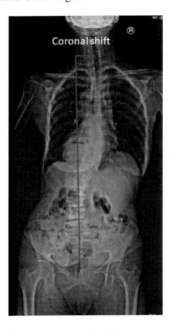

Figure 5. Coronal shift, the distance between center of C7 body to center sacral vertical line.

Measurement of Sagittal Parameters

Upright LA film is crucial to measure all sagittal parameters of the spine. These include the thoracic kyphosis angle, lumbar lordosis angle, sagittal balance of the spine, and pelvis parameters. Some of these parameters seems unlikely to be applicable in an AIS patient, but in young patients there is often an issue related to spinal hyper or hypo kyphosis, and in adult and degenerative cases, the lumbar and pelvic parameters should always be considered in surgical decision making.

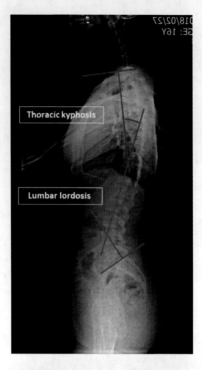

Figure 6. Upright lateral radiograph, useful sagittal parameters in scoliotic patient.

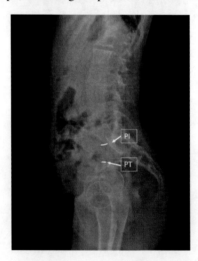

Figure 7. Pelvic parameters can be measured on an upright lateral x ray, pelvic incidence (PI) and pelvic tilt (PT).

The measurement of thoracic kyphosis and lumbar lordosis is done according to the Cobb method. In the thoracic spine, the normal sagittal curvature is kyphotic. The superior endplate of T1 (if visible) or T4/T5 and inferior endplate of T12 can be taken to measure thoracic kyphosis. The apex of thoracic kyphosis is at T6 or T7. If T4 or T5 has been taken for measurement, 10-15 degrees should be added on to get the real thoracic kyphosis [13-14] (Figure 6). The mean value of T1-T12 kyphosis has been reported 41.5 ± 9.9 degrees [15]. Other important kyphosis angles are T2-T5, T10-L2 angle, which are useful in Lenke classification. Lumbar lordosis is also variable between people. Because L5-S1 disk counts about 40% of lumbar lordosis, lumbar lordosis should be measured from superior endplate of L1 to superior endplate of S1 (Figure 6). The mean value of lumbar lordosis has been reported 55.4 ± 11.2 degrees [14].

Global Sagittal balance mainly refers to the sagittal vertical axis (SVA) which is defined as the linear offset of C7 in regard to the posterosuperior corner of S1[15]. Sagittal pelvic parameters are also useful in adult and mainly degenerative kyphoscoliosis. The most important measurements are pelvic incidence (PI) and pelvic tilt (PT) [16-17] (Figure 7). A low pelvic incidence decreases sacral-slope and the lumbar lordosis becomes flat. A high incidence (>62°) increases sacral-slope and the lordosis became more prominent [18].

Measurement of Vertebral Rotation

There are two commonly preferred methods for analyzing vertebral rotation. It is useful to determine the apical vertebral rotation. In the method of Nash and Moe, the vertebral body is divided into six segments, and grades from 0 to 4+ are assigned depending on the location of the pedicle within these segments (Figure 8). Since the concave pedicle disappears early in rotation, the convex pedicle, easily visible through a wide range or rotation, is used for the measurement. Zero rotation means that there is no asymmetry in either the position or shape of either pedicle; 1+ rotation indicates medial migration of the convex pedicle and slight flattening of the ovality of both pedicles; 2+ rotation signifies further migration of the convex pedicle into the second vertebral segment while the concave pedicle gradually becomes indistinct; 3+ rotation occurs when the convex pedicle reaches the mid-line and is completely within the third segment; 4+ rotation is passing of convex pedicle through the mid-line into the fourth segment on the concave side of the body [19] (Figure 8). The Perdriolle torsionmeter is a template that can measure the amount of vertebral rotation on a spinal x-ray. The pedicles offset and the edges of the vertebral body are marked, and then rotation can be measured with the Pedriolle torsionmeter (Figure 9) [20]. However, this still has limitations in inter-observer and intra-observer reliability, particularly when using it in curves greater than 30 degrees [21].

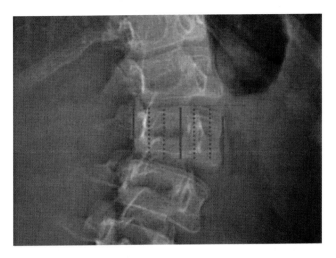

Figure 8. In the method of Nash and Moe, the apical vertebral body is divided into six segments then according to the appearance of the convex pedicle, the type of the rotation will be measured.

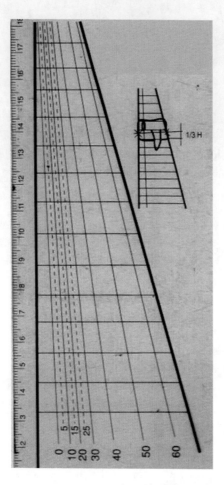

Figure 9. *Left*, Perdriolle torsionometer. *Right*, the template outer margins are fitted over the vertebra's lateral borders. The line intersecting the center of the convex pedicle shadow shows the amount of vertebral rotation.

Maturity Radiologic Evaluation

One other essential radiologic examination is the evaluation of bone maturity. It is critical to have an estimation of a patient's potential future growth because this will significantly affect scoliosis progression. There are controversies regarding how to evaluate bone maturity. The Risser sign or iliac crest apophysis ossification is a popular-but not accurate [22] indicator of spine maturity and prediction of the progression of a scoliotic curve (Figure 10). In the management of scoliosis, no treatment to prevent an increase in the scoliotic curve is needed for an individual who has a closed iliac apophysis. Conversely, the patient who has no visible iliac apophysis at all will require a sort of management from observation to surgery to prevent deformity progression.

Sanders et al. [23] proposed a simplified skeletal maturity staging system from the Tanner-Whitehouse III and Greulich and Pyle systems. This system uses hand radiograph to establish the skeletal maturity stage, which is then correlated with scoliosis progression based on skeletal maturity and curve magnitude in a predictive model (Figure 11). Sitoula et al. [24] in their recent study showed a strong predictive correlation between Sanders stage and initial Cobb angle for probability of curve progression in idiopathic scoliosis.

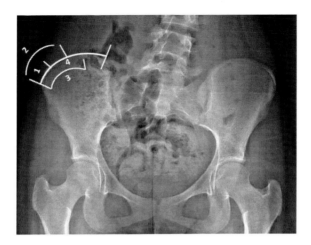

Figure 10. The Risser sign or iliac crest apophysis ossification in grade 4 patient, it proceeds from grade 0 (no ossification) to grade 4 (all four quadrants show ossification of the iliac apophysis). In Risser grade 5, the ossified apophysis has fused completely to the ilium, therefore, the patient is skeletally mature.

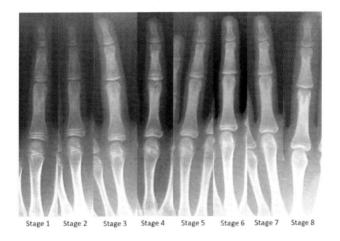

Figure 11. Skeletal maturity classification of Sanders. Stage 1, juvenile slow; stage (the epiphysis is not as wide as the metaphysis is especially noticeable at the middle phalanx); stage 2, preadolescent (Tanner 2) (The epiphyses are as wide as their metaphyses); stage 3, adolescent rapid-early (Tanner 2 to 3, Risser 0)(The epiphysis has a small bend over the metaphyseal edge, metacarpal head is wider than its metaphysis); stage 4: adolescent rapid-late (Tanner 3, Risser 0)(The distal phalangeal physis is beginning to close); stage 5, adolescent steady-early (Risser 0)(all of the distal phalangeal physes are closed); stage 6, adolescent steady-late (Risser > 0)(some of the proximal and middle phalangeal physes are closing); stage 7, early mature(all of hand physes are closed, except for those of the distal parts of the radius and ulna); stage 8, mature stage (Risser 5)(closure of all physes).

Magnetic Resonance Imaging

Aside from its controversial indications, it is very useful to evaluate neurocentral abnormalities such as syringomyelia, tethered cord, Arnold-Chiari malformation, and tumors. Routine MR imaging for a typical AIS patients is not indicated. Atypical AIS is considered when there is rapid curve progression or excessive thoracic kyphosis, left thoracic curves, significant coronal shift, or early onset scoliosis [25]. The most important indications for MR imaging is abnormal neurologic findings and a painful scoliosis (Figure 12).

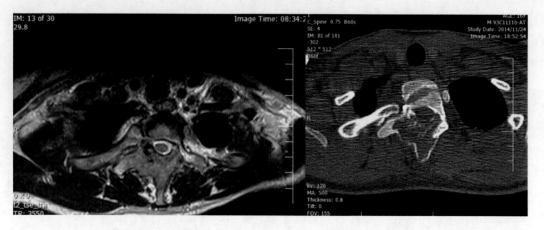

Figure 12. Shows MRI and CT images of a destructive lesion at T2 vertebra which produced a painful scoliosis in a 16 year old girl.

Computed Tomography

Though not a routine pre-operative evaluation of scoliosis, can be used in congenital curves and very severe idiopathic scoliosis when a Vertebral Column Resection is planned. It shows vertebral anomalies as well as intra-canal bony spicules especially when combined with myelography in very severe cases (more than 70 degrees scoliosis) [26].

REFERENCES

[1] Cheung KMC, Luk KDK. 1997. "Prediction of correction of scoliosis with use of the fulcrum bending radiographs." *J Bone Joint Surg*, 79(8), 1144-50. (Cheung 1997,1146).

[2] Cheung KM, Natarajan D, Samartzis D, Wong YW, Cheung WY, Luk KD. 2010. "Predictability of the fulcrum bending radiograph in scoliosis correction with alternate-level pedicle screw fixation." *J Bone Joint Surery* 1;92(1):169-76. (Cheung 2010, 169).

[3] Klepps SJ, Lenke LG, Bridwell K H, Bassett GS, Whorton J. 2001. "Prospective comparison of flexibility radiographs in adolescent idiopathic scoliosis." *Spine* 26(5): E74-E79. (Klepps 2001, E75).

[4] Marks M, Stanford C, Newton P. 2009. Which lateral radiographic positioning technique provides the most reliable and functional representation of a patient's sagittal balance? *Spine* 34(9), 949-54. (Marks 2009, 950).

[5] Cobb J. 1948 "Outline for the study of scoliosis." *AAOS Instr Course Lect* 5: 261–75. (Cobb 1948, 267).

[6] Tanure MC, Pinheiro AP, Oliveira AS. 2010. "Reliability assessment of Cobb angle measurements using manual and digital methods." *The spine journal* 10(9): 769-774. (Tanure 2010, 772).

[7] Chan AC, Morrison DG, Nguyen DV, Hill DL, Parent E, Lou EH. 2014. "Intra-and Interobserver Reliability of the Cobb Angle–Vertebral Rotation Angle–Spinous Process Angle for Adolescent Idiopathic Scoliosis" *Spine deformity* 2(3):168-75. (Chan 2014, 171).

[8] Gstoettner M, Sekyra K, Walochnik N, Winter P, Wachter R, Bach CM. 2007. "Inter- and intraobserver reliability assessment of the Cobb angle: manual versus digital measurement tools." *Eur Spine J* 16:1587-92. (Gstoettner 2007, 1589).

[9] Kuklo TR, Potter BK, O'brien MF, Schroeder TM, Lenke LG, Polly Jr DW. 2005. "Reliability analysis for digital adolescent idiopathic scoliosis measurements." *J Spinal Disord Tech* 18:15-9. (Kuklo 2005, 17).

[10] Karami M, Maleki A, Mazda K. (2016). "Assessment of coronal radiographic parameters of the spine in the treatment of adolescent idiopathic scoliosis." *Archives of Bone and Joint Surgery* 4(4): 376-80. (Karami 2016, 377).

[11] Lenke LG, Bridwell KH, Baldus C, Blanke K. 1992. "Preventing decompensation in King type II curves treated with Cotrel-Dubousset instrumentation. Strict guidelines for selective thoracic fusion." *Spine* 17(Suppl 8): S274. (Lenke 1992, S274).

[12] Behensky H, Cole AA, Freeman BJ, Grevitt MP, Mehdian HS, Webb JK. 2007. "Fixed lumbar apical vertebral rotation predicts spinal decompensation in Lenke type 3C adolescent idiopathic scoliosis after selective posterior thoracic correction and fusion." *Eur Spine J.* 16(10): 1570-8. (Behensky 2007, 1576).

[13] Gelb DE, Lenke LG, Bridwell KH, Blanke K, McEnery KW. 1995. "An analysis of sagittal spinal alignment in 100 asymptomatic middle and older aged volunteers." *Spine* (Phila Pa 1976) 20:1351–8. (Gelb 1995, 1355).

[14] Hasegawa K, Okamoto M, Hatsushikano S, Shimoda H, Ono M, Watanabe K. 2016. "Normative values of spino-pelvic sagittal alignment, balance, age, and health-related quality of life in a cohort of healthy adult subjects." *Eur Spine J.* 25(11): 3675-86. (Hasegawa 2016, 3680).

[15] Schwab FJ, Blondel B, Bess S, Hostin R, Shaffrey CI, Smith JS, Boachie-Adjei O, Burton DC, Akbarnia BA, Mundis GM, Ames CP. 2013 "Radiographical spinopelvic parameters and disability in the setting of adult spinal deformity." *Spine* 38: E803–E812. (Schwab 2013, E809).

[16] Legaye J, Duval-Beaupere G, Hecquet J, Marty C. 1998. "Pelvic incidence: a fundamental pelvic parameter for three-dimensional regulation of spinal sagittal curves." *Eur Spine J.* 7:99–103. (Legaye 1998, 101).

[17] During J, Goudfrooij H, Keessen W, Beeker TW, Crowe A. 1985. "Toward standards for posture. Postural characteristics of the lower back system in normal and pathologic conditions." *Spine* 10:83–7. (During 1985, 85).

[18] Boulay C, Tardieu C, Hecquet J, Benaim C, Mouilleseaux B, Marty C, Prat-Pradal D, Legaye J, Duval-Beaupère G, Pélissier J. 2006. "Sagittal alignment of spine and pelvis regulated by pelvic incidence: standard values and prediction of lordosis." *Eur Spine J.* 15(4): 415-22. (Boulay 2006, 419).

[19] Nash, CL, Moe JH. 1969. "A study of vertebral rotation." *J Bone Joint Surg Am*, 51(2): 223-9. (Nash 1969, 225).

[20] Richards BS. 1992. "Measurement error in assessment of vertebral rotation using the Perdriolle torsionmeter." *Spine* 17(5): 513-17. (Richards 1992, 516).

[21] Ömeroğlu H, Özekin O, Biçimoğlu A. 1996. "Measurement of vertebral rotation in idiopathic scoliosis using the Perdriolle torsionmeter: a clinical study on intraobserver and interobserver error." *Eur Spine J.* 5(3): 167-71. (Ömeroğlu 1996, 169).

[22] Shuren N, Kasser JR, Emans JB, Rand F. 1992. "Reevaluation of the use of the Risser sign in idiopathic scoliosis." *Spine* 17: 359 – 61. (Shuren 1992, 360).

[23] Sanders JO, Khoury JG, Kishan S, Browne RH, Mooney III JF, Arnold KD, McConnell SJ, Bauman JA, Finegold DN. 2008. "Predicting scoliosis progression from skeletal maturity: a simplifi ed classifi cation during adolescence." *J Bone Joint Surg* Am 90: 540 – 53. (Sanders 2008, 548).

[24] Sitoula P, Verma K, Holmes Jr L, Gabos PG, Sanders JO, Yorgova P, Neiss G, Rogers K, Shah SA. 2015. "Prediction of curve progression in idiopathic scoliosis: validation of the sanders skeletal maturity staging system." *Spine* 40(13): 1006-13. (Sitoula 2015, 1010).

[25] Karami, M., Sagheb, S., & Mazda, K. 2014. "Evaluation of coronal shift as an indicator of neuroaxial abnormalities in adolescent idiopathic scoliosis: a prospective study." *Scoliosis* 9(1): 9. (Karami 2014. 9).

[26] O'brien MF, Lenke LG, Bridwell KH, Blanke K, Baldus C. 1994. "Preoperative spinal canal investigation in adolescent idiopathic scoliosis curves > or =70 degrees." *Spine* 19:1606-10. (O'brien 1994, 1608).

In: Scoliosis: Diagnosis, Classification and Management Options ISBN: 978-1-53614-464-2
Editors: F. Canavese, A. Andreacchio and H. Xu © 2018 Nova Science Publishers, Inc.

Chapter 25

RASTERSTEREOGRAPHY FOR THE FOLLOW-UP OF AIS PATIENTS

Anne Tabard-Fougère[1,2,]*, PhD, Charlotte de Bodman[2,3], MD, Alice Bonnefoy-Mazure[1], PhD and Romain Dayer[2,3], MD

[1]Willy Taillard Laboratory of Kinesiology,
Geneva University Hospitals and Geneva University, Geneva, Switzerland
[2]Division of Paediatric Orthopaedics,
Geneva University Hospitals and Geneva University, Geneva, Switzerland
[3]Pediatric Orthopedics and Traumatology Unit, Lausanne University Hospital,
Lausanne, Switzerland

ABSTRACT

Scoliosis is a three-dimensional spine deformity. The most frequent scoliosis type is adolescent idiopathic scoliosis (AIS), with no clear specific underlying cause and risk of curve progression with growth. Treatment is based on curve magnitude and residual growth progression. The gold standard examination to monitor curve progression is standard postero-anterior radiography, which lead to frequent radiation exposure and an increase of mortality due to cancer. A promising radiation-free measurement tool is rasterstereography. It consists to evaluate scoliosis curve based on surface toppography of the skin of the back. Rasterstereography could help to reduce radiation exposure for monitoring of curve progression. The present chapter briefly details the history and the techniques of rasterstereography, describes the existing literature about the reliability and variability of rasterstereography and suggests some clinical applications and perpespectives for future studies.

Keywords: rasterstereography, surface topography, adolescent idiopathic scoliosis

---

* Corresponding Author Email: anne.tabard@hcuge.ch.

INTRODUCTION

Scoliosis is a lateral deviation and axial rotation of the spine leading to a three-dimensional (3D) spine deformity [1]. Most of the time, scoliosis is idiopathic with an absence of specific cause [2] and main risk of progression is during the pubertal adolescent growth spurt [3]. Adolescent Idiopathic Scoliosis (AIS) is diagnosed from 10 years of age. The treatment of patients with AIS is based on the risk of curve progression [4]. Different methods can be used to monitore AIS progression including conventional radiography (RX), low-dose stereography (EOS), surface topography, and 3D ultrasound [5]. There is unfortunately a lack of a consensus algorithm to know when each imaging method should be used [6].

The gold standard for the initial diagnosis and longitudinal monitoring is a two-dimensional (2D) postero-anterior full-length spine X-ray (XR) [7]. The potential for evolution during pubertal growth requires frequent radiological assessments, which can have negative long-term effects on young patients [8–10]. Repeated use of XR in the context has been associated with a five times higher cancer rate as reported in a 25-years longitudinal study [11]. The mean radiation dose evaluated was 0.8 to 1.4 mSv per examination and 2.4 to 5.6 mSv/year, and endometrial and breast cancers were more frequent [11].

However, AIS patients have a normal life expectancy with few associated long-term physical disorders other than moderate back pain and cosmetic concerns [12]. In this context it appears mandatory to reduce irradiation exposure of growing AIS patients [6]. The reduction of these irradiations is a major health challenge for these growing patients.

A low dose XR solution was developed in recent years with the EOS® System (Biospace Med, Paris, France), which provides reduced irradiation (theoretically by 8-10 compared to standard radiographs) [13, 14] with an image quality comparable to conventional XR [15]. This measurement tool uses an ultra-sensitive multi-wire proportional chamber detector to detect XR and performed simultaneously antero-posteror and lateral images. The EOS® System was validated in the clinical setting in order to follow the evolution of AIS patients [16–18]. A recent case series reported however that the total radiation exposure was only moderately reduced (50.6%) to skeletally immature scoliosis patients [19]. In addition, the EOS® System is significantly more expensive than standard RX system. Thus, the accessibility of this low dose system is limited.

A radiation-free method, developed by Drerup and Hierholzer in the 1980s, named rastersstereography [20, 21], seemed an interesting radiation-free alternative system for the assessment and observation of spinal deformity. This system based on surface topography is non-invasive and is using only an electric light source, a video camera and a computer. The current main application of rastersstereography is in research to measure and monitor spine deformities in AIS patients [22–26], but the recommendations for clinical application are not clear. The present chapter briefly detailles the history and the techniques of rastersstereography, describes the existing literature about the reliability and variability of rastersstereography and suggests some clinical applications and perpespectives for future studies.

HISTORY AND TECHNICS OF RASTERSTEREOGRAPHY

The clinical examination of a patient with scoliosis is most often based on the detection and measurement of landmarks on the back surface such as: pelvis tilt, trunk imbalance, waistline asymmetry, shoulder tilt difference, rib hump and lumbar hump. These specific anatomical landmarks are defined by skeletal structures detectable on the body surface. The determination of these points can be obtained using photogrammetric technique as the Moiré topography [27].

This specific technique is based on the analysis of the surface shape using the surface curvature. This physical phenomemon occurs when a set of curves overlap another set of curves, forming a new group [28]. For this, the shape of surface analysed is created by the projection and the alternation of clear and dark fringes on the object surface [29]. To obtain these curves deformations and pattern shape surface, only a camera, a light source and a grating are necessary. In the literature, it appears that the positioning of the camera and light source can vary [30, 31].

In the medical context, Takasaki was the first to propose the use of this approach for the analysis of the surface human body [32].

From there a method called rasterstereography has been developed and proposed by Drerup and Hierholzer in order to observe and analyse more specificaly posture and spinal deformities [20, 33–35]. As described before, this method uses a radiation-free technique projecting horizontal fringes on the surface of the patient's back and then analysing the distorsion of these projected fringes (Figure 1). For this, static images of the lines are recorded, digitized and then the distorsion of the fringes are used to produce a three-dimensional image of the back surface that is correlated with underlying spinal curve deformities [36].

Actually several systems have been developed based in this free radiation technology as: Formetric system [25], Integrated Shape Imaging System version 2 (ISIS2) [37], Inspeck system [38], as well as the Quantec spinal imaging system [39].

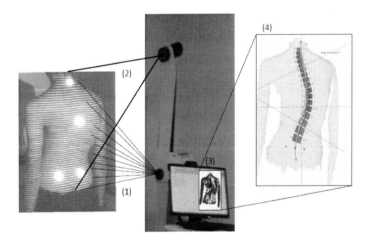

Figure 1. Set up of rasterstereography system (Formetric 4D Diers). 1) Parallel light lines projected, 2) Photo capture, 3) 3D spine modeling using surface topography, 4) Computation of scoliosis angle among other parameters.

The diffences between these systems is often due to the patient back skin preparation. Indeed, some systems require additional external markers glued directly on the skin [37, 39]. These additional markers enable to detect precisely specific bony structure on the back shape. Others systems detect the bony landmarks automatically [36]. This automatic detection limits the need for an experienced operator [37] and error due to the palpation [36].

RELIABILITY AND VALIDITY OF RASTERSTEREOGRAPHY

In current practice, the therapeutic choice of AIS treatment is mainly determined by changes in the Cobb angle [40], a 2D measurement of spinal deformity performed on a postero-anterior XR [41]. In this context, a reliable measurement of Cobb angle is necessary. The margin of error of Cobb angle measurement performed on XR is generally considered around 5° [42–44]. Based on this value Morrisy et al. [43] defined a 10° of change between two successive radiographs to determine progression.

The inter- and intra-observer reliability of rasterstereography in the evaluation of scoliosis angle on AIS patients were demonstrated to be high with respectively 1.0° and 0.3° mean of difference and intraclass correlation coefficient between 70% and 85% [26]. Similar results were observed on healthy participants on spinal parameters in sagittal and frontal planes [45–47].

A recent systematic review reported 12 studies evaluated the validity and accuracy of rasterstereography compared with XR [48]. Among them, three studies reported the Cobb angle in AIS patients [49–51] with also two additional recent studies [25, 26]. In comparison with XR they evaluated strong correlation and average difference between 5.8° and 7.0° of Cobb angle in thoracic spine, between 8.8° and 9.4° of Cobb angle in lumbar spine [22, 25] and between 5.4° and 8.0° of Cobb angle in all spine levels [26, 49].

Several factors could explain these differences higher than 5°. First, the rasterstreography calculations are based on location of the left (DL) and right (DR) lumbar dimples associated with the posterior superior illiac spine [20], and the vertebral prominens typically located at C7 [21] as illustrated in Figure 2. The location of these anatomical points is dependant of patient's anatomy changes in soft tissue contour and of palpation error. These errors could also be due to high body mass index [46]. Thus, this variability could influence the angle calculation [52].

In addition, the patient positioning sway and breathing could influence the angle calculation [45,52]. To reduce this last source of variability, it is recommended to use the standard average value calculated from 12 images recorded during a single scan of 6s [52].

It seems that there is a no "ideal position" determined to use for the patient evaluation. It is important to performed rasterstereography assessment in similar position than XR in order to compare measurements. The principal positions used on XR are the "clavical" and "straight out" postures [53, 54].

The "clavical" position is a validated radiological position of reference [53]. The patient bends his elbows, wrists and fingers and places the dorsal surface of the 2nd phalanges of the last two fingers in contact with the collarbones. This posture has been reported to be the most representative of a patient's functional balance while still allowing adequate lateral radiographic visualization of the spine in AIS patients [55].

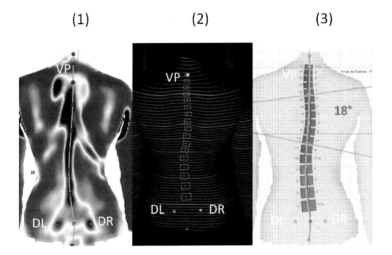

Figure 2. Illustration of rasterstereography (Formetric 4D Diers) scoliosis angle calculation. 1) View of 3D back reconstruction with convex areas in red and concave areas in blue, 2) View of the back with grid of lines projected, 3) View of scoliosis angle measurement. VP is vertebra prominent, DL and DR are respectively left and right dimples.

The "straight out" posture has likewise been radiologically validated [53, 54]. The patient brings his arms forward and place his hands on a support in such a way that the forearms were horizontal.

De Seze et al. [56] compared an upright posture known as "folding" with the "clavical" and "straight out" postures. The "folding" posture aim was to highlight the thoracic rib hump. The patient bends his shoulders, elbows and wrists so that the dorsal surface of the wrist would be in contact with the chin, while the ulnar sides of the forearms would be in contact with each other up to the elbows.

De Seze et al. [56] evaluated similar inter-observer reproducibility of these positions in comparison with two standard radiological postures. However, the "folding" position provided higher thoracic gibbosity values than those calculated in the other two positions. Furthermore, De Seze et al. [56] compared these postures on sagittal curve parameters and rib hump. However, it could be interesting to evaluate their influence on scoliosis angle and on major curve Cobb angle prior to made posture recommendation.

Currently the clavicle posture, which is considered the more representative of a patient's functional balance [55], seems to be the most appropriate posture to be used.

CLINICAL APPLICATIONS

According to the SOSORT 2012 guidelines to reduce irradiation, consensus statement 9 and 10 stated that non-radiographic modalities, such as physical examination, scoliometer readings, and surface topography, should be used first to detect curve progression in scoliosis patients and that when physical examination, scoliometer readings, and surface topography are used appropriately in the follow-up evaluation of the scoliosis patient, the number of subsequent radiographs can be reduced [6].

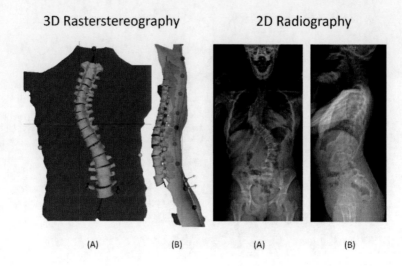

Figure 3. example of a 3D rasterstereography (Formetric 4D Diers) and a 2D radiography (EOS®) images obtained from the same AIS patient. *(A) Antero-posterio view; (B) lateral view.*

The high reliability of rasterstereography to evaluate the 3D spine deformity support its potential use for the longitudinal assessment of scoliosis progression [26, 45–47]. According to the currently available litterature results, we could suggest that rasterstereography will not fully replace XR evaluation, but it can significantly improve the radiation-free monitoring of the evolution of scoliosis with no limits of use, no risks for patients and at lower price than XR. However, the first XR evaluation remains necessary to assess morphology of the vertebra and exclude speficic scoliosis, like congenital scoliosis [6]. To definitively validate the use of rasterstereography in the monitoring of AIS, it is now required to evaluate the accuracy of this system to detect a scoliosis curve progression during patient follow-up.

Finally, measurement of scoliosis angle with 3D rasterstereography could improve evaluation of AIS, which is a 3D spine deformity of the spine (1) usually evaluated in a 2D fashion with conventional XR as illustrated Figure 3.

PERSPECTIVES

The challenge for future research is to determine the accuracy of rasterstereography to detect accurately scoliosis curve progression during follow-up of growing AIS patients. This last point should also be specifically evaluated in patients treated with a corrective rigid brace. Futhermore, it could be interesting to determinate when a clinically meaningful changes of scoliosis curve has occured using rasterstereography.

In addition we can speculate that curve progression evaluation using rasterstereography for patients treated with a corrective rigid brace could be overlooked. Indeed the in-brace correction could modify the back surface by pressing on anatomical points but the true spine curvature could still progress.

It seems also necessary to validate the use of rasterstereography in patients with high body fat percent, or with back skin scars. The influence of sex and age should also be evaluated in future research.

Finally, rasterstereography could be an interesting radiation-free tool for diagnosis and monitoring of other pathologies with thoracic spine and/or rib cage deformities such as Scheuermann kyphosis, pectus excavatum and carinatum.

As an alternative to rasterstereography to reduce radiation exposure of AIS patients, 3D-ultrasound (US) has been proposed to assess scoliosis curves [57, 58] and vertebral rotation [59–61]. The first method proposed consist of applying ultrasonic digitization to identify spinous processes and evaluated spinal curvature using the Ferguson method [58]. Another method proposed is to use spinous process and vertebral laminal as landmarks [59, 61]. More recently, Ungi et al. proposed to use US with a tracked transducer to determine spinal curves using transverse processes as landmarks [57]. This method was showed to determine a Cobb angle which strongly correlated with XR in pediatric and adults phantoms. The flat tranductor of the US did not fully contact the skin in patients with large humps [60] of with winged scapula [62]. The scoliosis curve and vertebral rotations were strongly correlated with XR with very good intra- and inter-observer reliability in AIS patients [60, 62, 63]. However,. one limitation of US is the poor image quality on patients with high body mass index (>25 kg.m-2) or with large Cobb angle (>50°) [62]. Additionally, US underestimated the Cobb angle in comparison to XR [62].

These radiation-free and accessible systems could help to reduce radiation exposure in AIS patients. US is at an earlier stage of development. Rasterstereography is a faster and less operator dependant radiation-free system than US and presents a promising potential to reduce radiation exposure in diagnosis and monitoring of AIS patients.

REFERENCES

[1] Perdriolle, R., Vidal, J. Morphology of scoliosis: three-dimensional evolution., *Orthopedics*. 10 (1987) 909–15.

[2] Kleinberg, S. The operative treatment of scoliosis, *Arch. Surg*. 5 (1922) 631.

[3] Riseborough, R., Edward J. and Wynne-Davies, A Genetic Survey of Idiopathic Scoliosis in, *J. Bone Jt. Surg. Br*. 55–A (1973) 974–982.

[4] Lonstein, J. E., Carlson, J. M. The prediction of curve progression in untreated idiopathic scoliosis during growth., *J. Bone Joint Surg. Am*. 66 (1984) 1061–71.

[5] Ng, S. Y., Bettany-Saltikov, J. Imaging in the Diagnosis and Monitoring of Children with Idiopathic Scoliosis, *Open Orthop. J*. 11 (2017) 1500–1520.

[6] Knott, P., Pappo, E., Cameron, M., DeMauroy, J. C., Rivard, C., Kotwicki, T., Zaina, F., Wynne, J., Stikeleather, L., Bettany-Saltikov, J., Grivas, T. B., Durmala, J., Maruyama, T., Negrini, S., O'Brien, J. P., Rigo, M. SOSORT 2012 consensus paper: Reducing x-ray exposure in pediatric patients with scoliosis, *Scoliosis*. 9 (2014) 1–9.

[7] Raso, V. J., Lou, E., Hill, D. L., Mahood, J., Moreau, M. J., Durdle, G. Trunk distorsion in adolescent idiopathic scoliosis, *J. Pediatr. Orthop*. 18 (1998) 222–226.

[8] Hoffman, D. A., Lonstein, J. E., Morin, M. M., Visscher, W., Harris, B. S. H., Boice, J. D. Breast Cancer in Women With Scoliosis Exposed to Multiple Diagnostic X Rays, *JNCI J. Natl. Cancer Inst*. 81 (1989) 1307–1312.

[9] Levy, A. R., Goldberg, M. S., Hanley, J. A., Mayo, N. E., Poitras, B. Projecting the lifetime risk of cancer from exposure to diagnostic ionizing radiation for adolescent idiopathic scoliosis., *Health Phys.* 66 (1994) 621–33.

[10] Nash, C. L., Gregg, E. C., Brown, R. H., Pillai, K. Risks of exposure to X-rays in patients undergoing long-term treatment for scoliosis., *J. Bone Joint Surg. Am.* 61 (1979) 371–374.

[11] Simony, E., Hansen, J., Christensen, S. B., Carreon, L. Y., Andersen, M. O. Incidence of cancer in adolescent idiopathic scoliosis patients treated 25 years previously, *Eur. Spine J.* 25 (2016) 3366–3370.

[12] Weinstein, S. L., Dolan, L. A., Spratt, K. F., Peterson, K. K., Spoonamore, M. J., Ponseti, I. V. Health and Function of Patients With Untreated Idiopathic Scoliosis, *JAMA.* 289 (2003) 559–567.

[13] Champain, S., Benchikh, K., Nogier, A., Mazel, C., De Guise, J., Skalli, W. Validation of new clinical quantitative analysis software applicable in spine orthopaedic studies, *Eur. Spine J.* 15 (2006) 982–991.

[14] Dubousset, J., Charpak, G., Dorion, I., Skalli, W., Lavaste, F., Deguise, J., Kalifa, G., Ferey, S. [A new 2D and 3D imaging approach to musculoskeletal physiology and pathology with low-dose radiation and the standing position: the EOS system]., *Bull. Acad. Natl. Med.* 189 (2005) 287-97-300.

[15] Deschênes, S., Charron, G., Beaudoin, G., Labelle, H., Dubois, J., Miron, M. C., Parent, S.Diagnostic imaging of spinal deformities: Reducing patients radiation dose with a new slot-scanning X-ray imager, *Spine* (Phila. Pa. 1976). 35 (2010) 989–994.

[16] Boissière, L., Bourghli, A., Vital, J. M., Gille, O., Obeid, I. The lumbar lordosis index: a new ratio to detect spinal malalignment with a therapeutic impact for sagittal balance correction decisions in adult scoliosis surgery., *Eur. Spine J.* 22 (2013) 1339–45.

[17] Somoskeöy, S., Tunyogi-Csapó, M., Bogyó, C., Illés, T. Clinical validation of coronal and sagittal spinal curve measurements based on three-dimensional vertebra vector parameters., *Spine J.* 12 (2012) 960–8.

[18] Somoskeöy, S., Tunyogi-Csapó, M., Bogyó, C., Illés, T. Accuracy and reliability of coronal and sagittal spinal curvature data based on patient-specific three-dimensional models created by the EOS 2D/3D imaging system., *Spine J.* 12 (2012) 1052–9.

[19] Luo, T. D., Stans, A. A., Schueler, B. A., Larson, A. N. Cumulative Radiation Exposure With EOS Imaging Compared With Standard Spine Radiographs, *Spine Deform.* 3 (2015) 144–150.

[20] Drerup, B., Hierholzer, E. Automatic localization of anatomical landmarks on the back surface and construction of a body-fixed coordinate system., *J. Biomech.* 20 (1987) 961–70.

[21] Drerup, B., Hierholzer, E. Objective determination of anatomical landmarks on the body surface: measurement of the vertebra prominens from surface curvature., *J. Biomech.* 18 (1985) 467–474.

[22] Frerich, J. M., Hertzler, K., Knott, P., Mardjetko, S. Comparison of radiographic and surface topography measurements in adolescents with idiopathic scoliosis., *Open Orthop. J.* 6 (2012) 261–5.

[23] Hackenberg, L., Hierholzer, E., Bullmann, V., Liljenqvist, U., Götze, C. Rasterstereographic analysis of axial back surface rotation in standing versus forward bending posture in idiopathic scoliosis, *Eur. Spine J.* 15 (2006) 1144–9.

[24] Hackenberg, L., Hierholzer, E., Pötzl, W., Götze, C. U. Liljenqvist, Rasterstereographic back shape analysis in idiopathic scoliosis after anterior correction and fusion, *Clin. Biomech.* 18 (2003) 1–8.

[25] Knott, P., Sturm, P., Lonner, B., Cahill, P., Betsch, M., McCarthy, R., Kelly, M., Lenke, L., Betz, R. Multicenter Comparison of 3D Spinal Measurements Using Surface Topography with Those from Conventional Radiography, *Spine Deform.* 4 (2016) 98–103.

[26] Tabard-Fougère, A., Bonnefoy-Mazure, A., Hanquinet, S., Lascombes, P., Armand, S., Dayer, R., Tabard-Fougere, A., Bonnefoy-Mazure, A., Hanquinet, S., Lascombes, P., Armand, S., Dayer, R. Validity and Reliability of Spine Rasterstereography in Patients with Adolescent Idiopathic Scoliosis, *Spine* (Phila Pa 1976). 41 (2016) 1–9.

[27] Willner, S. Moiré topography-A method for school screening of scoliosis, *Arch. Orthop. Trauma. Surg.* 95 (1979) 181–185.

[28] Oster, G. Moiré pattern, in: S. Parker (Ed.), *Opt. Source B. - Sci. Ref. Ser.*, McGraw-Hill, USA, 1988: pp. 379–381.

[29] Batouche, M., Benlamri, R. A computer vision system for diagnosing scoliosis, in: IEEE (Ed.), *IEEE Int. Conf. Pervasive Comput. Commun.*, 1994: pp. 2623–2628.

[30] Porto, F., Gurgel, J. L., Russomano, T., Farinatti, P. D. T. V. Moiré topography: Characteristics and clinical application, *Gait Posture.* 32 (2010) 422–424.

[31] Lim, J. S., Kim, J., Chung, M. S. Automatic shadow moiré topography: a moving-light-source method, *Opt. Lett.* 14 (1989) 1252.

[32] Takasaki, H. Moiré Topography, *Appl. Opt.* 9 (1970) 1467.

[33] Drerup, B., Principles of measurement of vertebral rotation from frontal projections of the pedicles., *J. Biomech.* 17 (1984) 923–35.

[34] Drerup, B. Improvements in measuring vertebral rotation from the projections of the pedicles., *J. Biomech.* 18 (1985) 369–78.

[35] Drerup, B., Hierholzer, E. Assessment of scoliotic deformity from back shape asymmetry using an improved mathematical model, *Clin. Biomech.* 11 (1996) 376–383.

[36] Drerup, B. Rasterstereographic measurement of scoliotic deformity, *Scoliosis.* 9 (2014) 1–14.

[37] Berryman, F., Pynsent, P., Fairbank, J., Disney, S. A new system for measuring three-dimensional back shape in scoliosis., *Eur. Spine J.* 17 (2008) 663–72.

[38] Pazos, V., Cheriet, F., Song, L., Labelle, H., Dansereau, J. Accuracy assessment of human trunk surface 3D reconstructions from an optical digitising system, *Med. Biol. Eng.* Comput. 43 (2005) 11–15.

[39] Goldberg, C. J., Kaliszer, M., Moore, D. P., Fogarty, E. E., Dowling, F. E. Surface Topography, Cobb Angles, and Cosmetic Change in Scoliosis, *Spine* (Phila. Pa. 1976). 26 (2001) E55–E63.

[40] Richards, B. S., Bernstein, R. M., D'Amato, C. R., Thompson, G. H. Standardization of criteria for adolescent idiopathic scoliosis brace studies: SRS Committee on Bracing and Nonoperative Management, *Spine* (Phila. Pa. 1976). 30 (2005) 2068–2075.

[41] Cobb, J. Outline for the study of scoliosis, Am Acad Orthop Surg. 7 (1948) 261–275.

[42] He, J. W., Yan, Z. H., Liu, J., Yu, Z. K., Wang, X. Y., Bai, G. H., Ye, X. J., Zhang, X. Accuracy and repeatability of a new method for measuring scoliosis curvature., *Spine* (Phila. Pa. 1976). 34 (2009) E323–E329.

[43] Morrissy, R. T., Goldsmith, G. S., Hall, E. C., Kehl, D., Cowie, G. H. Measurement of the Cobb angle on radiographs of patients who have scoliosis. Evaluation of intrinsic error., *J. Bone Joint Surg. Am.* 72 (1990) 320–7.

[44] Pruijs, J. E. H., Hageman, M. A. P. E., Keessen, W., van der Meer, R., van Wieringen, J. C. Variation in Cobb angle measurements in scoliosis, *Skeletal Radiol.* 23 (1994) 517–520.

[45] Guidetti, L., Bonavolontà, V., Tito, A., Reis, V. M., Gallotta, M. C., Baldari, C. Intra- and interday reliability of spine rasterstereography., *Biomed Res. Int.* 2013 (2013) 745480.

[46] Mohokum, M., Mendoza, S., Udo, W., Sitter, H., Paletta, J. R., Skwara, A., Melvin, M., Mohokum, M., Sylvia, M., Mendoza, S., Udo, W., Sitter, H., Paletta, J. R., Skwara, A. Reproducibility of rasterstereography for kyphotic and lordotic angles, trunk length, and trunk inclination: a reliability study., *Spine* (Phila. Pa. 1976). 35 (2010) 1353–1358.

[47] Schroeder, J., Reer, R., Braumann, K. M. Video raster stereography back shape reconstruction: a reliability study for sagittal, frontal, and transversal plane parameters, *Eur. Spine J.* 24 (2014) 262–269.

[48] Mohokum, M., Schülein, S., Skwara, A. The validity of rasterstereography: A systematic review, *Orthop. Rev.* (Pavia). 7 (2015) 68–73.

[49] Drerup, B., Hierholzer, E. Back shape measurement using video rasterstereography and three-dimensional reconstruction of spinal shape., *Clin. Biomech.* (Bristol, Avon). 9 (1994) 28–36.

[50] Schulte, T. L., Hierholzer, E., Boerke, A., Lerner, T., Liljenqvist, U., Bullmann, V., Hackenberg, L. Raster stereography versus radiography in the long-term follow-up of idiopathic scoliosis., *J. Spinal Disord. Tech.* 21 (2008) 23–8.

[51] Liljenqvist, U., Halm, H., Hierholzer, E., Drerup, B., Weiland, M.; 3-Dimensional surface measurement of spinal deformities with video rasterstereography., *Zeitschrift Für Orthopädie Und Ihre Grenzgebiete.* 136 (1) 57–64.

[52] Degenhardt, B., Starks, Z., Bhatia, S., Franklin, G. A. Appraisal of the DIERS method for calculating postural measurements: An observational study, *Scoliosis Spinal Disord.* 12 (2017) 1–11.

[53] Horton, W. C., Brown, C. W., Bridwell, K. H., Glassman, S. D., Suk, S. I., Cha, C. W. Is there an optimal patient stance for obtaining a lateral 36" radiograph?: A critical comparison of three techniques, *Spine* (Phila. Pa. 1976). 30 (2005) 427–433.

[54] Stahnara, P., DeMauroy, J., Dran, G., Gonon, G., Castanzo, G., Dimnet, J., Pasquet, A. Reciprocal Angulation of Vertebral Bodies in a Sagittal Plane: Approact to References for the Evaluationo f Kyphosis and Lordosis, *Spine* (Phila. Pa. 1976). 7 (1982) 335.

[55] Faro, F. D., Marks, M. C., Pawelek, J., Newton, P. O. Evaluation of a functional position for lateral radiograph acquisition in adolescent idiopathic scoliosis., *Spine* (Phila. Pa. 1976). 29 (2004) 2284–2289.

[56] De Sèze, M., Randriaminahisoa, T., Gaunelle, A., de Korvin, G., Mazaux, J. M. Inter-observer reproducibility of back surface topography parameters allowing assessment of scoliotic thoracic gibbosity and comparison with two standard postures, *Ann. Phys. Rehabil. Med.* 56 (2013) 599–612.

[57] Ungi, T., King, F., Kempston, M., Keri, Z., Lasso, A., Mousavi, P., Rudan, J., Borschneck, D. P., Fichtinger, G. Spinal curvature measurement by tracked ultrasound snapshots, *Ultrasound Med. Biol.* 40 (2014) 447–454.

[58] Letts, M., Quanbury, A., Gouw, G., Kolsun, W., Letts, E. Computerized ultrasonic digitization in the measurement of spinal curvature, *Spine* (Phila. Pa. 1976). 13 (1988) 1106–1110.

[59] Chen, W., Lou, E. H. M., Le, L. H. Using ultrasound imaging to identify landmarks in vertebra models to assess spinal deformity, in: *Proc. Annu. Int. Conf. IEEE Eng. Med. Biol. Soc. EMBS*, 2011: pp. 8495–8498.

[60] Wang, Q., Li, M., Lou, E. H. M., Chu, W. C. W., ping Lam, T., Cheng, J. C. Y., sang Wong, M. Validity study of vertebral rotation measurement using 3-D ultrasound in adolescent idiopathic scoliosis, *Ultrasound Med. Biol.* 42 (2016) 1473–1481.

[61] Suzuki, S., Yamamuro, T., Shikata, J., Shimizu, K., Hirokazu, I. Ultrasound Measurement of Vertebral Rotation in Idiopathic Scoliosis, *J. Bone Jt. Surg.* 71–B (1989) 252–255.

[62] Zheng, Y. P., Lee, T. T. Y., Lai, K. K. L., Yip, B. H. K., Zhou, G. Q., Jiang, W. W., Cheung, J. C. W., Wong, M. S., Ng, B. K. W., Cheng, J. C. Y., Lam, T. P. A reliability and validity study for Scolioscan: a radiation-free scoliosis assessment system using 3D ultrasound imaging, Scoliosis *Spinal Disord.* 11 (2016) 13.

[63] Khodaei, M., Hill, D., Zheng, R., Le, L. H., Lou, E. H. M. Intra- and inter-rater reliability of spinal flexibility measurements using ultrasonic (US) images for non-surgical candidates with adolescent idiopathic scoliosis: a pilot study, *Eur. Spine J.* (2018) 1–9.

In: Scoliosis: Diagnosis, Classification and Management Options   ISBN: 978-1-53614-464-2
Editors: F. Canavese, A. Andreacchio and H. Xu   © 2018 Nova Science Publishers, Inc.

Chapter 26

ANESTHESIA CONSIDERATIONS AND PAIN MANAGEMENT IN CHILDREN UNDERGOING SCOLIOSIS SURGERY

Marie Granier[1,2,*] and Xing Rong Song[2]
[1]Department of Anesthesia, University Hospital Estaing, Clermont Ferrand, France
[2]1Department of Pediatric Anesthesia, Guang Zhou Women and Children Medical Center, Guangzhou, China

ABSTRACT

Scoliosis surgery is a major procedure. Care for children with spinal deformities starts well before their admission for surgery.

The approach to scoliosis surgery is multidisciplinary: several teams must work together to assure the best possible outcome and to decrease the risk of possible complications.

This chapter aims to provide an overview of the anesthetic approach to patients undergoing spinal surgery for scoliosis as well as to give some key-information regarding principles and strategies of pain management in these patients.

Keyword: scoliosis surgery, anesthesia, children, adolescents, pain

INTRODUCTION

Care for children with spinal deformities starts well before their admission for surgery. Scoliosis surgery requires a multidisciplinary approach; several teams must work together to assure the best possible outcome and to decrease the risk of complications [1-11].

The anesthesia management starts with a careful preoperative evaluation. The major intra-operative challenges include the maintenance of safe positioning, fluid and temperature balance,

---

[*] Corresponding Author Email: marigranier@yahoo.fr.

blood conservation and spinal cord function monitoring. On the other hand, adequate analgesia and ventilation are the primary issues of concern in the postoperative period to allow early awakening and extubation [1, 2, 5, 8].

Anesthesia management has the following aims:

1) To *evaluate*
   - the location and degree of spinal deformity;
   - the etiology of the scoliosis;
   - the patients exercise tolerance, respiratory function;
   - the presence of any comorbidities.
2) To *define* an effective and safe blood saving strategy;
3) To *control* postoperative pain.

PRE-OPERATIVE EVALUATION

The anesthetic management must begin with a focused pre-operative evaluation.

Before surgery, the anesthesiologist should know about the surgical approach, anterior, posterior or combined, as well as the number of levels to be fused and the location of instrumented fusion, i.e., thoracic (T1-T12), lumbar (L1-L5), sacral (S1 and below) or cervical (C1-C7). Although the procedure is rarely performed, it is also important to know if a thoracoplasty (partial rib resection to decrease the gibbous) is planned.

The scoliosis can be idiopathic (most frequent form; more than 90% of cases, mostly females) or secondary to neuromuscular disease, tumor, infections or injury. Gathering this information is extremely important as anesthesia management and postoperative treatment have different specificities. Moreover, patients with scoliosis secondary to neuromuscular disease have a higher incidence of complications and assessment of cardiorespiratory status is more difficult [2, 6, 8-11].

Cardio-Respiratory and Neurologic Assessment

A physical exam of the cardiorespiratory system should determine the presence of dyspnea, increased work of breathing, tachypnea, wheezing, or signs of right heart failure.

For most patients with idiopathic scoliosis a good exercise tolerance is the best guide to cardiorespiratory status. Preoperative assessment of patients with neuromuscular disease or immobility is more challenging as these patients are neither able to give a history of exercise tolerance nor to perform spirometry adequately.

Two main factors significantly affect respiratory function in scoliosis patients: the degree of the curve (Cobb angle) and the association of neuromuscular disease.

When the Cobb Angle exceeds 65 degrees, respiratory function is likely to be compromised. Pulmonary function testing may demonstrate the characteristic pattern of restrictive lung disease with decreased vital capacity, reduced functional residual capacity, and diminished total lung volume. Usually, the greatest reduction is in vital capacity. The alterations in lung volumes are caused by changes in chest wall compliance and the resting position of the thoracic cage, rather than parenchymal changes or lower airway obstruction [1].

The primary abnormality in pulmonary gas exchange is ventilation-perfusion maldistribution. As the scoliotic deformity progresses, the work of breathing increases and alveolar hypoventilation predominates. Therefore, these patients may develop hypoxemia, hypercapnia and progress to pulmonary hypertension and respiratory failure.

Cardiomyopathy complicates many progressive muscle diseases such as DMD, myotonic dystrophy and other myopathies.

Preoperative neurologic deficits, if any, should be carefully sought and recorded, in all patients.

Laboratory Studies

Based on the severity of the curve and the degree of respiratory impairment and other organ involvement, the following preoperative laboratory studies should be considered:

- Chest radiograph;
- Pulmonary function testing;
- Electrocardiogram;
- Echocardiography;
- Pharmacological stress echocardiography.

- *Blood test*
    - Full count blood cells,
    - Arterial blood gases,
    - Coagulation Studies: Platelet count, Prothrombin time (PT) and Partial thromboplastin time (PTT)
    - Electrolyte panel +/- Liver function
    - ABO blood group +/- Blood cross-match

Nutrition

Increased prevalence of malnutrition in patients with neuromuscular scoliosis is a significant concern and one that needs to be evaluated preoperatively. In particular, if patients are malnourished and have low BMI and body weight, gastrostomy should be considered. Patients with weight below 40 kg are at risk of developing postoperative complications while patients below 20 kg are at very high risk of developing postoperative complications.

Determining the point at which the risks of surgical complications outweigh the benefits of scoliosis surgery is difficult, particularly in patients whose life expectancy is limited by the progressive nature of the disease.

The use of invasive monitoring lines and catheters along with postoperative analgesia plan should be explained fully to the patient and family at that time.

Patients and families may benefit from talking to patients who have been through the procedure.

INTRAOPERATIVE MANAGEMENT

Positioning and Monitoring Devices

In addition to standard ASA monitors, an arterial catheter for blood pressure monitoring, lab draws and pulse pressure variation monitoring is important. This is ideally placed in the upper extremity to allow for easy access to the cannula during surgery. Two large peripheral IV cannula are sited. A central venous cannula is placed if there is significant comorbidity (e.g., neuromuscular disease), or if there is inadequate peripheral access. Central access may be useful for administration of vasoactive infusions, fluid administration, and for postoperative care. Patients who are anticipated to require intensive care unit admission postoperatively should have a central line inserted for surgery.

A urinary catheter is used to monitor urine output.

Two forced air-warming blankets are used to maintain normothermia. One is placed on the upper extremities and one on the lower extremities below the buttocks [1].

Extra care is taken when positioning these patients in the prone position to compulsively avoid compression of eyes/face and abdomen/genitalia, and to maintain neutral extremity position, particularly avoiding hyperextension of the shoulders. Pressure points should be well padded (elbows, pelvis, knees, ankles) [1].

ANESTHESIA

The aim of anesthesia is to maintain a stable anesthetic depth allowing for intraoperative neurophysiological monitoring and this can be achieved using various anesthetic techniques.

Anesthetic agents and physiologic perturbations may interfere with SSEP and MEP signals. The best anesthetic technique is the one that provides quiet and perpetual anesthetic effect avoiding bolus dosing, over rapid bolus doses in order to avoid marked fluctuations in recording the Eps.

Good communication between the neurophysiology team, anesthesiologists and surgeons is critically important, tailoring the administered anesthetics to those known to least affect the quality of electrophysiological monitoring.

Anesthetic Effects on Somato-Sensory Evoked Potentials (SSEP)

Volatile anesthetics produce a dose-dependent increase in latency and decrease in amplitude. Up to 0.5-1 MAC of a volatile anesthetic in the presence of nitrous oxide is compatible with adequate monitoring of SSEPs. However there is a high degree of inter-individual variability of response, and the overall quality of the SSEP is superior in the absence of volatile anesthetics and nitrous oxide. Intravenous agents have minimal effects on cortical SSEPs, except etomidate and ketamine, which actually increase SSEP signal amplitude. Continuous infusion of propofol is well tolerated. Muscle relaxants improve SSEP recording because they suppress EMG activity and provide a "cleaner" background, however NMB will of course obliterate MEPs. High doses of continuously infused opioids are compatible with

SSEP monitoring, but bolus doses of opioids and other sedatives should be avoided during critical stages of surgery to eliminate transient effects on the SSEP that may be confused with spinal cord compromise [4-8].

Anesthetic Effects on Motor-Evoked Potentials (MEP)

MEPs are extremely sensitive to the inhibitory effects of volatile anesthetics. Nitrous oxide, although less suppressive than other inhaled agents, demonstrates a synergistic effect on amplitude depression when combined with other anesthetics. Helenius et al. showed that pregabalin can be used preoperatively, and it does not interfere with the intraoperative spinal cord monitoring. Calderon et al. reported that a single bolus of clonidine (1-2 microg/Kg) severely interferes with neuromonitoring of the spinal cord motor pathways [4-8].

BLOOD LOSS AND BLOOD SAVING STRATEGIES

Due to the large area of decorticated bone exposed, spinal surgery is typically associated with extensive blood loss and perioperative transfusion.

Blood loss is related to length of procedure and number of segments fused.

Pre-operative recombinant erythropoietin (rEPO) treatment should be discussed, depending on the blood sample results.

Erythropoietin therapy is systematically associated with iron supplementation.

The use of blood saving strategies such as recombinant Erythropoietin (rEPO) and Antifibrinolytic therapy (AFT), resulted in a reduction of perioperative autologous blood transfusion. The healthy teen with idiopathic scoliosis usually will not require transfusion in the operating room. Children with other etiologies of scoliosis will almost always require intraoperative blood transfusion [1, 9].

Children with neuromuscular disease are at increased risk of excessive blood loss.

Red blood cell scavenging ("Cell Saver") is used for all patients undergoing spinal fusion surgery who do not have malignancies. Intraoperative cell salvage is mandatory for this type of surgery. Blood is collected, anti-coagulated, filtered, centrifuged and re-suspended in saline. Approximately 50% of blood loss can be salvaged and swab washing has been shown to recover a significant amount of red cells.

PAIN MANAGEMENT

Good postoperative pain control is essential and requires a multimodal approach. Postoperative pain control after posterior spinal fusion is an essential component in the care of patients after scoliosis surgery. The multimodal analgesic therapy includes IV opioids via patient-controlled analgesia (PCA), epidural infusion of opioids with or without local anesthetic, or intrathecal (IT) morphine, NSAIDs and Paracetamol. Intravenous patient-controlled analgesia (IV-PCA) and oral opioids remain the standard of care at most institutions. Regional anesthetic modalities such as continuous epidural infusions of local anesthetic [epidural analgesia (EPI)] and/or opioid and intrathecal morphine (ITM) have been explored and have shown improved postoperative pain control [1, 10, 11].

In spite of a vast array of therapeutic options available for control of post spinal surgery pain, none of them can be individually labeled as the most effective form of treatment. A multimodal approach using different agents and routes seems the best option to provide postsurgical pain relief. Beyond drugs, the non-pharmacological pain treatment as relaxation, hypnosis, massage, musicotherapy, etc. may help to control pain [1].

REFERENCES

[1] *Guidelines for the Anesthetic Management of Patients with Scoliosis Undergoing Posterior Spinal Fusion Surgery*. Lucile Packard Children's Hospital Stanford, USA.
[2] Zentner, J., Albrecht, T., et al. Influence of halothane, enflurane, and isoflurane on motor evoked potentials. *Neurosurg.*, 1992; 31: 298 - 305.
[3] Calancie, B., Klose, K., Baier, S., Green, B. Isoflurane-induced attenuation of motor evoked potentials caused by electrical motor cortex stimulation during surgery. *J. Neurosurg.*, 1991; 74: 897 - 904.
[4] Deletis, V., Sala, F. Intraoperative neurophysiological monitoring of the spinal cord during spinal cord and spine surgery: a review focus on the corticospinal tracts. *Clin. Neurophysiol.*, 2008; 119: 248 - 64.
[5] Glover, C. D., Carling, N. P. Neuromonitoring for scoliosis surgery. *Anesthesiol. Clin.*, 2014; 32: 101 - 114.
[6] Nuwer, M., Emerson, R., Galloway, G., Legatt, A., Lopez, J., Minahan, R., et al. Evidence-based guideline update: intraoperative spinalmonitoring with somatosensory and transcranial electricalmotor evoked potentials. *J. Clin. Neurophysiol.*, 2002; 29: 101 - 108.
[7] Helenius, L., Puhakka, A., Manner, T., Pajulo, O., Helenius, I. Preoperative pregabalin has no effect on intraoperative neurophysiological monitoring in adolescents undergoing posterior spinal fusion for spinal deformities: a double-blind, randomized, placebo-controlled clinical trial. *EPOS Annual Meeting, Oslo, Norway*, April 2018.
[8] Calderón, P. et al. Clonidine administration during intraoperative monitoring for pediatric scoliosis surgery: Effects on central and peripheral motor responses. *Neurophysiologie Clinique/Clinical Neurophysiology*, 2017; DOI: 10.1016/ j.neucli.2017.11.001.
[9] Edler, A., Murray, D. J., Forbes, R. B. Blood loss during posterior spinal fusion surgery in patients with neuromuscular disease: is there an increased risk? *Paediatr. Anaesth.*, 2003; 13: 818 - 22.
[10] Ravish, M., Muldowne, B., Becker, A., et al. Pain Management in Patients With Adolescent Idiopathic Scoliosis Undergoing Posterior Spinal Fusion: Combined Intrathecal Morphine and Continuous Epidural Versus PCA. *J. Pediatr. Orthop.*, 2012; 32: 799 - 804.
[11] Eschertzhuber, S., Hohlrieder, M., Keller, C. et al. Comparison of high- and low-dose intrathecal morphine for spinal fusion in children. *Br. J. Anaesth.*, 2008; 100: 538 - 543.

Chapter 27

EXPERIMENTAL ANIMAL MODELS IN SCOLIOSIS: INCIDENCE AND DIAGNOSIS OF IDIOPATHIC AND CONGENITAL SCOLIOSIS IN RHESUS MONKEY (*MACACA MULATTA*) THROUGH EVOKED POTENTIALS AND IMAGING STUDIES

Alejandra Ibáñez-Contreras[1,*]*, David Ducoing-Gonzalez*[2]*,*
Janine Cardoso[1] *and Braulio Hernández-Godínez*[1]

[1]Investigación Biomédica Aplicada (INBIOMA) S.A.S de C.V.
Ciudad de México, México
[2]Hospital Sedna S.A. de C.V. Ciudad de México, México

ABSTRACT

Scoliosis is a deformity of the spine characterized by the rotation of the vertebral bodies, altogether with the structural malformation of these. It affects the periferal nervous system, ligaments, joints and skeletal muscles. It has been described as a disabling and painful disease, which is produced by various factors, making it difficult to elucidate the etiology. Scoliosis is divided into congenital (CE) and idiopathic (IE). Congenital escoliosis is defined as lateral curvatures of the spine caused by the abnormal development of vertebral bodies. It is associated with neuromuscular abnormalities, which may be genetic, as well as by the compensation of different lower limb lengths. Idiopathic scoliosis is defined as the lateral curvature of the spine without a specific cause, presenting a higher incidence in the population in contrast to EC. To date the IE etiology is unknown, so different animal models have been developed to simulate the defect and to determine possible treatment options. Since these model, new information has come to light, that terrestrial quadruped animals rarely present scoliosis naturally in the spine. However, in our monkey colony using different diagnostic techniques, both image and neurophysiological studies, showing that quadruped animals can development a true scoliosos with all morphologic and physiologic alterations. We come to the conclusion that

---

[*] Corresponding Author Email: ibanez.alejandra@hotmail.com.

Rhesus monkey makes an excellent model for the study of idiopathic and congenital scoliosis, and has a wide similarity with humans.

Keywords: idiopathic scoliosis, congenital scoliosis, evoked potentials, computed axial tomography, *Macaca mulatta*

INTRODUCTION

The normal and abnormal vertebral development has been studied in the last 200 years. At increasing levels as the techniques of biological research have evolved. Spinal disorders have been evaluated both from a clinical and experimental point of view, with the purpose of creating new treatment options as well as to understand the etiology and effects that these alterations can generate in the organism (Kallemeier et al. 2006; Giardo et al. 2011; Stokes et al. 2011).

Degenerative diseases of the spine have evolved into an economical burden, due to the high investment in diagnosis and treatment, as well as the familiar and business economic repercussions due to lack of work and rehabilitation (Boswell and Ciruna 2017).

Degenerative spine disease comprises several abnormalities: osteoporosis, arthritis, hernia of the discs, spondylosis, narrowing of the vertebral foramen and IE, are some of the etiologies. The degenerative changes in intervertebral space by disc collapse and facetary arthrosis, alter load patterns of the vertebral bodies and spinal associated structures, introducing greater stress in the facet joints, spinal ligaments, tendons and crossing neurological tissues, contributing to futher deterioration (Hernandez- Godinez et al. 2012; Boswell and Ciruna 2017; Buser et al. 2018).

In particular, scoliosis is a spine deformity characterized by a lateral deviation in the frontal plane, accompanied by a rotation of the vertebral bodies and a displacement from midline to lateral. It affects the nervous system, ligaments, joints and the muscular and skeletal systems (Werneck et al. 2008; Odent et al. 2011; Bobyn et al. 2015).

Scoliosis has been described as an orthopedic disorder that occurs as a result of various aetiologies: genetic, congenital, inflammatory, degenerative, iatrogenic, neuromuscular disorders and asymmmetric or abnormal growth; making it hard to diagnose its accurate etiology (Janssen et al. 2011; Girardo et al. 2011; Dede et al. 2011; Boswell and Ciruna 2017).

Clinical scoliosis is divided into congenital or idiopathic. Congenital scoliosis (CS) is defined as lateral curvatures of the spine caused by the anomalous development of the vertebral bodies during the first six weeks of intrauterine growth (Bobbin et al. 2015). The incidence is 0.13-0.5 of 1000 live births of the world population (Hayes et al. 2014). Idiopathic scoliosis (IS) accounts for 75% of cases of scoliosis. IS, is defined as a lateral curvature of the spine with an axial twist without a determined cause and exhibits a greater incidence than congenital scoliosis. The IS affects 3% of children worldwide, requiring some type of clinical intervention throughout life (Hayes et al. 2014). The IS associated with alterations in respiratory mechanics, because it modifies the position of the ribs, diminishing anteroposterior thoracic diameter. This deformity also causes compression of certain pulmonary zones thus reducing the number of vascular units per pulmonary acinus. (Hernández-Godínez et al. 2012).

The skeletal deformities produced by the IS are well characterized in humans, and they include: the lateral deviation of more than 10° in the transverse-frontal plane and the inversion of the lordosis in the sagittal plane, without a determined cause. However, its etiology is still unclear, and metabolic, hormonal, mechanical and genetic factors have been proposed (Odent et al. 2011; Hayes et al. 2014; Bobyn et al. 2015). In general, IS presents in adolescence (AIS) as a three-dimensional rotation of the spine that has a propensity to increase in magnitude according to sexual maturity, being more severe in women (Hayes et al. 2014). Idiopathic scoliosis is classified as: infantile (zero to three years), juvenile (three years to eleven) and adolescent (eleven years and older) (Giampietro et al. 2003; Gonzalez- Miranda et al. 2016). Similarly, degenerative or de novo scoliosis has been identified, which is characterized by the deviation of the column resulting from a progressive degeneration in adulthood (García -Ramos et al. 2015).

Research on the etiology of idiopathic scoliosis has focused on multiple areas and has demonstrated the complex pathophysiology of this disorder: connective tissue abnormalities, abnormal biomechanical forces, neurophysiological predisposition, genetics and increased calmodulin or decreased melatonin during puberty (Girardo et al. 2011; Ouellet and Odent 2013; Boswell and Ciruna 2017).

Although great progress has been made in recent years in terms of knowledge of its pathogenesis and biomechanics, which has allowed to make important contributions regarding the conservative and surgical treatment; this has not happened in the knowledge of its etiology which still remains unknown. As the etiology of clinical scoliosis is not known to date, a considerable number of surgical approaches in different animal models have been used to induce this disease to find out about is possible origin, etiology and treatment.

EXPERIMENTAL ANIMAL MODELS IN SCOLIOSIS

Many hypotheses have been established to evaluate the etiology and pathogenesis of scoliosis in animal models. Historically, IS had only been described in humans. Spinal deformities described in other animal species are typically classified as congenital (James 1970; Cheung et al. 2005; Gorman and Breden 2009). Considering that the spontaneous appearance of scoliosis in animals is rare, great efforts are required to achieved and develop scoliotic animal models (Bobyn et al. 2015). It has been documented that quadruped animals rarely display natural spontaneous scoliotic rachis deviations, thus determining that the bipedal position could be a determining factor for the appearance of the IS. Consequently, it has been accepted that the mechanisms involved in IS have a direct relationship with the axial load in the erect posture along the spine to produce skeletal deformity (Hayes et al. 2014; Bobyn et al. 2015; Zhang et al. 2017). It has been suggested that in the human species, the bipedal posture gave rise to anatomical modifications generating compensatory changes that have proved to be functionally inadequate throughout human life. This adaptation has resulted in excessive tension in the lumbosacral region, producing accelerated aging and degenerative changes on the column (Jinkins 2001). In the case of quadruped animals, the structure of their vertebral column and its center of gravity are different from humans and do not have the same axial load, because it is distributed between the scapular and pelvic girdles, decreasing tension as length of the spine (Hernández-Godínez et al. 2012; Hayes et al. 2014; Boswell and Ciruna 2017).

Scarse data from veterinary clinical cases has been collected from domestic quadrupeds (mainly dogs, horses and rabbits), but they have not resulted in a predictable animal model

(Ouellet and Odent 2013). Similarly, the bipedal position in the case of chickens, has become a very popular animal model in the investigation of scoliosis, however the anatomical restrictions on spinal mobility are probably protective and avoid the full range of scoliotic curvatures seen in humans (Hayes et al. 2014).

The procedures for inducing scoliosis have varied from systemic to local interventions in a wide variety of animal species. The procedures for creating the spinal deformity were initially performed in small animals and, more recently, in large species (goats, mini pigs and yorkshire pigs) (Odent et al. 2011).

The diversity of animal species and techniques to induce scoliosis is very wide, including teratogenic models of scoliosis induction through the use of endocrine or pharmacological treatments. In other techniques, neuromuscular types of scoliosis have been induced by the section of nerve roots of spinal muscles, surgical techniques through immobilization, as well as rib resection and/or muscle relaxation, anchoring procedures, etc (Turgot et al. 2003; Kallemeier et al. 2006; Fagan et al. 2009; Zhang et al. 2009, Zhang et al. 2017). Most scoliosis models have been developed around techniques designed to create a mechanical asymmetry in the spine (Bobyn et al. 2015). On the other hand, the genetic models seek to reproduce the conditions that could predisposed scoliotic deformity These models have a great predictive value, which favors the early and preventive intervention of the scoliotic curve, offering also a directed and much more specific idea to determine the genetic factors involved in the deformity (Bobyn et al. 2015).

Genetic Models

Through different studies a genetic predisposition for the appearance of the IS has been suggested. The genetic models seek to reproduce the conditions that can predispose an individual to scoliotic deformity (Bobyn et al. 2015). Chromosomes 1, 6, 7, 8, 12 and 14 have been linked to adolescent IS. However, in this context, few studies have used animal models to study the genetics of IS (Boswell and Ciruna 2017). A central principle of most scoliotic models is the concept that bipedalism is a requirement for the development of scoliosis, however the genetic models have proven that bipedalism is not a necessary feature (Bobbin et al. 2015). Among the animal models that have been used, genetically altered mice with known deformities of the spine or tail (scoliotic phenotypes) are found to identify possible loci related to IS or human IE (Giampietro et al. 2003). Mice represent one of the least used animal species in the genetic model scoliosis. However, the ability to generate transgenic mice provides the opportunity to study the function of several genes involved, but only in vivo (Bobyn et al. 2015). An example of these mice genetically altered is the Ky mouse (Blanco et al. 2001). It has been reported that the loci of the mutations responsible for deformities in mice have analogues in humans, including the Pax1, Dll3, Wnt3a, Ky, Lmx1a, Fbn-2 and Sim2 (Giampetro et al. 2003, 2005, 2006, 2008, 2013).

On the other hand, the use of teleosts has been documented as a model for polygenetic inheritance with female predominance of greater spinal deformity, similar to IS in humans (Figure 1). The investigation of Gorman and Breden (2009) suggest that although this deformity may arise in the absence of a bipedal march, since the biomechanical forces acting on the guppy's spine may in fact be similar to those of the human being (Bobyn et al. 2015; Boswell and Ciruna 2017). In the teleost's, the axial load, as in humans, acts along the crania-caudal axis, but is independent of gravity, instead it originates in the force of movement in the compass of the tail pushing the animal through the dense medium of water. The result is a compression force along this axis (Gorman and Breden 2009; Bobyn et al. 2015). Therefore, similar biomechanical forces along the spinal column can make the fish more susceptible to late-onset spinal curvatures.

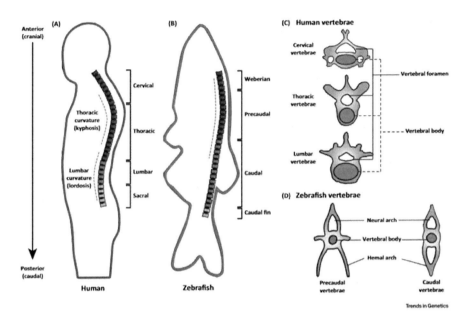

Figure 1. Functional Organization of the Spine. A) The human spine comprises 30 evenly spaced vertebrae that connect at the base of the skull and traverse the body to the pelvis. B) Organization and structure of the zebrafish spine exhibit similarities to that of humans. Adult zebrafish have between 29 and 33 vertebrae in total. C) In each region, vertebrae number, size, and structure differ to accommodate various rotational and loadbearing forces traversing the spinal column. D) Zebrafish vertebrae display bony arches on both dorsal and ventral surfaces, but lack complex processes seen in human vertebrae (Boswell and Ciruna 2017).

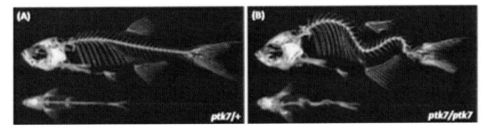

Figure 2. Visualization and analysis of Idiopathic Spinal deformity in adult Zebrafish by Microcomputed Tomography (micro CT). A) Lateral micro CT image of ptk7 heterozygous sibling and B) ptk7 mutant zebrafish (dorsal view in lower left corner). These mutant fish exhibit defining features of idiopathic scoliosis (IS), including non-visible vertebral defects during curve onset, complex 3D rotational deformity of the spine, and late onset of spinal curvature (Boswell and Ciruna 2017).

On the other hand, the recent revolution in the inverse genetic approaches, including the specific induced lesions and the technologies of gene editing in the zebra fish genome, have allowed us to know the genes that participate in the development of scoliosis, so that the recessive mutation in Kinesin family member 6 (Kif6), causes the development of isolated spinal curvatures in the absence of vertebral malformations. In fact, the first genetically defined development model of IS was characterized by protein tyrosine kinase 7 (ptk7) in the mutated zebra fish (Figure 2) (Boswell and Ciruna 2017).

Neuroendocrine Models

Melatonin Deficiency

One of the most used models and therefore studied in the evaluation of the pathophysiology of scoliosis is in pinealectomy chickens (Kanemura et al. 1997; Turgut et al. 2003, 2006; Fu et al. 2011; Girardo et al. 2011). The term pinealectomy (PINX) refers to the surgical ablation of the pineal gland (Man et al. 2014). The progression of scoliosis after pinealectomy was first developed in chickens by Thillard et al. in 1959. The animals underwent an ileectomy at birth and they developed a high incidence of spinal deformity, between 52% and 100%. Based on this, it was not until Machida and Duboussett popularized this model by establishing the morphological correlation in IS (Machida et al. 1993, 1995, 1997; Man, et al. 2014). This model raises the hypothesis that melatonin (neuroendocrine protein) plays an important role in the development of scoliosis. The model was validated by administering melatonin or serotonin to pinealectomized chickens and these did not develop scoliotic curvatures (Machida et al. 1993). However, when this model is extrapolated to mammals, pinealectomy rats only develop scoliosis as long as they are forced to maintain a bipedal posture, which indirectly confirms that the axial load of the spinal column plays an important role in the development of scoliosis. In this context we have evaluated the C57BL/6J mouse which is naturally deficient in melatonin, where scoliosis only develops when forced to a bipedal posture. (O´Kelly et al. 1999; Machida et al. 1999, 2005, 2006). Cheung et al. (2005) tried to reproduce these findings in a bipedal nonhuman primate model with surgical pinealectomy and showing a decrease in the melatonin level. None of the 18 study monkeys developed scoliosis in a mean follow up period of 28 months.

Alterations in Growth

Alterations in growth are found within the etiopathology of IS. It has been described that a mismatch between anterior spinal growth in relation to posterior spinal growth may be the triggering factor for the lordoescoliotic deformity observed in adolescent IS. In this case, one of the most used models is the Knockout FGFR3 mouse, mainly due to the presence of skeletal anomalies (McDonald et al. 2001; Bobyn et al. 2015).

Neurological Models

Starting from the hypothesis that the scoliotic deformity is produced from a neuromuscular problem. Several authors have addressed the issue in different animal models. Pincott and Taffs 1982, demonstrated the development of scoliosis from an intraspinal injection of oral attenuated live poliomyelitis vaccine in monkeys. Spinal deformity developed incidentally after a virulence test protocol. The histological results of the spinal cord showed greater damage in the spinal medulla on the convex side, located in the posterior horn and the Clarke column where the afferent sensorile/propioceptive nerve endings entered the spinal medulla (Figure 3). Based on these findings, they concluded that the deformity was not caused by the poliovirus, but that it occurred due to an asymmetrical weakness of the paraspinal muscles produced by the loss of proprioceptive innervation. From these findings, the same research group performed a selective rhizotomy of the dorsal root. Pincott et al. (1984) suggested that true scoliosis can develop from asymmetrical spinal muscle weakness appearing after neurosensorial loss has occurred in animals; a fact proven in a study in which Cynomolgus monkeys (*Macaca fascicularis*) underwent a series of spinal nerve roots cuts, revealing that after surgery true scoliosis followed allowing the grading of lateral deviation of the spine and its axial twist, demonstrating also that the severity of scoliosis depended on the site and the number of nerve roots cut and observing similarly that the section of the lumbar dorsal spinal nerve root had a particular tendency to produce scoliosis.

The resulting scoliosis developed on the convex side towards the damaged site and its severity was directly proportional to the number of cutted nerve roots. Long curves were observed in the form of "C" similar to the neuromuscular curvatures that occur in humans suffering from cerebral palsy (Pincott et al. 1984).

On other hand, Arrotegui et al. (1990), investigated whether the damage of gracilis nucleus could develop scoliosis deformities in rats; they concluded that the interruption of the proprioceptive afferent can facilitate the development of scoliotic attitude in experimental animals. This study provides the experimental support that the gracilis nucleus can be a determining factor in IS.

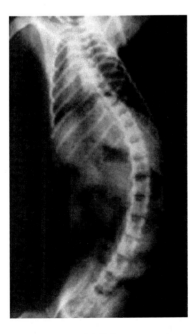

Figure 3. Examples of a neurological animal model. Direct posterior column cord injury post-intraspinal injection of polio virus in a monkey (Pincott and Taffs 1982). Taken from Ouellet and Odent 2013.

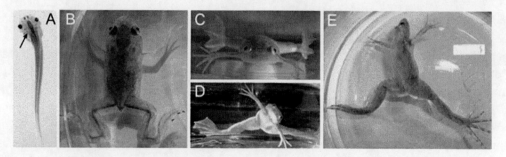

Figure 4. Spinal deformities in *Xenopus laevis* after removal of the left labyrinth. (A) Top view of larva illustrating the induced bending of the body/tail. Top and Front views of a young adult control frog (B, C) and after labyrinthine ablation (D, E). From Ouellet and Odent, 2013.

On the other hand, another neurological hypothesis linked to the alteration of the vestibular system has been postulated, it suggests that there is an imbalance in the neuronal activity of the descending pathways of the locomotor / postural control (Barrios and Arrotegui 1992; Lambert and Straka 2012; Catanzariti et al. 2014). Based on this hypothesis, De Waele et al. (1989) evaluated the effect of selective lesions on otolith receptors in which, finding that the lesion induced scoliotic curvatures with rotation towards the contralateral side. Head and spine radiographs after hemi-laberintectomy showed rotation of the head due to rotation of the cervical vertebrae and inclination of the head due to rotation of the thoracic vertebrae. Lambert et al. (2009) carried out the unilateral elimination of the labyrinthine organs in *Xenopus laevis* (African frog) in the larval stage, observing that after the metamorphosis, the spines of the young frogs had developed curvatures in the three planes, including the rotation along the longitudinal axis of the body with characteristics similar to the adolescent IS (Figure 4). However, when trying to perform the same experiment in mammals, the curvature in the column did not manifest. What was observed was an abnormal posture of the limbs. With this evidence, it is believed that the proprioceptive signals of the peripheral limbs of rodents replace the loss of the entrance of the inner ear, which generates the recovery of the abnormal posture. Based on the above Lambert et al. concluded that their scoliotic model in frogs developed spinal deformities because in these animals a persistent asymmetric tone occurs in the axial muscles and limbs during growth without compensatory peripheral proprioceptive feedback as developed in an environment without weight (water). As a consequence, during the metamorphosis, the mainly cartilaginous skeleton of the tadpoles is progressively deformed (Lambert et al. 2009, 2012).

Another neurological model used is the Ky mouse. This mouse is deficient in the Ky protein, which is considered crucial in the stability of the neuromuscular junctions and the ability of the muscles to grow and function normally. The Ky gene is located on chromosome 9 and encodes a new muscle protein (Blanco et al. 2001).

Mechanical Models

Various procedures have been developed to induce scoliotic deformities in different animal models. Within the great variety of experiments, these can be subdivided into external constraints, internal constraints and direct or indirect spinal attachments with or without tissue damage. For models with posterior anchoring, the need to perform a thoracic anchor has important drawbacks: high early mortality of animals and older animals are needed so that the period of exponential growth that results in a long period of study awaiting deformities is lost.

In particular, the effect of the thoracic wall procedure on the spinal deformity is also difficult to predict and can modulate the deformity variably. In addition, thoracic scars with extensive paraspinal fibrosis may limit our ability to test new methods of correction (Figure 5) (Smith and Dickson 1987; Kallemeier et al. 2006; Rooney et al. 2008; Odent et al. 2011; Janssen et al. 2011; Silva et al. 2012; Ouellet and Odent 2013; Moal et al. 2013; Bobyn et al. 2015; Barrios et al. 2018; Hachem et al. 2017; Zhang et al. 2017).

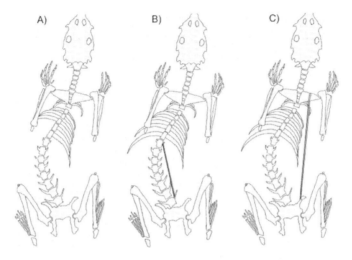

Figure 5. Mechanical asymmetry along the spine of a quadruped can be created via (A) unilateral resection of ribs and costovertebral joint, (B) unilateral tethering between transverse processes of ipsilateral vertebrae, or (C) unilateral tethering between ipsilateral pelvis and scapula. Take from Bobyn et al. 2015.

In Table 1, the most common animal models used to produce scoliosis experimentally, as well as the procedures, are listed.

Table 1. Most common animal models

Type	Procedure	Animal Model	Reference
Prenatal Procedures			
	Maternal exposure to infectious agents	Sheep	Woods and Anderson 1992 Parsonson et al. 1977
	Maternal exposure to carbon monoxide	Mouse Chicken	Farley et al. 2006 Farley et al. 2001 Alexander and Tuan 2003
	Vitamin deficiency	Rats	Li et al. 2012 Thomas and Cheng 1952
	Surgery scoliosis in utero through a hysterotomy	Lamb	Kent and Zingg 1974 Kent et al. 1978
	Injection of teratogenic chemicals in embryos	Chicken Rat Mouse	Duraiswami 1952 Murphy et al. 1957 Singh et al. 1993 Nogami and Ingalls 1967
	Unilateral removal of the labyrinthine end organs	Frog	Lambert et al. 2013 Lambert et al. 2009

Table 1. (Continued)

Type	Procedure	Animal Model	Reference
Postnatal Procedures			
	Systemic interventions		
	Pinealectomy	Chicken	Beuerlein et al. 2001 Bagnall et al. 1999 Thillard 1959 Machida et al. 1993, 1994, 1995, 1997 Wang et al. 1997 Kanemura et al. 1997 Turgut et al. 2006 Fu et al. 2011 Girardo et al. 2011 Man et al. 2014 O´Kelly et al. 1999 Aota et al. 2013 Akel et al. 2009 Poon et al. 2006 Coillard and Rivard 1996
		Rats	O´Kelly et al. 1999 Machida et al. 1999, 2005, 2006 Oyama et al. 2006
		Primate	Cheung et al. 2005 a, b Shangguan et al. 2009
		Salmon	Fjelldal et al. 2004
		Hamster	O´Kelly et al. 1999
	Long time exposure to intense light	Chicken	Nette et al. 2002
	Brainstem damage	Rabbit	Barrios et al. 1987 De Salis et al. 1980
	Vitamin deficiency	Rat	Ponseti 1957 Kitamura et al. 1965
Local procedures			
	Damage to the spinal column		
	Unilateral resection transverse processes and facet joints	Rabbit	Werneck et al. 2008 Pal et al. 1991
	Unilateral epiphysiodesis	Pig	Zhang et al. 2008, 2011 Cil et al. 2005 Beguiristain et al. 1980 Coillard et al. 1999
	Anterior destabilization and insertion of a wedge-shape resin disc	Cow	Shono et al. 1991

Type	Procedure	Animal Model	Reference
	Unilateral growth modulation of end plate with implanted electrodes	Rabbit	Dodge et al. 2010
	Damage to the neural tissues		
	Unilateral resection of the phrenic nerves	Rabbit	Agadir et al. 1990 Langenskiold and Michelsson 1959, 1961, 1962 Von Lesser 1888
	Intercostal nerve resection	Rabbit Rat Goat	Langenskiold and Michelsson 1961 Miles 1947 Robin 1966 Agadir et al. 1988, 1990 Sevastik et al. 1990 a, b, 1993 Schwartzman and Miles 1945 Birgard 1935.
	Rhizotomy	Rabbit Primate	Liszka 1961 Suk et al. 1989 Alexander et al. 1972 Pincott 1984
	Surgical damage of spinal cord	Rabbit Dog Primate	Barrios et al. 1987 De Salis et al. 1980 Chuma et al. 1997 Pincott and Taffs 1982
	Damage to the surrounding tissue		
	Unilateral resection of spinal ligaments	Rabbit	Pal et al. 1991 Langenskiold and Michelsson 1961, 1962
	Hemilaminectomy	Rabbit Pig	Langenskiold and Michelsson 1962
	Bilateral rib osteotomies plus unilateral fixation of overriding ribs	Rabbit	Sevastikoglou et al. 1978 Sevastik et al. 1984
	Unilateral rib resections	Chicken Rabbit	Deguchi et al. 1995 Robin 1996 Langenskiold and Michelsson 1959, 1961, 1962 Agadir et al. 1988 Thometz et al. 2000
	Bilateral resection of dorsal ribs	Primate	Pincott 1982
	Unilateral resection of paravertebral muscles	Rabbit Primate	Pal et al. 1991 Smith and Dickson 1987 Langenskiold and Michelsson 1962 Miles 1947 Pincott et al. 1982

Table 1. (Continued)

Type	Procedure	Animal Model	Reference
	Gradual rib elongation	Pig	Langenskiold and Michelsson 1962
		Rabbit	Sevastik et al. 1990 a, b.
	Unilateral electrical muscle stimulation	Rabbit	Kowalski et al. 2001 Willers et al. 1995
	Arterial ablation	Pig	De Salis et al. 1980
	Immobilization and tethering		
	Tying together of transfer processes with bilateral cauterization of the lamine	Rabbit	Somerville 1952 Lawton et al. 1985 Dickson 1985 Smith and Dickson 1987 Langenskiold and Michelsson 1961
	Forcing a scoliosis position using a casto or extension splint	Rabbit	Poussa et al. 1991 Hakkarainen 1981 Silva et al. 2012
	Unilateral tethering of the spinous apophysis and transverse apophysis	Rabbit	Carpintero et al. 1997
	Scapula-to-pelvis tethering	Rabbit Rat	Kallemeier et al. 2006 Sarwark et al. 1988
	Forcing a scoliotic position using an external fixation apparatus	Rat	Mente et al. 1997 Stokes et al. 2006 Aronsson et al. 2010 Stokes et al. 2008
	Posterior asymmetric tether from T5 to L1 laminae with rib resection	Goat	Braun and Akyuz 2005 Braun et al. 2003, 2004, 2005 a, b, 2006 a, b, c, d.
	Unilateral tethering with a rod or stainless-steel wire	Pig Goat	Laffosse et al. 2009, 2010 Patel et al. 2010, 2011 Schwab et al. 2009 Accadbled et al. 2010 Odent et al. 2011 Zhang et al. 2009
	Unilateral anterolateral flexible tether or shape memory alloy staples over consecutive vertebrae	Pig Goat Cow	Newton et al. 2008, 2011 Hunt et al. 2010 Newton et al. 2005
	Modulation of spinal growth using nickel-titanium coil springs	Dog	Zhang et al. 2017
Genetic Models		Mouse Teleost´s	Bobyn et al. 2015 Blanco et al. 2001 Giampetro et al. 2003 Gorman et al. 2009 Boswell and Ciruna 2017 Hayes et al. 2014 Grimes et al. 2016

Adapted from Janssen et al. 2011.

METHODS

Animals

As part of the annual screening in the non-human primates (NHP) unit of INBIOMA S.A.S de C.V., different clinical studies were done in forty rhesus monkeys (*Macaca mulatta*). In the study population, we noted several age-associated vertebral spine pathologies among the older animals, particularly those older than 9 years. The screened population of 4 years of age and younger did not present any sort of osteopathy, with the exception of a 2-year-old female, that showed gait alterations, mainly in the hind limbs, a clumsy gait and slight claudication in the right hind limb.

Among the 47% of monkeys showing some osteopathology (Hernandez-Godínez et al. 2011). In this particular way scoliosis affecting 10% of population studied. Based on these findings, we proceeded to perform clinical and imaging studies for the prescient diagnosis of this condition, in which idiopathic scoliosis was determined in the case of 3 adults and, the presence of scoliosis congenita in an infant Rhesus monkey. From these findings several studies were conducted to characterize and describe the severity of scoliosis.

All animal procedures were strictly carried out according to Mexican Official Ethics Standard NOM-062-ZOO-1999 and the Guide for the Care and Use of Experimental Animals (National Research Council Institute for Laboratory Animal Research, U.S., 1996) and the American Society of Primatologists (Principles for the Ethical treatment of Non-Humans Primates). It was approved by the Internal Committee for the Care and Use of Laboratory Animals (ICCULA) and the Research Ethics Commissions by INBIOMA S.A.S de C.V.

The monkeys live in five corral-type cages made of concrete floors covered with ceramic tiles. Roofs offer secure protection from weather and the doors are equipped with padlocks to ensure the safety of both animals and handlers. Each cage has automatic water dispensers with food containers placed outside to prevent contact with feces and urine.

Radiological Examination

We performed lateral left/right and ventrodorsal x-ray films of the vertebral column (C1-S1) using fluoroscopy equipment model Siemens® Siregraphs CF (Siemens Medical Solutions USA, Malvern, PA), as well as a computerized tridimensional tomography (CAT) scans with three-dimensional computerized equipment model Siemmens® 3D (Somaton Sensation, 3D model, Siemens Medical Solutions USA, Malvern, PA). The imaging studies were based on the Mexican health legislation NOM-157-SSA1-1996 and were performed in the Imaging Unit of Hospital General Dr. Manuel Gea González S.S., Mexico.

Neurophysiological Studies

Evoked potentials of the somatosensory pathway (SEPTN) were recorded in the Neurophysiology Laboratory at INBIOMA S.A.S de C.V., using a NEURONICA 5® computer for evoked potentials (EP) (Neuronic®; Havana, Cuba). Silver chloride (Ag-Cl) cutaneous disc electrodes with 5 millimeters in diameter were used (Natus Medical Inc.). Before the electrodes placement, asepsis of the area was performed, cleaning with neutral soap and water. Disc electrodes were placed according to the international 10/20 systems, with impedance less than 5 Kω (Hernández-Godínez et al. 2012, 2014; Ibáñez-Contreras et al. 2017). The duration of registration was performed in 20 minutes and monkeys were not given an extra dose of anesthetic.

To monitor the SSEPMN, electrodes were placed at the cubital fossa (CF) (-), the Erb point (-), the seventh cervical vertebra (C7) (-), and the contralateral somatosensory cortex (C3' or C4') (-), of the stimulated limb, referenced to Fz (+). The ground was placed on the mastoids. To record the SSEPTN, electrodes were placed at the following derivations: the popliteal fossa (PF) (-), the fifth lumbar vertebra (L5) (-), the third thoracic vertebra (T3) (-), and the contralateral somatosensory cortex (C3' or C4') (-), of the stimulated limb, also referenced to Fz with the ground placed on the mastoids. The stimulus was a squared monophasic electric pulse of 100 µseg of duration at a stimulation frequency of 0.5-1.1 stimuli/sec applied behind the internal malleolus. A total of 250 stimuli were averaged and the response was replicated at least once to ensure events reproducibility. The filters utilized were 5-2,500 Hz with an intensity of 1.5 mÅ (Hernández-Godinez et al. 2011, 2012, 2014; Ibáñez-Contreras et al. 2016, 2017).

Physiological Parameters

Physiological parameters were monitored, included heart rate, respiratory frequency, arterial oxygen saturation, and systolic/diastolic pressure with an Ohmeda Cardiocap/5® (Datex-Ohmeda Inc., Louis-ville, KY, USA). These procedures were executed without animal sedation using a restraining chair for non-human primates (Primate Products ®, Immokalee, FL, USA; IRIRIO – Macaque Restrainer).

CASE PRESENTATION: CONGENITAL SCOLIOSIS

In this particular case the NHP was born by cesarean section at 23 weeks of gestation and kept with another infant monkey in individual stainless-steel boxes specially designed to NHP. After the end of the lactation period, it was housed in group cages (previously described). Alterations in the gait were observed when introduced to a group cage.

In the radiologic studies, a compensatory scoliosis in the lumbar zone was observed caused by the absence of the right wing of the ilium (Figure 6).

The SEPTN was performed as previously described. In this study we observed a wave that remained constant and defined in all neural generators of the somatosensory pathway and presents an enlargement of the latencies from L5 to the cortex, mainly in the left afference, correlating with the imaging studies (Figure 7). Showed the obtained latencies for P1 in both derivations: left and right.

This finding contribute to the description of the CS in this animal species. By having few reports of CS in NHP, the finding itself is considered as incidental while monitoring the health status of the captive animals. The results of this work were published in Journal of Medical Primatology in 2013 by Solis Chavez et al. 2013.

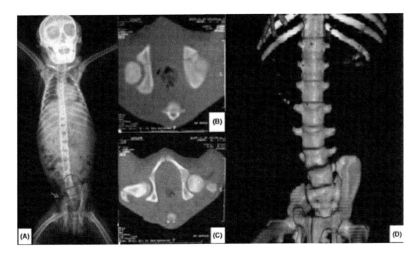

Figure 6. (A) Ventral-dorsal radiograph of the spine of Rhesus monkey female with 3 years old, with congenital scoliosis, with an arrow showing the compensatory scoliosis, she also had absence of right wing of the ilium. (B) and (c) Axial spine. Note the malformation of the hip joint. (D) Computerized axial tomography (CAT) of Rhesus monkey with congenital scoliosis (Solís Chavez et al. 2013).

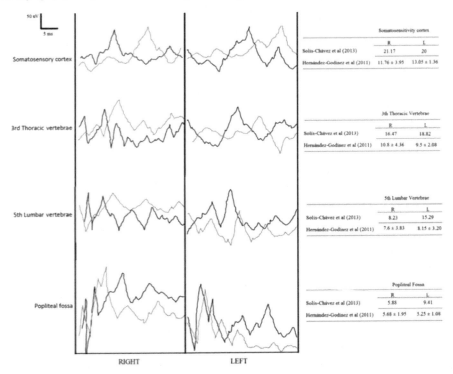

Figure 7. Somatosensory Evoked Potentials Tibial Nerve (SEPTN). In black shows the response obtained from the electrical activity of the monkeys without scoliosis, in gray shows elongated response of the monkey with congenital scoliosis. L, left afferencies; R, right afferencias (Solis-Chavez et al. 2013).

CASE PRESENTATION: IDIOPHATIC SCOLIOSIS

This study was carried out in the three macaques with true thoracic scoliosis. Animals consisted of one 21-year-old female weighing 7700g and two 23-year-old males with an average weight of 8500g. No information on the exact date of osteopathology presentation could be obtained. Results were compared with a control group of animals with no spinal abnormalities and included one 25-year-old female weighing 8230g and two 20-year-old males with an average weight of 10,500g.

Our results were published in *Journal of Medical Primatology* (2012) by Hernandez-Godinez et al. (2012). Table 2 shows results of the evaluation of physiological parameters. In this examination, the two-sided *P value* showed significant differences ($P < 0.05$) in respiratory rate and diastolic pressure.

Changes in the respiratory system occurring due to various degrees of scoliotic curvatures can be grouped into three different forms: Compromise of vital aerial mechanics, gasometrical dysfunction and pulmonary hypertension.

Colomina and Godet (2005) described that advanced phases of human scoliosis are related to restrictive respiratory function resulting in shallow breathing, concomitant with grossly underdeveloped pulmonary acinar structures because of the chronically compromised lungs, a mild to severe thoracic deformity impairing normal vascular development where pulmonary space constraints may have affected airway branching patterns that participate in gas exchange. Rhesus monkeys do not exhibit the same physiopathology observed in humans, because a rather normal breathing was observed in this study, lacking notorious deficiencies such as a restricted or shallow breathing owing to the fact that the mean RR recorded in the scoliotic monkeys was lower than that of the non-scoliotic animals. The remarkable differences between the human reports and our study, apparently rests merely on unique corrective–adaptive postural changes that quadruped species assume derived from true scoliosis, which in turn minimizes thoracic deformity and consequently circumvents or limits pulmonary compression.

Regarding the cardiovascular alterations related to true scoliosis, it is assumed that these are the result of severe displacement of the mediastinal structures affecting the pericardium and great vessels. From the evaluation of X-rays, a left cardiomegaly was noted in a male with scoliosis as a possible associated pathology, as suggested by Gillingham et al. (2006), Herrera-Soto et al. (2006), and Kawakami et al. (1995) that indicated that in humans, congenital heart conditions are risk factors increasing the development of this disease. In this evaluation, no significant differences were reported regarding the heart rate parameters among scoliotic and non-scoliotic monkeys as described in Table 2, although statistically significant differences were observed for the DPs ($P = 0.027$). Colomina and Godet (2005) discovered that a dysfunction of the cardiovascular system can be primarily related to severe distortion of the blood vessel's morphology which in turn simulates a chronic form of constrictive pericarditis. From these structural changes, significant differences were specifically encountered in the arterial blood pressure of the scoliotic monkeys (Table 2), where both systolic and DPs were lower 95.6 ± 9.07 and 59.6 ± 10.26 mmHg, respectively, in comparison with the healthy monkeys displaying 114.8 ± 15.89 mmHg systolic and 77 ± 7.48 mmHg of DPs, thus interpreting this to be a deficient ventricular filling in the scoliotic monkeys as a consequence of the heart's diminished capacity to increase cardiac output secondary to preventricular filling in the presence of coexisting cardiomyopathies.

Table 2. Evaluation of physiological parameters in scoliotic and non-scoliotic Rhesus macaques

Physiological parameters	Health condition	Mean SD	P
Heart rate (HR, bpm)	Scoliotic	141.8 ± 6.53	0.194
	Non-Scoliotic	142.4 ± 0.54	
Respiratory rate (RR, rpm)	Scoliotic	17.0 ± 2.54	0.025
	Non-Scoliotic	21.2 ± 1.48	
Body temperature (°C)	Scoliotic	37.34 ± 0.43	0.170
	Non-Scoliotic	37.78 ± 0.45	
Oxygen saturation (SpO2, %)	Scoliotic	95 ± 1.87	0.054
	Non-Scoliotic	97.8 ± 2.04	
Systolic pressure (SP, mmHg)	Scoliotic	95.6 ± 9.07	0.059
	Non-Scoliotic	114.8 ± 15.89	
Diastolic pressure (DP, mmHg)	Scoliotic	59.6 ± 10.26	0.027
	Non-Scoliotic	77.0 ± 7.48	

Note: SPSS for Windows 16 software (SPSS, Chicago, IL, USA) was used. A P value of <0.05 defined statistical significance. We used a non-parametric test for two independent samples, Mann–Whitney U test. Degrees of freedom and central tendency measures were documented, comparing the results of evaluations in monkeys with scoliosis in relationship to the control group.

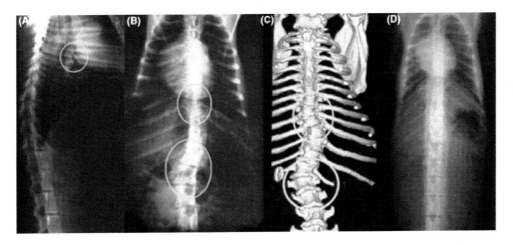

Figure 8. (A) Right lateral radiograph of the spine of Rhesus monkey male with 21-year-old. The radiography shows a posterior-anterior view with diminished heart space and dilated aorta. (B) A ventral-dorsal chest radiograph of Rhesus monkey male with 21-year-old with idiopathic scoliosis. The radiography shows a normal thorax with right rotoscoliosis in the thoracic column. Cardiophrenic sinus and costo-diaphragmatic recesses free. Pleura not visible. Lung fields with increased density in hilum. Enlarged cardiac silhouette with an augment in the size of left atrium. (C) Computerized axial tomography were taken (C1 to S1). (D) Barrel chest thorax with normal cercoepithecoid form and normal size. Soft tissue without alterations. Bone tissue with adequate density, diaphgram with cardiophrenic sinus and costodiaphragmatic recess free. Pleura not visible. Lung fields clear (Hernández – Godinez et al. 20102).

	P1			P2		
	Right afferency latencies (mseg)			Right afferency latencies (mseg)		
	Scoliotic monkeys	Non-scoliotic monkeys		Scoliotic monkeys	Non-scoliotic monkeys	
	Mean ± SD	Mean ± SD	P	Mean ± SD	Mean ± SD	P
Superior cortex (C4)	17.85 ± 7.66	16.66 ± 1.21	0.827	28.78 ± 11.21	24.02 ± 3.46	0.269
Cervical (C7)	11.89 ± 2.90	13.02 ± 3.24	0.513	19.67 ± 4.33	21.20 ± 3.96	0.519
Erb's point	10.34 ± 4.07	9.99 ± 4.15	0.271	17.26 ± 5.75	15.48 ± 5.07	0.760
Anterior cubital fossa	5.71 ± 0.45	5.73 ± 1.63	0.347	11.51 ± 0.70	10.46 ± 1.53	0.376
	P1			P2		
	Left afferency latencies (mseg)			Left afferency latencies (mseg)		
	Scoliotic monkeys	Non-scoliotic monkeys	P	Scoliotic monkeys	Non-scoliotic monkeys	P
	Mean ± SD	Mean ± SD		Mean ± SD	Mean ± SD	
Superior cortex (C4)	20.82 ± 4.13	18.77 ± 2.24	0.076	28.52 ± 6.76	27.51 ± 3.51	0.657
Cervical (C7)	14.98 ± 0.60	13.96 ± 4.76	0.192	23.44 ± 1.81	21.91 ± 6.16	0.519
Erb's point	12.43 ± 1.97	8.75 ± 1.04	0.049	19.66 ± 3.05	14.76 ± 0.60	0.067
Anterior cubital fossa	7.00 ± 0.20	7.86 ± 1.79	0.907	12.66 ± 0.50	12.76 ± 1.03	0.656

SD, standard deviation; fd, freedom degrees, in all cases the fd were 4; P, significant value of P.

Figure 9. Upper limb afferencies and somatosensory-evoked potentials (SEPMN) of Rhesus Monkeys (*Macaca mulatta*).

	P1			P2		
	Right afferency latencies (mseg)			Right afferency latencies (mseg)		
	Scoliotic monkeys	Non-scoliotic monkeys		Scoliotic monkeys	Non-scoliotic monkeys	
	Mean ± SD	Mean ± SD	P	Mean ± SD	Mean ± SD	P
Inferior cortex (C4)	27.20 ± 7.76	16.53 ± 3.01	0.458	39.16 ± 16.00	23.10 ± 2.38	0.059
Thoracic (T3)	20.35 ± 4.05	11.80 ± 1.51	0.040	31.82 ± 12.64	16.80 ± 3.10	0.055
Lumbar (L5)	14.50 ± 3.32	8.93 ± 1.14	0.510	20.94 ± 7.74	16.27 ± 3.30	0.128
Popliteal fossa	5.90 ± 1.84	7.47 ± 2.44	0.376	16.92 ± 2.54	13.60 ± 1.83	0.127
	P1			P2		
	Left afferency latencies (mseg)			Left afferency latencies (mseg)		
	Scoliotic monkeys	Non-scoliotic monkeys	P	Scoliotic monkeys	Non-scoliotic monkeys	P
	Mean ± SD	Mean ± SD		Mean ± SD	Mean ± SD	
Inferior cortex (C4)	30.79 ± 6.73	19.53 ± 4.15	0.127	40.58 ± 16.95	28.03 ± 3.15	0.275
Thoracic (T3)	21.96 ± 2.52	13.67 ± 0.42	0.030	33.40 ± 12.81	21.80 ± 1.22	0.352
Lumbar (L5)	14.71 ± 7.07	10.67 ± 1.80	0.513	23.42 ± 11.58	15.20 ± 2.00	0.534
Popliteal fossa	6.11 ± 1.81	7.73 ± 1.36	0.127	13.11 ± 4.48	14.07 ± 3.64	0.827

SD, standard deviation; fd, freedom degrees, in all cases the fd were 4; P, significant value of P.

Figure 10. Lower limb and somatosensory evoked potentials (SEPTN) of Rhesus Monkeys (*Macaca mulatta*).

During the neurophysiologic evaluation, significant differences were noted in P1 for the thoracic derivative in both afferencies (P = 0.040 for the right afferency and P = 0.030 for the left afferency). Figures 9 and 10 show comparative results of both groups in terms of their neurophysiological response upon stimulation of the upper and lower limbs. In both cases, longer latencies were observed in the scoliotic monkeys when compared with normal animals. It is important to emphasize that in all cases, the scoliotic curvature was right-sided and for that reason consistent with the lengthening of both afferencies observed at the thoracic region, revealing a lesion on the somatosensory pathways possibly derived from congenital stenosis of the rachidial canal due to medullar compression. As for the upper limbs, a difference at the Erb's point for the left afferency in P1 was reported (P = 0.049); in this case, observed as a response to spinal morphological changes acting against the functional status of the locomotor system and consequence of the spine's rotation at the thoracic level; a condition leading to late postural deformity at the scapular girdle as compensatory to improve locomotion affected by this osteopathology.

CONCLUSION

It is clear that the use of different diagnostic tools complements the knowledge of the pathophysiology of many diseases. In the case of scoliosis in Rhesus monkeys it was fundamental to describe how this osteopathology involves different systems, starting from the fact that idiopathic scoliosis is not reported in quadrupeds, much less in non-human primates. For this reason, it was essential to evaluate all the changes generated from the involvement of different systems, allowing to establish the relationship between idiopathic scoliosis in rhesus monkeys and the presence of heart disease, manifesting with changes in blood pressure. In addition, the applicability of non-invasive neurophysiological tools such as the somatosensory evoked potentials is provided, allowing to observe the relationship that exists between the results of the radiologic films and the delays in the electrical conductivity of the somatosensory pathway when observed being compromised by the degree of deviation and deformity of the spine.

REFERENCES

Accadbled, F., Laffose, J. M., Odent, T., Gomez-Brouchet, A., Sales de Gauzy, J., Swider, P. 2010. Influence of growth modulation on the effective permeability of the vertebral end plate. A porcine experimental scoliosis model. *Clinical Biomechanics* (Bristol Avon). 26 (4): 337-342. doi: 10.1016/j.clinbiomech.2010.11.007.

Agadir, M., Sevastik, B., Sevastik, J., Persson, A., Isberg, B. 1988. Induction of scoliosis in the growing rabbit by unilateral rib-growth stimulation. *Spine* (Phila Pa 1976). 13 (9): 1065-1069. PMID: 3206301

Agadir, M., Sevastik, B., Reinholt, F. P., Perbeck, L., Sevastik, J. 1990. Vascular changes in the chest wall after unilateral resection of the intercostal nerves in the growing rabbit. *Journal of Orthopeaedic research*. 8 (2): 283-290. PMID: 2303962.

Akel, I., Kocak, O., Bozkurt, G., Alanay, A., Marcucio, R., Acaroglu, E. 2009. The effect of calmodulin antagonists on experimental scoliosis: a pinealectomized chicken model. *Spine* (PhilaPa 1976). 34 (6): 533-538. DOI: 10.1097/BRS.0b013e31818be0b1.

Alexander, P. G., Tuan, R. S. 2003. Carbon monoxide-induced axial skeletal dysmorphogenesis in the chick embryo. Birth Defects Research. Part A. *Clinical and Molecular Teratology*. 67(4): 219-230. DOI: 10.1002/bdra.10041.

Aota, Y., Terayama, H., Saito, T., Itoh, M. 2013. Pinealectomy in a broiler chicken model impairs endochondral ossification and induces rapid cancellous bone loss. *Spine Journal*. 13 (11): 1607-1616. doi: 10.1016/j.spinee.2013.05.017.

Aronsson, D. D., Stokes, I. A., Mc Bride, C. 2010. The role of remodeling and asymmetric growth in vertebral wedging. *Studies in health technology Informatics*. 158: 11-15. PMID: 20543392.

Arrotegui, J. I., Barrios, C., Cano, G. F. 1990. Interrupción de aferencias propioceptivas a nivel de la segunda neurona, inducen escoliosis en ratas. [Interruption of proprioceptive afferents at the level of the second neuron, induce scoliosis in rats.] *Revista Española de Cirugía y Osteología*. 9: 681-685. http://hdl.handle.net/10550/56614.

Bagnall, K. M., Raso, V. J., Moreau, M., Mahood, J. K., Wang, X., Zhao, J. 1999. The effects of melatonin therapy on the development of scoliosis after pinealectomy in the chicken. *Journal of Bone and Joint Surgery American*. 81: 191-199. PMID: 10073582.

Barrios, C., Tuñon, M. T., De Salis, J. A., Bequiristain, J. L., Cañadell, J. 1987. Scoliosis induced by medullary damage: an experimental study in rabbits. *Spine*. 12; 433-439. PMID: 3306965.

Barrios, C., Arrotegui, J. I. 1992. Experimental kyphoscoliosis induced in rats by selective brain stem damage. *International Orthopaedics*. 16 (2): 146-151. PMID: 1428313.

Barrios, C., Lloris, J. M., Alonso, J., Maruenda, B., Burgos, J., Llombart-Blanco, R., Gil, L., Bisbal, V. 2018. Novel porcine experimental model of severe progressive thoracic scoliosis with compensatory curves induced by interpedicular bent rigid temporary tethering. *Journal of orthopaedic research*. 36 (1): 174-182. doi: 10.1002/jor.23617.

Beguiristain, J. L., De Salis, J., Oriaifo, A., Cañadell, J. 1980. Experimental scoliosis by epiphysiodesis in pigs. *International Orthopaedics*. 3 (4): 317-321. PMID: 7399773.

Beuerlein, M., Wilson, J., Moreau, M., Raso, V. J., Mahood, J., Wang, X., Greenhill, B., Bagnall, K. M. 2001. The critical stage of pinealectomy surgery after which scoliosis is produced in young chickens. *Spine* (Phila Pa 1976). 26 (3): 237-240. PMID: 11224858.

Bisgard, J. D. 1935. Experimental thoracogenic scoliosis. *Journal of Thoracic Surgery*. 4: 435.

Blanco, G., Coulton, G. R, Biggin, A., Grainge, C., Moss, J., Barrett, M., Berguin, A., Marechal, G., Skynner, m., Van Mier, P., Nikitopoulou, A., Kraus, M., Mason, R. M., Brown, S. D. 2001. The kyphoscoliosis (ky) mouse is deficient in hypertrophic responses and is caused by a mutation in a novel muscle-specific protein. *Human Molecular Genetic*. 10 (1): 9-16. PMID: 11136708.

Bobyn, J. D., Little, D. G., Gray, R., Schindeler, A. 2015. Animal models of scoliosis. *Journal of Orthopaedic Research*. 33 (4): 458-467. DOI: 10.1002/jor.22797.

Boswell, C. W., Ciruna, B. 2017. Understanding Idiopathic Scoliosis: A New Zebrafish School of Thought. *Trends in Genetic*. 33 (3): 183-196. DOI: 10.1016/j.tig.2017.01.001.

Brodner, W., Krepler, P., Nicolakis, M., Langer, M., Kaider, A., Lack, W., Waldhauser, F. 2000. Melatonin and adolescent idiopathic scoliosis. *Journal of Bone Joint and Surgery British*. 82(3): 399-403. PMID: 10813177.

Braun, J. T., Ogilvie, J. W., Akyuz, E., Brodke, D. S., Bachus, K. N., Stefko, R. M. 2003. Experimental scoliosis in an immature goat model: a method that creates idiopathic-type deformity with minimal violation of the spinal elements along the curve. *Spine (Phila Pa 1976)*. 28 (19): 2198-2203. DOI: 10.1097/01.BRS.0000085095.37311.46.

Braun, J. T., Ogilvie, J. W., Akyuz, E., Brodke, D. S., Bachus, K. N. 2004. Fusionless scoliosis correction using a shape memory alloy staple in the anterior thoracic spine of the immature goat. *Spine (Phila Pa 1976)*. 29 (18): 1980-1989. PMID: 15371698.

Braun, J. T., and Akyuz, E. 2005. Prediction of curve progression in a goat scoliosis model. *Journal of Spinal Disorders and techniques.* 18 (3): 272-276. PMID: 15905773.

Braun, J. T., Akyuz, E., Ogilvie, J. W., Bachus, K. N. 2005. The efficacy and integrity of shape memory alloy staples and bone anchors with ligament tethers in the fusionless treatment of experimental scoliosis. *Journal of Bone and Joint Surgery American Volumen.* 87 (9): 2038-2051. DOI: 10.2106/JBJS.D.02103.

Braun, J. T., Akyuz, E., Udall, H., Ogilvie, J. W., Brodke, D. S., Bachus, K. N. 2006. Three-dimensional analysis of 2 fusionless scoliosis treatments: a flexible ligament tether versus a rigid-shape memory alloy staple. *Spine (Phila Pa 1976).* 31 (3): 262-268. DOI: 10.1097/01.brs.0000197569.13266.fe.

Braun, J. T., Hoffman, M., Akyuz, E., Ogilvie, J. W., Brodke, D. S., Bachus, K. N. 2006. Mechanical modulation of vertebral growth in the fusionless treatment of progressive scoliosis in an experimental model. *Spine (Phila Pa 1976).* 31 (12): 1314-1320. DOI:10.1097/01.brs.0000218662.78165.b1.

Braun, J. T., Ogilvie, J. W., Akyuz, E., Brodke, D. S., Bachus, K. N. 2006. Creation of an experimental idiopathic-type scoliosis in an immature goat model using a flexible posterior asymmetric tether. *Spine (Phil Pa 1976).* 31 (13): 1410.1414. DOI:10.1097/01.brs.0000219869.01599.6b.

Braun, J. T., Hines, J. L., Akyuz, E., Vallera, C., Ogilvie, J.W. 2006. Relative versus absolute modulation of growth in the fusionless treatment of experimental scoliosis. *Spine (Phila PA 1976).* 31 (16): 1776-1782. DOI:10.1097/01.brs.0000227263.43060.50.

Buser, Z., Ortega, B., D'Oro, A., Pannell, W., Cohen, J. R., Wang, J., Wang, J. C. (2018). Spine Degenerative Conditions and Their Treatments: National Trends in the United States of America. *Global Spine Journal*, 8(1), 57–67. DOI: 10.1177/2192568217696688.

Carpintero, P., Mesa, M., Garcia, J., Carpintero, A. 1997. Scoliosis induced by asymmetric lordosis and rotation: an experimental study. *Spine* (Phila Pa 1976). 22 (19): 2202-2206. PMID: 9346139.

Catanzariti, J. F., Agnani, O., Guyot, M. A., Wlodyka-Demaille, S., Khenioui, H., Donze, C. 2014. Does adolescent idiopathic scoliosis relate to vestibular disorders? A systematic review. *Annals of Physical Rehabilitation Medicine.* 57 (6-7): 465-479. DOI: 10.1016/j.rehab.2014.04.003.

Cheung, K. M., Wang, T., Poon, A. M., Carl, A., Tranmer, B., Hu, Y., Luk, K. D., Leong, J. C. 2005. The effect of pinealectomy on scoliosis development in young nonhuman primates. *Spine (Phila Pa 1976).* 30 (18): 2009-2013. PMID: 16166887.

Chuma, A., Kitahara, H., Minami, S., Goto, S., Takaso, M., Moriya, H. 1997. Structural scoliosis model in dogs with experimentally induced syringomyelia. *Spine (Phila Pa 1976).* 22 (6): 589-594. PMID: 9089930.

Coillard C., and Rivard C. H. 1996. Vertebral deformities and scoliosis. *European Spine Journal.* 5: 91-100. PMID: 8724188.

Coillard, C., Rhalmi, S., Rivard, C. H. Experimental scoliosis in the minipig: study of vertebral deformations. *Annales de Chirurgie.* 53 (8): 773-780. PMID: 10584389.

Colomina, M. J., and Godet, C. 2005. Anestesia para la cirugía de la escoliosis. Estudio preoperatorio y seleccion de pacientes de riesgo en la cirugia de las enfermedades raquideas. [Anesthesia for scoliosis surgery. Preoperative study and selection of patients at risk in the surgery of spinal diseases.] *Revista Española de Anestesiologia y Reanimación.* 52: 24-43.

Deguchi, M., Kawakami, N., Kanemura, T., Mimatsu, K., Iwata, H. 1995. Experimental scoliosis induced by rib resection in chickens. *Journal of Spinal Disorders.* 8 (3): 179-185. PMID: 7670207.

De Salis, J. Beguiristain, J. L., Cañadell, J. 1980. The production of experimental scoliosis by selective arterial ablation. *International Orthopaedics*; 3: 311-315. PMID: 7399772.

De Waele, C., Graf, W., Josset, P., Vidal, P. P. 1989. A radiological analysis of the postural syndromes following hemilabyrinthectomy and selective canal and otolith lesions in the guinea pig. *Experimental Brain Research.* 77 (1):166–182. PMID: 2792260.

Dede, O., Akel, I., Demirkiran, G., Yalcin, N., Marcucio, R., Acaroglu, E. 2011. Is decreased bone mineral density associated with development of scoliosis? A bipedal osteopenic rat model. *Scoliosis.* 6 (1): 24. DOI: 10.1186/1748-7161-6-24.

Dickon, R. A. 1985. Thoracic lordoscoliosis in neurofibromatosis: treatment by a Harrington rod with sublaminar wiring. Report of two cases. *Journal of Bone and Joint Surgery American Volumen.* 67 (5): 822-823. PMID: 3922991.

Dodge, G. R., Bowen, Jr., Jeong, C. 2010. Vertebral growth modulation by electrical current in an animal model: potential treatment for scoliosis. *Journal of pediatric orthopedics.* 30 (4): 365-370. DOI: 10.1097/BPO.0b013e3181d8fa74.

Duraiswami, P. K. 1952. Experimental causation of congenital skeletal defects and its significance in orthopaedic surgery. *Journal of Bone Joint and Surgery British Volumen.* 34-B: 646-698. PMID: 12999957.

Fagan, A. B., Kennaway, D. J., Oakley, A. P. 2009. Pinealectomy in the chicken: a good model of scoliosis? *Europena Spine Journal.* 18 (8): 1154-1159. DOI: 1007/s00586-009-0927-7.

Farley, F. A., Loder, R. T., Nolan, B. T., Dillon, M. T., Frankenburg, E. P., Kaciroti, N. A., Miller, J. D., Goldstein, S. A., Hensinger, R. N. 2001. Mouse model for thoracic congenital scoliosis. *Journal of Pediatric Orthopedics.* 21(4): 537-540. PMID: 11433171.

Farley, F. A., Hall, J., Goldstein, S. A. 2006. Characteristics of congenital scoliosis in a mouse model. *Journal of Pediatric Orthopedics.* 26 (3): 341-346. DOI: 10.1097/01.bpo.0000203011.58529.d8.

Fjelldal, P. G., Grotmol, S., Kryvi, H., Gjerdet, N. R., Taranger, G. L., Hansen, T., Porter, M. J., Totland, G. K. 2004. Pinealectomy induces malformation of the spine and reduces the mechanical strength of the vertebrae in Atlantic salmon, Salmo salar. *Journal of Pineal Research.* 36 (2): 132-139. DOI: doi.org/10.1046/j.1600-079X.2003.00109.x.

Fu, G., Yoshihara, H., Kawakami, N., Goto, M., Tsuji, T., Ohara, T., Imagama, S. 2011. Microcomputed tomographic evaluation of vertebral microarchitecture in pinealectomized scoliosis chickens. *Journal of Pediatric Orthopedics Part B.* 20 (6): 382-388. DOI: 10.1097/BPB.0b013e3283474c6e.

García-Ramos C-L., Obil-Chavarría C. A., Zárate-Kalfópulos B., Rosales-Olivares L. M., Alpizar-Aguirre A., Reyes-Sánchez A. A. 2015. Escoliosis degenerativa del adulto. [Degenerative scoliosis of the adult.] *Acta Ortopedica Mexicana.* 29 (2): 127-138. ISSN 2306-4102.

Giampietro, P. F., Blank, R. D., Raggio, C. L., Merchant, S., Jacobsen, F. S., Faciszewski, T., Shukla, S. K., Greenlee, A. R., Reynolds, C., Schowalter, DB. 2003. Congenital and idiopathic scoliosis: clinical and genetic aspects. *Clinical Medicine Research.* 1(2):125-136. PMID: 15931299.

Giampietro, P. F., Raggio, C.L., Reynolds, C.E., Shukla, S. K., McPherson, E., Ghebranious, N., Jacobsen, F. S., Kumar, V., Faciszewski, T., Pauli, R. M., Rasmussen, K., Burmester,

J. K., Zaleski, C., Merchant, S., David, D., Weber, J. L., Glurich, I., Blank, R. D. 2005. An analysis of PAX1 in the development of vertebral malformations. *Clinical Genetics.* 68 (5): 448–453. DOI: 10.1111/j.1399-0004.2005.00520.x.

Giampietro, P. F., Raggio, C. L., Reynolds, C., Ghebranious, N., Burmester, J. K., Glurich, I., Rasmussen, K., McPherson, E., Pauli, R. M., Shukla, S. K., Merchant, S., Jacobsen, F. S., Faciszewski, T., Blank, R. D. 2006. DLL3 as a candidate for vertebral malformations. *American Journal of Medical Genetics.* Part A. 140 (22): 2447–2453. DOI: 10.1002/ajmg.a.31509.

Giampietro, P. F., Dunwoodie, S. L., Kusumi, K., Pourquié, O., Tassy, O., Offiah, A. C., Cornier, A. S., Alman, B. A., Blank, R. D., Raggio, C. L., Glurich, I., Turnpenny, P. D. 2008. Molecular diagnosis of vertebral segmentation disorders in humans. *Expert Opinion on Medical Diagnostics.* 2 (10): 1107–1121. DOI: 10.1517/17530059.2.10.1107.

Giampietro, P. F., Raggio, C. L., Blank, R. D., McCarty, C., Broeckel, U., Pickart, M. A. 2013. Clinical, genetic and environmental factors associated with congenital vertebral malformation. *Molecular Syndromology.* 4: 94-105. DOI: 10.1159/000345329.

Gillingham, B. L., Fan, R. A., Akbarnia, B. A. 2006. Early onset idiopathic scoliosis. *Journal of American Academie ON Orthopaedics and Surgery.* 14: 101-112.

Girardo, M., Bettini, N., Dema, E., Cervellati, S. 2011. The role of melatonin in the pathogenesis of adolescent idiopathic scoliosis (AIS). *Europena Spine Journal.* 20 (Suppl 1): S68-S74. DOI: 1007/s00586-011-1750-5.

González-Miranda, A., Riquelme-García, O., Moyano-Ortega, G., Viveros-Montoro, A., Largo-Aramburu, C., Del Cañizo-López, J. F., García-Barreno, P. 2016. Use of paravertebral injection of botulinum toxin to control scoliosis progression in pinealectomized chicken: the spine as a tensegrity system. *Cirugía Plática Ibero-Latinoamericana.* 42 (2): 121-130. DOI: 10.4321/s0376-78922016000200005.

Gorman, K. F., Breden, F. 2009. Idiopathic-type scoliosis is not exclusive to bipedalism. *Medical Hypotheses.* 72 (3): 348-352. DOI: 10.1016/j.mehy.2008.09.052.

Hachem, B., Aubin, C. E., Parent, S. 2017. Porcine spine finite element model: a complementary tool to experimental scoliosis fusionless instrumentation. *European Spine Journal.* 26 (6): 1610-1617. DOI: 10.1007/s00586-016-4940-3.

Hakkarainen, S. 1981. Experimental scoliosis: production of structural scoliosis by immobilization of young rabbits in a scoliotic position. *Acta Orthoaedica Scandinavica Supplementum.* 192: 1-5. PMID: 6945791.

Hayes, M., Gao, X., Yu, L. X., Paria, N., Henkelman, R. M., Wise, C. A., Ciruba, B. 2014. ptK7 mutant zebrafish models of congenital and idiopathic scoliosis implicate dysregulated Wnt signalling in disease. *Nature communications.* 5: 4777. DOI: 10.1038/ncomms5777.

Hernández-Godínez B, Bonilla-Jaime H, Poblano A, Arteaga-Silva M, Bautista-Rodríguez MA, Solís-Chávez S, Heras-Romero Y, Tena-Betancourt E, Ibáñez-Contreras A. Ontogeny of Somatosensory Evoked Potentials of Median and Tibial Nerves in Rhesus Monkeys (Macaca mulatta): Influence of Dissociative Anesthetic Mixtures under Captivity Conditions. Capítulo 3. In *Monkeys: Brain development, Social & hormonal mechanisms and Zoonotic diseases.* Editorial Nova Science Publishers, Inc. USA, 2014, pp 51-78.

Hernández-Godínez, B., Ibáñez-Contreras, A., Reyes-Pantoja, S., Durand-Rivera, A., Galvan-Montaño, A., Perdigón-Castañeda, G., Climent-Palmer, M. C., Tena-Betancourt, E. 2012. Preliminary studies of neurosensory and cardiopulmonary health compromise in captive-bred Rhesus macaques (Macaca mulatta) suffering scoliosis. *Journal of Medical Primatology*. 41 (3):163-171. doi: 10.1111/j.1600-0684.2012.00539. x.

Hernández-Godínez, B., Ibáñez-Contreras, A., Durand-Rivera, A., Reyes-Pantoja, S. A., Ramírez-Hernández, R., Rodríguez-Guzmán, P., Tena-Betancourt, E. 2011. Somatosensory evoked potentials of median and tibial nerves in rhesus monkeys (Macaca mulatta) under captivity: influence of ontogenic status in neonatal, infant, young, adult, and senile stages. *Journal of Medical Primatology*. 40 (2):79-87. doi: 10.1111/j.1600-0684.2010.00458. x.

Herrera-Soto, J. A., Van der Have, K. L., Barry-Lane, P., Woo, A. 2006. Spinal deformity after combined thoracotomy and sternotomy for congenital heart disease. *Journal of Pediatric Orthopaedics*. 26: 211-215.

Hunt, K. J., Braun, J. T., Christensen, B. A. 2010. The effect of two clinically relevant fusionless scoliosis implant strategies on the health of the intervertebral disc: analysis in an immature goat model. *Spine (Phila Pa 1976)*. 35 (4): 371-377. DOI: 10.1097/BRS.0b013e3181b962a4.

Ibáñez-Contreras, A., Hernández-Arciga, U., Poblano, A., Arteaga-Silva, M., Hernández-Godínez, B., Mendoza-Cuevas, G. I., Toledo-Pérez, R., Alarcón-Aguilar, A., González-Puertos, V. Y., Konigsberg, M. 2017. Electrical activity of sensory pathways in female and male geriatric Rhesus monkeys (Macaca mulatta), and its relation to oxidative stress. *Experimental Gerontology*. 101:80-94. doi: 10.1016/j.exger.2017.11.003.

Ibáñez-Contreras, A., Poblano, A., Arteaga-Silva, M., Hernández-Godínez, B., Hernández-Arciga, U., Toledo, R., Königsberg, M. 2016. Visual, auditive and somatosensory pathways alterations in geriatric rhesus monkeys (Macaca mulatta). *Journal of Medical Primatology*. 45 (2): 92-102. doi: 10.1111/jmp.12211

James, J. I. 1970. The etiology of scoliosis. *Journal of Bone and Joint Surgery. British volume*. 52 (3): 410-419. PMID: 4724275.

Janssen, M. M., de Wilde, R. F., Kouwenhoven, J. W., Castelein, R. M. 2011. Experimental animal models in scoliosis research: a review of the literature. *Spine*. 11 (4): 347-358. DOI: 10.1016/j.spinee.2011.03.010.

Jinkins, J. R. 2001. Acquired degenerative changes of the intervertebral segments at and suprajacent to the lumbosacral junction. A radioanatomic analysis of the nondiskal structures of the spinal column and perispinal soft tissues. *Radiologic clinics of North America*. 39 (1): 73-99. PMID: 11221507.

Kallemeier, P. M., Buttermann, G. R., Beaubien, B. P., Chen, X., Polga, D. J., Lew, W. D., Wood, K. B. 2006. Validation, reliability, and complications of a tethering scoliosis model in the rabbit. *Europena Spine Journal*. 15 (4): 449-456. DOI: 10.1007/s00586-005-1032-1

Kanemura, T., Kawakami, N., Deguchi, M., Mimatsu, K., Iwata, H. 1997. Natural course of experimental scoliosis in pinealectomized chickens. *Spine*. 22 (14):1563–1567. PMID: 9253089.

Kawakami, N., Mimatsu, K., Deguchi, M., Kato, F., Maki, S. 1995. Scoliosis and congenital heart disease. *Spine (Phila Pa 1976)*. 20: 1252-1255. PMID: 7660233.

Kent, G. M., Zingg, W. 1974. Experimental scoliosis in fetal lambs. *Surgical Forum*. 25 (0):75-77. PMID: 4474719.

Kent, G. M., Zingg, W., Armstrong, D. 1978. Muscle changes in lambs with surgically created scoliosis produced in utero. *Canadian Journal of Neurological Science*. 5 (3): 283-287. PMID: 698893.

Kitamura, S., Ohara, S., Suwa, T., and Nakagawa, K. 1965. Studies on vitamin requirements of rainbow trout, Salmo Gairdneri-I. On the ascorbic acid, *Bull Jap Soc Fish*. 31: No. 10.

Kowalski, I. M., Szarek, J., Zarzycki, D., Rymarczyk, A. Experimental scoliosis in the course of unilateral surface electrostimulation of the paravertebral muscles in rabbits: effects according to stimulation period. *European Spine Journal*. 10 (6): 490-494. PMID: 11806388.

Laffosse, J. M., Accadbled, F., Odent, T., Cachon, T., Gomez-Brouchet, A., Ambard, D., Viquier, E., Sales de Gauzy, J., Swider, P. 2009. Influence of asymetric tether on the macroscopic permeability of vertebral plate. *European Spine Journal*. 18 (12): 1971-1977. DOI: 10.1007/s00586-009-1140-4.

Laffosse, J. M., Accadbled, F., Bonnevialle, N., Gomez-Brouchet, A., de Gauzy, J., Swider, P. 2010. Remodeling of vertebral endplate subchondral bone in scoliosis: a micro-CT analysis in a porcine model. *Clinical Biomechanics* (Bristol, Avon). 25 (7): 636-641. DOI: 10.1016/j.clinbiomech.2010.04.011.

Lambert, F. M., Malinvaud, D., Glaunès, J., Bergot, C., Straka, H., Vidal, P. P. 2009. Vestibular Asymmetry as the Cause of Idiopathic Scoliosis: A Possible Answer from Xenopus. *The Journal of Neuroscience*. 29 (40): 12477–12483. DOI: 10.1523/JNEUROSCI.2583-09.2009.

Lambert, F. M., Straka, H. 2012. The frog vestibular system as a model for lesion-induced plasticity: basic neural principles and implications for posture control. *Frontiers in Neurology*. 3; 3: 42. DOI: 10.3389/fneur.2012.00042.

Lambert, F. M., Malinvaud, D., Gratacap, M., Straka, H., Vidal, P. P. 2013. Restricted neural plasticity in vestibulospinal pathways after unilateral labyrinthectomy as the origin for scoliotic deformations. *Journal of Neuroscience*. 33 (16): 6845-6856. DOI: 10.1523/JNEUROSCI.4842-12.2013.

Langenskiold, A., Michelsson, J. E. 1959. Experimental scoliosis. *Acta Orthopaedica Scandinavica*. 29: 158-159. PMID: 14413930.

Langenskiold, A., Michelsson, J. E. 1961. Experimental progressive scoliosis in the rabbit. *Journal of Bone and Joint Surgery British volume*. 43-B: 116-120. PMID: 13831176.

Langenskiold, A., Michelsson, J. E. 1962. The pathogenesis of experimental progressive scoliosis. *Acta Orthopaedica Scandinavica. Supplementum*. 59: 1-26. PMID: 13928602.

Li, Z., Shen, J., Wu, W. K., Wang, X., Liang, J., Qiu, G., Liu, J. 2012. Vitamin A deficiency induces congenital spinal deformities in rats. *PLoS One*. 7 (10): e46565. DOI: 10.1371/journal.pone.0046565.

Liszka, O. Spinal cord mechanisms leading to scoliosis in animal. *Acta medica Polona*. 2: 45-63. PMID: 14465851.

Machida, M., Dubousset, J., Imamura, Y., Iwaya, T., Yamada, T., Kimura, J. 1993. An experimental study in chickens for the pathogenesis of idiopathic scoliosis. *Spine (Phila Pa 1976)*. 18 (12): 1609–1615. DOI: 10.3390/ijms150916484.

Machida, M., Dubousset, J., Imamura, Y., Iwaya, T., Yamada, T., Kimura, J. 1995. Role of melatonin deficiency in the development of scoliosis in pinealectomised chickens. *Journal of Bone and Joint Surgery. British volume*. 77 (1):134–138. PMID: 7822371.

Machida, M., Miyashita, Y., Murai, I., Dubousset, J., Yamada, T., Kimura, J. 1997. Role of serotonin for scoliotic deformity in pinealectomized chicken. *Spine* 22: 1297-1301. PMID: 9201831.

Machida, M., Murai, I., Miyashita, Y., Dubousset, J., Yamada, T., Kimura, J. 1999. Pathogenesis of idiopathic scoliosis. Experimental study in rats. *Spine (Phila Pa 1976).* 24 (19): 1985-1999. PMID: 10528372.

Machida, M., Saito, M., Dubousset, J., Yamada, T., Kimura, J., Shibasaki, K. 2005. Pathological mechanism of idiopathic scoliosis: Experimental scoliosis in pinealectomized rats. *European Spine Journal.* 14 (9): 843–848. DOI: 10.1007/s00586-004-0806-1.

Machida, M., Dubousset, J., Yamada, T., Kimura, J., Saito, M., Shiraishi, T., Yamagishi, M. 2006. Experimental scoliosis in melatonin-deficient C57BL/6J mice without pinealectomy. *Journal of Pineal Research.* 41 (1): 1–7. DOI: 10.1111/j.1600-079X.2005.00312. x.

Man, G. C., Wang, W. W., Yim, A. P., Wong, J. H., Ng, T. B., Lam, T. P., Lee, S. K., Ng, B. K., Wang, C. C., Qiu, Y., Cheng, C. Y. 2014. A review of pinealectomy-induced melatonin-deficient animal models for the study of etiopathogenesis of adolescent idiopathic scoliosis. *International Journal of Molecular Science.* 15(9): 16484-16499. DOI: 10.3390/ijms150916484.

McDonald, M. P., Miller, K. M., Li, C., Deng, C., Crawley, J. N. 2001. Motor deficits in fibroblast growth factor receptor-3 null mutant mice. *Behavioral Pharmacology.* 12 (6-7): 477-486. PMID: 11742142.

Mente, P. L., Stokes, I. A., Spence, H., Aronsson, D. D. 1997. Progression of vertebral wedging in an asymmetrically loaded rat tail model. *Spine (Phila Pa 1976).* 22 (12): 1292-1296. PMID: 9201830.

Murphy, M. L., Dagg, C. P., Karnofsky, D. A. 1957. Comparison of teratogenic chemicals in the rat and chick embryos; an exhibit with additions for publication. *Pediatrics.* 19 (4 pt 1): 701-714. PMID: 13419444.

Moal, B., Schwab, F., Demakakos, J., Lafage, R., Riviere, P., Patel, A., Lafage, V. 2013. The impact of a corrective tether on a scoliosis porcine model: a detailed 3D analysis with a 20 weeks follow-up. *European Spine Journal.* 22 (8): 1800-1899. DOI: 10.1007/s00586-013-2743-3.

Nette, F., Dolynchuk, K., Wang, X., Daniel, A., Demianczuk, C., Moteau, M., Raso, J., Mahood, J., Bagnall, K. 2002. The effects of exposure to intense, 24 h light on the development of scoliosis in young chickens. *Studies in health technology and informatics.* 91: 1-6. PMID: 15457683.

Newton, P. O., Faro, F. D., Farnsworth, C. L., Shapiro, G. S., Mohamad, F., Parent, S., Fricka, K. Multilevel spinal growth modulation with an anterolateral flexible tether in an immature bovine model. *Spine (Phila Pa 1976).* 30 (23): 2608-2613. PMID: 16319746.

Newton, P. O., Upasani, V. V., Farnsworth, C. L., Oka, R., Chambers, R. C., Dwek, J., Kim, J. R., Perry, A., Mahar, A. T. 2008. Spinal growth modulation with use of a tether in an immature porcine model. *Journal of Bone and Joint Surgery American volume.* 90 (12): 2695-2706. DOI: 10.2106/JBJS.G. 01424.

Newton, P. O., Farnsworth, C. L., Upasani, V. V., Chambers, R. C., Varley, E., Tsutsui, S. 2011. Effects of intraoperative tensioning of an anterolateral spinal tether on spinal growth modulation in a porcine model. *Spine (Phila Pa 1976).* 36 (2): 109-117. DOI: 10.1097/BRS. 0b013e3181cc8fce.

Nogami, H. and Ingalls, T. H. 1967. Pathogenesis of spinal malformations induced in the embryos of mice. *Journal of Bone Joint and Surgery.* 49A (8): 1551-1560. PMID: 4229794.

O'Kelly, C., Wang, X., Raso, J., Moreau, M., Mahood, J., Zhao, J., Bagnall, K. 1999. The production of scoliosis after pinealectomy in young chickens, rats, and hamsters. *Spine (Phila Pa 1976).* 24 (1): 35–43. PMID: 9921589.

Odent, T., Cachon, T., Peultier, B., Gournay, J., Jolivet, E., Elie, C., Abdoul, H., Viguier, E. 2011. Porcine model of early onset scoliosis based on animal growth created with posterior mini-invasive spinal offset tethering: a preliminary report. *Europena Spine Journal.* 20 (11): 1869-1876. DOI: 10.1007/s00586-011-1830-6.

Ouellet, J. Odent, T. 2013. Animal models for scoliosis research: state of the art, current concepts and futura perspective applications. *Europena Spine Journal.* 22 (Suppl 2): S81-S95. DOI: 10.1007/s00586-012-2396-7.

Oyama, J., Murai, I., Kanazawa, K., Machida, M. 2006. Bipedal ambulation induces experimental scoliosis in C57BL/6J mice with reduced plasma and pineal melatonin levels. *Journal of Pineal Research.* 40: 219-224. DOI: 10.1111/j.1600-079X.2005.00302.x.

Pal, G. P., Bhatt, R. H., Patel, V. S. 1991. Mechanism of production of experimental scoliosis in rabbits. *Spine (Phila Pa 1976).* 16 (2): 137-142. PMID: 2011768.

Parsonson, I. M., Della-Porta, A. J., Snowdon, W. A. 1977. Congenital abnormalities in newborn lambs after infection of pregnant sheep with Akabane virus. *Infection and immunity.* 15 (1): 254-262. PMID: 832900.

Patel, A., Schwab, F., Lafage,V., Patel, A., Obeidat, M. M., Farcy, J. P. 2010. Computed tomographic validation of the porcine model for thoracic scoliosis. *Spine (Phila Pa 1976).* 35 (1): 18-25. DOI: 10.1097/BRS. 0b013e3181b79169.

Patel, A., Schwab, F., Lafage, R., Lafage, V., Farey J. P. 2011. Does removing the spinal tether in a Porcine Scoliosis Model Result in Persistent Deformity? *Clinical Ortopedic Related Research.* 469: 1368-1374. DOI: 10.1007/s11999-010-1750-5.

Pincott, J. R., Taffs, L. F. 1982. Experimental scoliosis in primates: a neurological cause. *Journal of Bone and Joint Surgery. British volume.* 64: (4): 503-507. PMID: 6284765.

Pincott, J. R., Davies, J. S., Taff, L. F. 1984. Scoliosis caused by section of dorsal spinal nerve roots. *Journal of Bone and Joint Surgery. British volume.* 66 (1): 27-29. PMID: 6693473.

Ponseti, I. V. 1957. Skeletal lesions produced by aminonitriles. *Clinical Orthopedics.* 9: 131-144. PMID: 13447243.

Poon, A. M., Cheung, K. M, Lu, D. S., Leong, J. C. 2006. Changes in melatonin receptors in relation to the development of scoliosis in pinealectomized chickens. *Spine (Phila Pa 1976).* 31 (18): 2043-2047. DOI: 10.1097/01.brs.0000231796.49827.39.

Poussa, M., Schlenzka, D., Ritsilä, V. 1991. Scoliosis in growing rabbits induced with an extension splint. *Acta Orthopaedics Scandinavica.* 62 (2): 136-138. PMID: 2014723.

Robin, G. C. 1966. Experimental paralytic scoliosis. *Israel Journal of Medical Science.* 2 (2): 208-211. PMID: 5912554.

Robin, G. C., Stein, H. 1975. Experimental scoliosis in primates. Failure of a technique. *Journal of Bone and Joint Surgery British.* 57 (2):142-145. PMID: 806595.

Robin, G. C. 1996. Scoliosis induced by rib resection in Chickens. *Journal of spinal disorders.* 9 (4): 351. PMID: 8877966.

Rooney, G. E., Vaishya, S., Ameenuddin, S., Currier, B. L., Schiefer, T. K., Knight, A., Chen, B., Mishra, P. K., Spinner, R. J., Macura, S. I., Yaszemski, M. J., Windebank, A. J. 2008. Rigid fixation of the spinal column improves scaffold alignment and prevents scoliosis in the transected rat spinal cord. *Spine (Phila Pa 1976).* 33(24): E914-919. DOI: 10.1097/BRS.0b013e318186b2b1.

Sarwark, J. F., Dabney, K. W., Salzman, S. K, Wakabayashi, T., Kitada, H. K., Beauchamp, J. T., Beckman, A. L., Bunnell, W. P. 1988. Experimental scoliosis in the rat. I. Methodology, anatomic features and neurologic characterization. *Spine (Phila Pa 1976)*. 13 (5): 466-471. PMID: 3055339.

Schwab, F., Patel, A., Lafage, V., Farcy, J. P. 2009. A porcine model for progressive thoracic scoliosis. *Spine (Phila Pa 1976)*. 34 (11): E397-404. DOI: 10.1097/BRS.0b013e3181a27156.

Schwartzman, J. R., and Miles, M. 1945. Experimental production of scoliosis in rats and mice. *Journal of bone and joint surgery*. 27: 59.

Sevastik, J. A., Aaro, S., Normelli, H. Scoliosis. 1984. Experimental and clinical studies. *Clinical orthopaedics and related research*. 191: 27-34. PMID: 6499319.

Sevastik, J., Agadir, M., Sevastik, B. 1990. Effects of rib elongation on the spine. I. Distortion of the vertebral aligment in the rabbit. *Spine (Phila Pa 1976)*. 15 (8): 822-825. PMID: 2237633.

Sevastik, J., Agadir, M., Sevastik, B. 1990. Effects of rib elongation on the spine. II. Correction of scoliosis in the rabbit. *Spine (Phila Pa 1976)*. 15 (8): 826-829. PMID: 2237634.

Sevastik, B., Willers, U., Hedlund, R., Sevastik J., Kristjansson, S. 1993. Scoliosis induced immediately after mechanical medial rib elongation in the rabbit. *Spine (Phila Pa 1976)*. 18 (7): 923-926. PMID: 8316895.

Sevastikoglou, J. A., Aaro, S., Lindholm, T. S., Dahlborn, M. 1978. *Clinical Orthopaedics and Related Research*. 136: 282-286. PMID: 729296.

Shangguan, L., Fan, X., Luo, Z. 2009. The association between melatonin signaling dysfunction and idiopathic scoliosis. *Medical Hypotheses*. 72 (2): 228-229. DOI: 10.1016/j.mehy.2008.09.002.

Shono, Y., Kaneda, K., Yamamoto, I. 1991. A biomechanical analysis of Zielke, Kaneda and Cotrel- Dubousset instrumentations in thoracolumbar scoliosis. A calf spine model. *Spine (Phila Pa 1976)*. 16 (11): 1305-1311. PMID: 1750005.

Silva, C. A., Guirro R. R. J., Delfino, G. B., Arruda, E. J. Proposal of non-invasive experimental model to induce scoliosis in rats. *Revista Brasileira de Fisioterapia*, Sao Carlos. 16 (3): 254-260. ISSN: 1413-3555.

Singh, J., Aggison, L. Jr., Moore-Cheatum, L. 1993. Teratogenicity and developmental toxicity of carbon monoxide in protein-deficient mice. *Teratology*. 48 (2): 149-159. DOI: 10.1002/tera.1420480209.

Smith, R. M., Dickson, R. A. 1987. Experimental structural scoliosis. *Journal of Bone and Joint Surgery. British volume*. 69 (4): 576-581. PMID: 3611161.

Somerville, E. W. 1952. Rotational lordosis; the development of single curve. *Journal of Bone and joint Surgery British* Volume. 34-B (3): 421-727. PMID: 12999923.

Stilwell D. L. Jr., 1962. Structural deformities of vertebrae. Bone adaptation and modeling in experimental scoliosis and kyphosis. *Journal of Bone Joint and Surgery American* volume. 44-A: 611-634. PMID: 14037781.

Stokes, I. A., Aronsson, D. D., Clark, K. C., Roemhildt, M. L. 2006. Intervertebral disc adaptation to wedging deformation. *Studies in health technology Informatics*. 123: 182-187. PMID: 17108424.

Stokes, I. A., McBride, C., Aronsson, D. D. 2008. Intervertebral disc change in an animal model representing altered mechanics in scoliosis. *Studies in health technology Informatics*. 140: 273-277. PMID: 18810036.

Stokes, I. A., McBride, C., Aronsson, D. D., Roughley, P. J. 2011. Intervertebral disc changes with angulation, compression and reduced mobility simulating altered mechanical environment in scoliosis. *European Spine Journal.* 20 (10):1735-1744. DOI: 10.1007/s00586-011-1868-5.

Suk, S. I., Song, H. S., Lee, C. K. 1989. Scoliosis induced by anterior and posterior rhizotomy. *Spine (Phila Pa 1976).* 14 (7): 692-697. PMID: 2772717.

Thillard, M. J. 1959. Vertebral column deformities following epiphysectomy in the chick. *Comptes rendus hebdomadaires des seances de l'Academie des sciences.* 248 (8): 1238-1240. PMID: 13629950.

Thomas, B. H., and Cheng, D. W. 1952. Congenital abnormalities associated with vitamin E malnutrition. *Proc. Iowa.Sci.* 59: 218.

Thomas, S., Dave, P.K. 1985. Experimental scoliosis in monkeys. *Acta Orthopaedica Scandinavica.* 56 (1): 43–46. PMID: 3920863.

Thometz, J. G., Liu, X. C., Lyon, R. 2000. Three-dimensional rotations of the thoracic spine after distraction with and without rib resection: a kinematic evaluation of the apical vertebra in rabbits with induced scoliosis. *Journal of Spinal Disorders.* 13 (2): 108: 112. PMID: 10780684.

Turgut, M., Yenisey, C., Uysal, A., Bozkurt, M., Yurtseven, M. E. 2003. The effects of pineal gland transplantation on the production of spinal deformity and serum melatonin level following pinealectomy in the chicken. *Europena Spine Journal.* 12 (5); 487-494. DOI: 10.1007/s00586-003-0528-9.

Turgut, M., Basaloglu, H. K., Yenisey, C., Ozsunar, Y. 2006. Surgical pinealectomy accelerates intervertebral disc degeneration process in chicken. *European Spine Journal.* 15 (5): 605–612. DOI: 10.1007/s00586-005-0972-9.

Von Lesser, L. Experimentelles und klinisches über skoliose, [Experimental and clinical about scoliosis.] *Virchow Arch Path Anat.* 113; 10.

Wang, X., Jiang, H., Raso, J., Moreau, M., Madhoo, J., Zhao, J., Bagnall, K. 1997. Characterization of the scoliosis that develops after pinealectomy in the chicken and comparison with adolescent idiopathic scoliosis in humans. *Spine (Phila Pa 1976).* 22 (22): 2626-2635. PMID: 9399448.

Werneck, L. C., Cousseau, V. A., Graells, X. S., Werneck, M. C., Scola, R. H. 2008. Muscle study in experimental scoliosis in rabbits with costotransversectomy: evidence of ischemic process. *European Spine Journal.* 17 (5): 726-733. DOI: 10.1007/s00586-008-0598-9.

Willers, U. W., Sevastik, B., Hedlund, R., Sevastik, J. A., Kristjansson, S. 1995. Electrical muscle stimulation on the spine: Three-dimensional effects in rabbits. *Acta Ortopaedics Scandinavica.* 66 (5): 411-414. PMID: 7484119.

Woods, L. W., Anderson, M. L. 1992. Scoliosis and hydrocephalus in an ovine fetus infected with Toxoplasma gondii. *Journal of Veterinary Diagnostic Investigation.* 4(2): 220- 222. DOI: 10.1177/104063879200400227.

Zhang, H., and Sucato, D. J. 2008. Unilateral pedicle screw epiphysiodesis of the neurocentral synchondrosis. Production of idiopathic – like scoliosis in an immature animal model. *Journal of Bone and Joint Surgery. American volume.* 90 (11): 2460-2469. DOI: 10.2106/JBJS.G.01493.

Zhang, H., and Sucato, D. J. 2011. Neurocentral synchondrosis screws to create and correct experimental deformity: a pilot study. *Clinical orthopaedics and related research.* 469 (5): 1383-1390. DOI: 10.1007/s 11999-010-1587-y.

Zhang, Y. G., Zheng, G. Q., Zhang, X.S., Wang, Y. 2009. Scoliosis model created by pedicle screw tethering in immature goats. The Feasibility, Reliability, and Complications. *Spine*. 34 (21): 2305-2310. DOI: 10.1097/BRS.0b013e3181bfdd0.

Zhang, H. Y., Li, Q. Y., Wu, Z. H., Zhao, Y., Qiu, G. X. 2017. Lumbar scoliosis induction in juvenile dogs by three-dimensional modulation of spinal growth using nickel-titanium coil springs. *Chinese Medical Journal (Engl)*. 130 (21): 2579-2584. DOI: 10.4103/0366-6999.213910.

EDITORS CONTACT INFORMATION

Dr. Federico Canavese, MD, PhD, Prof
Head, Pediatric Spine and Orthopedic Surgery,
University Hospital of Clermont Ferrand,
Clermont Ferrand, France
Professor of Pediatric Orthopedic Surgery,
University of Auvergne, Faculty of Medicine,
Clermont Ferrand, France
Email: canavese_federico@yahoo.fr

Antonio Andreacchio, MD
Head, Pediatric Orthopaedic Department
"Regina Margherita" Children's Hospital
Torino, Italy
Email: a.andreacchio@libero.it

HongWen Xu, MD
Head, Department of Pediatric Orthopedic Surgery GuangZhou
Women and Children Medical Center
GuangZhou, China
Email: gzorthopedics@qq.com

LIST OF CONTRIBUTORS

Alaaeldin A. Ahmad
Ramallah, Palestine

Loai J. Aker
Nablus, Palestine

Erdem Aktas
Ankara, Turkey

Nicolas Amirghasemi
Geneva, Switzerland

Alexandre Ansorgue
Geneva, Switzerland

Alice Bonnefoy-Mazure
Geneva, Switzerland

François Bonnel
Montpellier, France

Janine Cardoso
Mexico City, Mexico

Mehmet Çetinkaya
Erzincan, Turkey

Suzanne Clements Martins
Almeda (CA), USA

Mattia Cravino
Torino, Italy

Ismail Daldal
Sakarya, Turkey

Romain Dayer
Geneva, Switzerland

Charlotte de Bodman
Geneva, Switzerland

Jacques Deslandes
Moulins, France

Alain Dimeglio
Montpellier, France

Jörg Drumm
Karlsbad, Germany

David Ducoing-Gonzalez
Mexico City, Mexico

Ron El-Hawary
Halifax (NS), Canada

Ali Eren
Gümüşhan, Turkey

Ismat Ghanem
Beirut, Lebanon

Marie Granier
Clermont Ferrand, France

List of Contributors

Yahia B. Hanbali
Nablus, Palestine

Braulio Hernandéz-Godínez
Mexico City, Mexico

Alejandra Ibáñez-Contreras
Mexico City, Mexico

Ashok Johari
Mumbai, India

Jun Jiang
Nanjing, China

Qiang Jie
Xi'an, China

André Kaelin
Geneva, Switzerland

Mohsen Karami
Teheran, Iran

Michèle Kläusler
Basel, Switzerland

Qingda Lu
Xi'an, China

Lorenza Marengo
Torino, Italy

Kedar Padhye
Halifax (NS), Canada

Vito Pavone
Catania, Italy

Xiaodong Qin
Nanjing, China

Maroun Rizkallah
Beirut, Lebanon

Michael Ruf
Karlsbad, Germany

Erich Rutz
Basel, Switzerland

Alpaslan Senkoylu
Ankara, Turkey

XingRong Song
Guangzhou, China

Fei Su
Xi'an, China

Anne Tabard-Fougère
Geneva, Switzerland

Gianluca Testa
Catania, Italy

Xiaowei Wang
Xi'an, China

Shujie Wang
Beijing, China

Zhaomin Zheng
Guangzhou, China

Zezhang Zhu
Nanjing, China

Qianyu Zhuang
Beijing, China

INDEX

A

a two-dimensional, 211, 366
accuracy, 20, 24, 26, 109, 201, 206, 298, 348, 368, 370, 372, 373
adding-on, vi, 204, 211, 212, 261, 262, 268, 269, 274, 275, 276, 283, 286, 287, 288, 289, 290, 291, 292
adding-on phenomenon, 261, 262, 275, 276, 292
adolescence, 26, 46, 110, 133, 135, 136, 153, 171, 194, 246, 364, 385
adolescent idiopathic scoliosis, 2, 4, 15, 24, 25, 32, 35, 36, 43, 47, 59, 60, 61, 85, 89, 104, 106, 132, 133, 134, 155, 156, 157, 162, 169, 170, 171, 172, 173, 175, 176, 191, 192, 193, 196, 199, 213, 214, 215, 217, 226, 227, 228, 231, 232, 240, 241, 243, 244, 253, 254, 255, 256, 257, 258, 259, 261, 262, 273, 274, 275, 276, 277, 291, 292, 304, 305, 320, 323, 335, 336, 342, 355, 362, 363, 364, 365, 371, 372, 373, 374, 375, 402, 403, 405, 408, 411
adult, 2, 3, 11, 14, 28, 36, 46, 70, 114, 136, 137, 170, 214, 245, 254, 255, 256, 257, 310, 320, 322, 328, 347, 357, 359, 363, 372, 387, 390, 404, 406
age, ix, 2, 3, 4, 5, 6, 7, 11, 13, 14, 15, 17, 19, 20, 21, 22, 23, 27, 28, 31, 32, 33, 36, 46, 47, 48, 49, 53, 54, 55, 57, 58, 62, 64, 70, 72, 75, 77, 79, 80, 85, 87, 94, 99, 101, 103, 104, 106, 108, 109, 114, 115, 117, 129, 136, 137, 149, 155, 159, 162, 169, 175, 176, 177, 178, 183, 186, 188, 192, 194, 201, 218, 231, 232, 248, 255, 257, 264, 268, 269, 317, 319, 320, 321, 322, 323, 325, 332, 334, 338, 363, 366, 370, 395
air-warming blankets, 380
alert, 143, 236, 308, 309, 312, 313, 314
allograft bone, 234, 305
alveolar hypoplasia, 6
alveoli, 6, 48, 175

anesthesia, vii, 49, 53, 56, 57, 60, 62, 63, 80, 91, 95, 178, 183, 189, 232, 309, 310, 377, 378, 380, 403
anesthetic approach, 377
angle, 9, 28, 31, 56, 59, 60, 75, 77, 83, 94, 98, 122, 124, 127, 129, 168, 200, 202, 203, 204, 207, 209, 214, 218, 234, 245, 246, 248, 249, 257, 262, 265, 268, 273, 278, 279, 287, 322, 325, 332, 334, 342, 356, 357, 358, 362, 367, 368, 369, 370, 371, 378
anterior, vi, 7, 12, 18, 29, 51, 65, 67, 73, 74, 77, 78, 80, 83, 85, 122, 138, 159, 160, 166, 175, 178, 180, 183, 184, 186, 189, 192, 195, 196, 206, 209, 214, 215, 217, 218, 219, 220, 221, 222, 224, 226, 227, 228, 229, 245, 246, 247, 248, 251, 255, 259, 273, 274, 278, 296, 309, 311, 325, 340, 341, 346, 354, 355, 365, 366, 368, 373, 378, 388, 392, 399, 402, 411
anterior approach, 217, 221, 227, 341
anterior correction, 218, 220, 221, 222, 224, 227, 274, 373
anterior release, 65, 221, 226, 341
anterior technique, 218
anterior vertebral body tethering, 85, 175, 196
anteverted, 246, 247
antibiotic, 76, 293, 299, 300, 304, 344
anticipation, 48, 101, 106, 107, 108
apical level, 37, 184
appearance, 21, 22, 53, 65, 102, 159, 201, 203, 210, 239, 262, 270, 271, 359, 385, 386
approach, 13, 20, 26, 33, 42, 84, 91, 114, 115, 116, 118, 119, 127, 130, 133, 135, 137, 138, 183, 189, 206, 214, 215, 219, 221, 228, 229, 231, 232, 233, 236, 237, 239, 240, 241, 251, 300, 308, 315, 316, 317, 331, 341, 343, 348, 350, 367, 372, 377, 381, 382
arm span, 4, 16, 104
Arnold Chiari malformation, 50, 71
arterial catheter, 380

arthrodesis, ix, 7, 8, 9, 11, 43, 46, 48, 58, 110, 150, 192, 193, 227, 254, 258, 276, 292, 294, 295, 296, 351
assessment, v, vii, 3, 5, 13, 16, 19, 20, 22, 23, 24, 25, 26, 36, 43, 58, 103, 105, 106, 107, 108, 110, 114, 117, 118, 123, 124, 125, 127, 144, 167, 172, 178, 191, 193, 201, 211, 212, 214, 228, 254, 256, 257, 274, 275, 291, 297, 305, 307, 310, 319, 323, 336, 353, 355, 362, 363, 366, 368, 370, 373, 374, 375, 378
asymmetry, 29, 123, 131, 132, 135, 136, 137, 141, 142, 144, 145, 150, 151, 156, 264, 323, 345, 359, 373, 386, 391, 407
axial, 50, 89, 118, 142, 186, 191, 243, 244, 247, 261, 262, 366, 372, 384, 385, 386, 388, 389, 390, 397, 399, 401

B

balance, 29, 31, 81, 94, 121, 122, 123, 124, 131, 139, 141, 143, 144, 146, 168, 201, 203, 205, 207, 228, 243, 244, 246, 248, 249, 250, 252, 253, 254, 255, 257, 258, 259, 261, 262, 266, 270, 273, 274, 278, 283, 284, 285, 322, 323, 324, 333, 335, 338, 340, 341, 355, 356, 357, 359, 362, 363, 368, 369, 372, 377
balanced, 107, 122, 187, 203, 219, 225, 243, 244, 261, 262, 267, 270, 271, 273, 278, 310, 323
balanced posture, 243, 244
band, 50, 51, 121, 147
bending films, 205, 219, 232, 355
biomechanical forces, 385, 386
biometric, 101, 102, 103, 106, 108
bipedalism, 121, 386, 405
bleeding, 293, 339, 342, 343
blood loss, 64, 65, 206, 231, 232, 239, 307, 312, 351, 381, 382
blood saving strategies, 381
blood test, 379
body habitus, 9, 46, 70, 156
body mass index (BMI), 15, 25, 232, 255, 368, 371, 379
body weight, 15, 62, 144, 379
bone age, 5, 13, 14, 17, 19, 20, 22, 23, 25, 101, 102, 103, 104, 105, 106, 107
bone graft, 234, 235, 299, 339, 342
Boston, 158, 160, 161, 162, 166, 169, 170, 171
brace, 1, 14, 15, 18, 19, 22, 29, 56, 59, 60, 98, 111, 119, 120, 126, 127, 128, 129, 131, 133, 134, 144, 146, 156, 157, 158, 159, 160, 161, 162, 163, 164, 165, 166, 167, 168, 169, 170, 171, 172, 173, 191, 192, 197, 199, 200, 213, 214, 291, 319, 323, 325, 326, 327, 370, 373

brace weaning, 19, 133, 158
bracing, 9, 14, 15, 17, 24, 54, 56, 60, 80, 114, 115, 116, 119, 123, 124, 125, 126, 127, 128, 129, 131, 133, 155, 156, 157, 158, 159, 160, 161, 163, 164, 168, 169, 170, 171, 172, 176, 191, 195, 213, 240, 319, 323, 324, 325, 327, 329, 331, 335, 343, 346, 350, 373
breathing, 6, 9, 46, 48, 49, 119, 135, 138, 141, 145, 147, 161, 324, 325, 329, 338, 347, 368, 378, 379, 398
bronchial tree, 6, 7, 70

C

calcaneal apophysis maturation classification, 23
calcaneal radiograph, 14, 23
cantilever procedure, 222
cardiac dysfunctions, 46, 70
cardiomyopathy, 379
cardio-respiratory, 114, 336, 343, 378
cartilage, 2, 18, 48, 104, 107, 138, 177, 186, 341, 355
casting, v, 9, 45, 46, 47, 48, 49, 51, 53, 54, 55, 56, 57, 58, 59, 60, 61, 66, 82, 116
cell saver, 381
central sacral vertical line, 37, 41, 203, 207, 267
cerebral palsy, 4, 10, 31, 34, 36, 120, 319, 320, 321, 322, 324, 328, 329, 330, 331, 332, 333, 335, 338, 389
cervical sagittal alignment, 247, 249, 256, 257
cervicothoracic junction, 249
cervico-thoraco-lumbo-sacral orthosis (CTLSO), 159
Charleston, 161, 162, 170, 172
Chêneau, 161, 171
chest kinematics, 49
chest radiograph, 379, 399
children, vii, ix, 2, 3, 4, 5, 7, 9, 10, 11, 12, 16, 19, 26, 27, 31, 32, 34, 46, 48, 49, 53, 54, 55, 56, 57, 62, 66, 67, 69, 70, 71, 75, 76, 78, 79, 80, 81, 82, 83, 84, 85, 87, 89, 92, 94, 97, 99, 102, 103, 104, 109, 110, 115, 120, 131, 140, 156, 175, 177, 178, 181, 182, 193, 194, 195, 196, 218, 239, 241, 252, 259, 293, 294, 295, 304, 305, 319, 320, 321, 322, 324, 325, 328, 329, 333, 334, 335, 338, 342, 343, 344, 345, 346, 347, 348, 349, 350, 352, 371, 377, 381, 382, 384, 413
chronic obstructive pulmonary diseases, 46
chronological age, 5, 13, 18, 19, 23, 102, 104
circumference, 1, 6, 14, 48
classification, v, 13, 14, 21, 22, 25, 26, 27, 28, 29, 31, 33, 35, 36, 37, 39, 42, 43, 76, 82, 100, 110, 114, 133, 150, 172, 177, 194, 201, 204, 218, 227,

246, 254, 256, 268, 269, 276, 280, 287, 289, 292, 295, 319, 320, 344, 361

classification system, 28, 29, 35, 36, 37, 39, 42, 43, 82, 268

clavicle-rib cage intersection difference, 262, 263

clavicular angle, 262, 263

clavicular tilt angle difference, 262, 263

cobalt chrome, 236

Cobb angle, 40, 41, 56, 65, 72, 75, 77, 94, 97, 106, 114, 121, 123, 125, 126, 127, 129, 136, 137, 138, 139, 157, 167, 182, 183, 188, 190, 200, 201, 202, 203, 204, 209, 218, 232, 267, 268, 269, 319, 320, 322, 325, 326, 327, 332, 334, 341, 356, 357, 360, 362, 363, 368, 369, 371, 374, 378

coccyx, 147, 247, 249, 343

comfortable seating, 340

co-morbidities, 53, 70, 71, 335, 336

compensatory curves, 218, 219, 402

compliance, 28, 94, 125, 127, 128, 144, 156, 158, 159, 161, 162, 167, 169, 176, 192, 379

complication(s), vi, 14, 29, 46, 47, 54, 56, 59, 61, 65, 66, 67, 69, 70, 71, 72, 73, 75, 76, 77, 79, 80, 81, 82, 83, 84, 85, 87, 89, 92, 93, 94, 95, 96, 97, 98, 99, 100, 129, 130, 132, 150, 159, 175, 176, 183, 187, 217, 220, 231, 239, 240, 255, 283, 287, 294, 295, 296, 305, 308, 317, 324, 328, 331, 332, 336, 338, 341, 342, 343, 347, 349, 377, 378, 379, 406, 412

compression, 6, 28, 50, 54, 88, 93, 122, 128, 129, 142, 182, 210, 218, 219, 273, 283, 380, 384, 387, 398, 401, 411

computed axial tomography, 384

computed tomography, 8, 58, 193, 353, 362

congenital, vii, 1, 9, 10, 12, 27, 28, 29, 33, 34, 36, 48, 49, 56, 57, 60, 65, 67, 71, 75, 77, 79, 83, 87, 115, 178, 181, 183, 194, 195, 294, 295, 355, 362, 370, 383, 384, 385, 396, 397, 398, 400, 404, 405, 406, 407, 409, 411

congenital bars, 48

congenital scoliosis, 1, 9, 10, 12, 33, 34, 56, 60, 65, 67, 77, 79, 83, 178, 181, 194, 295, 370, 384, 397, 404

conservative, vi, 45, 46, 47, 56, 59, 70, 115, 116, 123, 131, 132, 135, 137, 138, 150, 155, 156, 163, 169, 170, 171, 191, 201, 240, 300, 319, 323, 324, 325, 328, 329, 331, 344, 385

contouring, 80, 87, 250

convex compression, 222

Cor Pulmonale, 2, 10, 47, 193, 329

coracoid height difference, 262, 263, 278, 279

coronal, 37, 39, 40, 42, 43, 64, 75, 79, 82, 89, 92, 94, 97, 119, 131, 178, 188, 189, 201, 203, 204, 205, 206, 207, 208, 211, 213, 217, 220, 226, 243, 244, 247, 250, 252, 261, 262, 265, 269, 273, 355, 356, 357, 361, 363, 364, 372

coronal and the sagittal plane, 39

correction maneuver, 218, 221

corrective forces, 54, 156, 159, 312, 340

crankshaft, 7, 12, 48, 49, 95, 107, 194, 341, 343, 350

C-reactive protein (CRP), 297

CT scan, 6, 11, 203, 234, 353

curve pattern, 35, 37, 39, 41, 42, 59, 138, 155, 160, 206, 213, 269, 274, 276, 292, 334, 338, 339

curve progression, 13, 14, 16, 17, 19, 22, 23, 31, 53, 54, 56, 57, 70, 101, 102, 104, 106, 107, 133, 156, 157, 158, 161, 162, 163, 170, 177, 178, 200, 201, 214, 302, 304, 306, 324, 334, 335, 360, 361, 364, 365, 366, 369, 370, 371, 403

curve type, 37, 38, 39, 40, 41, 138, 204, 218, 334

D

debridement, 65, 95, 293, 294, 300, 301, 302, 303, 304

deep infection(s), vi, 76, 293, 294, 298, 300, 302, 305, 306, 342

deep venous thrombosis, 240

definitive treatment, 53, 261, 262

deformity correction, 61, 64, 72, 186, 187, 200, 231, 236, 243, 244, 247, 249, 251, 252, 257, 307, 308, 312, 316

delayed deep surgical site infections, 240

delaying tactic, 53, 56, 58

density, 15, 67, 118, 136, 250, 251, 258, 259, 298, 355, 399, 404

derotation, 45, 47, 49, 50, 57, 58, 60, 71, 165, 200, 204, 205, 213, 215, 217, 218, 220, 226, 236, 238, 259, 273

descending neurogenic-evoked potentials, 308, 309

development, 1, 3, 5, 6, 7, 9, 10, 14, 15, 18, 19, 26, 28, 29, 33, 46, 47, 48, 82, 102, 109, 115, 116, 120, 121, 136, 137, 140, 141, 149, 161, 162, 176, 177, 178, 191, 193, 217, 221, 269, 270, 283, 286, 288, 293, 311, 317, 320, 332, 333, 371, 383, 384, 386, 387, 388, 389, 398, 402, 403, 404, 405, 407, 408, 409, 410

disadvantages, 159

disc disease, 114, 221

discomfort, 65, 116, 128, 159, 296, 335

dislocated hip, 321, 333

distal radius and ulna (DRU), 21, 22, 25, 26

distortion, 2, 46, 47, 49, 116, 176, 398, 410

dizziness, 65

domino effect, 2, 47, 176

double shelled braces, 325

DRU classification, 21, 22

duration, 15, 56, 65, 66, 75, 79, 97, 115, 130, 297, 300, 308, 309, 396
dyspnea, 46, 70, 378

E

early onset, 1, 2, 4, 5, 7, 9, 10, 27, 28, 31, 32, 33, 34, 45, 46, 47, 48, 49, 53, 55, 56, 58, 69, 71, 82, 83, 84, 85, 95, 98, 115, 361, 405, 409
early onset scoliosis (EOS), v, 1, 2, 4, 5, 9, 10, 27, 28, 31, 32, 33, 34, 45, 47, 49, 53, 54, 55, 56, 58, 59, 69, 70, 71, 75, 76, 79, 80, 81, 82, 83, 84, 85, 87, 88, 89, 91, 92, 93, 94, 95, 96, 97, 98, 115, 165, 361, 366, 370, 372, 409
early-onset spinal deformities, 27
echocardiography, 379
elbow ossification center, 13, 22
elbow radiograph, 22, 23, 106, 108
electrocardiogram, 379
elevation, 14, 142, 204, 263, 265, 266, 277, 283
elliptical, 6, 7
elongation, v, 45, 47, 49, 50, 57, 58, 60, 71, 118, 119, 122, 123, 138, 187, 188, 190, 394, 410
elongation derotation flexion, v, 45
end vertebra (EV), 38, 51, 52, 184, 189, 206, 219, 221, 268, 269, 270, 356, 357
endo-thoracic hump, 6
epidural infusion, 381
erythrocyte sedimentation rate (ESR), 297
etiology, 9, 15, 28, 36, 80, 81, 116, 295, 304, 331, 332, 378, 383, 384, 385, 406
evoked potentials, 318, 342, 382, 384, 395, 400
exercise, vi, 115, 116, 117, 118, 119, 120, 127, 132, 133, 135, 136, 137, 138, 139, 140, 141, 142, 143, 144, 145, 146, 147, 149, 151, 156, 163, 170, 378
expiratory congenital hypotonia, 48
exudation, 293, 297, 301

F

facet joints, 233, 235, 384, 392
fever, 293, 297, 298, 299
filum terminale, 50, 71
flexibility, 35, 37, 42, 94, 114, 115, 121, 129, 136, 149, 156, 161, 167, 182, 183, 203, 205, 206, 219, 232, 240, 246, 264, 267, 269, 270, 277, 278, 281, 282, 336, 339, 355, 362, 375
flexible, 37, 80, 99, 114, 125, 161, 162, 163, 172, 178, 186, 188, 196, 205, 218, 239, 240, 271, 281, 282, 283, 287, 394, 403, 408
flexion, 45, 47, 49, 50, 57, 58, 60, 121, 143, 145, 191, 247, 258, 321

fluoroscopy, 89, 178, 184, 189, 233, 234, 395
formation, 29, 30, 36, 296, 300, 302
fourth dimension, 5
frame, 49, 50, 51, 147
Fulcrum bending, 355
fused ribs, 10, 12, 48, 79, 83, 194
fusion levels, 35, 42, 43, 204, 206, 211, 268, 270, 276, 292, 339
fusionless, vi, 70, 85, 88, 89, 91, 93, 100, 175, 176, 178, 187, 191, 192, 195, 196, 197, 402, 403, 405, 406

G

gastroesophageal reflux disease, 338
gastro-intestinal assessment, 338
gastrostomy, 338, 379
Gelpi retractor, 234
genetic models, 386
gentle, 51, 53, 103
global sagittal balance, 244, 249
gold standard, 54, 65, 84, 353, 365, 366
gram-negative, 296, 300
Greulich and Pyle (GP), 19, 20, 105, 214, 256, 257, 360
gross motor function level, 332
growth modulation, 71, 80, 99, 182, 191, 196, 393, 401, 404, 408
growth parameters, 1, 9, 10, 13, 176
growth rods, 71, 72, 73, 75, 81, 82, 83, 84, 85
growth sparing, 46, 53, 55, 56, 69
growth spurt, 10, 11, 12, 16, 18, 21, 25, 101, 102, 103, 105, 106, 107, 108, 136, 177, 186, 194, 217, 366
guidelines, 35, 38, 124, 132, 137, 150, 214, 292, 335, 343, 363, 369, 382

H

halo traction, 61, 62, 67
halo-femoral, 61, 63, 65, 66, 67, 341
halo-gravity, 61, 62, 64, 65, 66, 67, 214, 341
halo-pelvis, 61, 63, 64
hand and wrist radiograph, 13, 19
heart failure, 324, 378
height, 2, 3, 4, 5, 7, 13, 14, 15, 16, 23, 24, 26, 46, 47, 49, 55, 65, 70, 72, 78, 79, 94, 102, 103, 104, 109, 110, 111, 129, 158, 160, 162, 176, 177, 183, 194, 214, 262, 263, 277, 278, 280, 283
hemiplegia, 320, 334
hemivertebra, 29, 48
hereditary, 252

hypercapnia, 379
hyperextension, 355, 380
hyperreflexia, 65
hypoventilation, 324, 338, 379

I

idiopathic scoliosis, 10, 12, 13, 15, 19, 24, 25, 27, 32, 33, 34, 36, 43, 58, 59, 60, 73, 85, 101, 103, 105, 106, 107, 114, 115, 116, 131, 132, 133, 134, 137, 155, 163, 169, 170, 171, 172, 173, 175, 178, 182, 188, 191, 192, 194, 195, 196, 197, 199, 214, 215, 216, 217, 227, 228, 240, 241, 255, 256, 257, 273, 274, 275, 276, 292, 294, 295, 296, 305, 323, 332, 342, 343, 360, 362, 363, 364, 371, 372, 373, 374, 378, 381, 383, 384, 385, 387, 395, 399, 401, 404, 405, 407, 408, 410
imbalance, vi, 123, 164, 169, 201, 203, 211, 221, 246, 247, 256, 262, 267, 277, 278, 283, 319, 320, 323, 332, 336, 338, 340, 356, 367, 390
imbalanced position, 334
implants, v, 72, 79, 80, 83, 84, 87, 88, 89, 96, 97, 99, 100, 178, 191, 236, 237, 294, 302, 304, 308
implants removal, 237
incidence, vii, 66, 71, 72, 81, 85, 129, 131, 170, 176, 187, 204, 205, 211, 215, 246, 247, 258, 261, 264, 266, 267, 268, 269, 273, 274, 289, 290, 293, 297, 307, 308, 319, 320, 321, 322, 328, 331, 332, 333, 342, 343, 344, 345, 346, 348, 358, 359, 363, 372, 378, 383,384, 388
incisions, 91, 189, 210, 231, 232, 233, 234, 235, 236, 237, 299
indication(s), v, vi, 24, 61, 69, 70, 81, 82, 115, 124, 125, 128, 132, 144, 155, 156, 158, 164, 175, 176, 178, 183, 188, 199, 200, 217, 218, 231, 232, 259, 266, 274, 298, 319, 324, 325, 336, 361
infantile, 1, 12, 28, 32, 34, 36, 45, 46, 51, 53, 54, 55, 56, 57, 58, 59, 69, 155, 193, 329, 385
infantile deformity, 69
infantile scoliosis, 28, 45, 55, 58, 59
infection(s), 54, 58, 65, 75, 76, 78, 79, 80, 81, 82, 91, 95, 97, 98, 130, 187, 239, 240, 241, 293, 294, 295, 296, 297, 298, 299, 300, 302, 304, 305, 306, 324, 331, 334, 339, 342, 343, 344, 378, 409
injury, 31, 34, 65, 67, 95, 99, 139, 186, 241, 308, 310, 329, 378, 389
instrumented fusion, 46, 74, 79, 200, 211, 217, 218, 222, 226, 340, 378
intraoperative intervention strategy, 307
intraoperative irrigation, 299
intraoperative management, 380
intraoperative neuromonitoring (IONM), 178, 183, 236, 307, 308, 310, 311, 312, 313, 314, 315, 316

intrathecal baclofen, 321, 328, 329, 333
ischemia, 308, 309, 312

J

Jarcho-Levin, 48, 79
Jeune, 48, 79
juvenile, vi, 12, 28, 32, 36, 45, 46, 48, 51, 53, 54, 56, 57, 58, 59, 60, 108, 175, 176, 188, 192, 196, 361, 385, 412
juvenile scoliosis, 28, 45, 46, 48, 57, 60

K

king classification, 35, 37, 38, 39, 42
kyphoscoliosis, 29, 66, 90, 94, 359, 402
kyphosis, 15, 25, 28, 29, 31, 33, 34, 42, 49, 64, 66, 67, 79, 80, 81, 88, 91, 93, 94, 95, 98, 116, 121, 129, 179, 182, 183, 204, 205, 207, 208, 211, 215, 218, 219, 222, 228, 245, 247, 248, 249, 250, 252, 253, 254, 258, 266, 322, 337, 340, 343, 349, 357, 358, 371, 374, 410

L

L1-L5, 3, 4, 53, 177, 378
laboratory studies, 379
landmarks, 167, 367, 368, 371, 372, 375
learning, 106, 125, 142, 144, 201, 232, 236, 239, 240
learning curve, 106, 201, 232, 236, 239, 240
Lenke, 33, 35, 38, 39, 40, 42, 43, 60, 66, 67, 134, 138, 150, 186, 196, 204, 205, 206, 208, 209, 210, 212, 213, 214, 215, 217, 218, 219, 220, 224, 225, 226, 227, 228, 233, 239, 240, 241, 245, 246, 247, 249, 251, 252, 253, 254, 255, 256, 257, 258, 259, 264, 265,266, 267, 268, 269, 270, 271, 273, 274, 275, 276, 278, 280, 282, 283, 284, 285, 286, 287, 290, 291, 292, 313, 315, 317, 341, 346, 349, 350, 351, 358, 362, 363, 364, 373
Lenke classification, 35, 39, 40, 42, 43, 204, 213, 245, 358
levels for fusions, 38
long C shape, 334
loosening, 65, 95, 178, 186, 187, 190
low dose, 353, 366
low risk, 54, 156
low weight, 46, 70
lower instrumented vertebra (LIV), 203, 204, 205, 206, 207, 208, 209, 210, 211, 247, 267, 268, 269, 270, 276, 283, 287, 288, 289, 290, 291
lumbar lordosis, 87, 116, 160, 203, 206, 207, 244, 245, 247, 252, 255, 322, 357, 358, 359, 372

lumbar spine modifier, 40, 41, 287
lung function, 47, 129, 203
lung parenchyma, 6, 7, 11, 46, 177
lungs development, 2, 6, 47
Lyon, 116, 119, 133, 160, 161, 411

M

Macaca mulatta, vii, 383, 384, 395, 400, 405, 406
magnet driven rods, 76
magnetic resonance imaging (MRI), 192, 253, 259, 353, 361
magnetic rod, 75, 81, 84
magnitude, 1, 9, 15, 22, 35, 37, 40, 48, 53, 56, 69, 70, 71, 78, 80, 85, 97, 101, 102, 106, 107, 109, 160, 178, 181, 182, 186, 195, 196, 199, 200, 201, 239, 264, 339, 360, 365, 385
major curve, 28, 37, 38, 40, 41, 42, 81, 188, 205, 206, 232, 235, 236, 341, 369
malnutrition, 338, 379, 411
management, vi, ix, 12, 14, 22, 25, 26, 28, 37, 53, 54, 56, 67, 69, 73, 80, 82, 83, 84, 91, 95, 99, 110, 115, 123, 130, 132, 139, 141, 142, 153, 161, 170, 171, 172, 173, 175, 190, 191, 192, 194, 201, 213, 214, 215, 232, 254, 270, 275, 300, 301, 307, 308, 312, 319, 328, 329, 330, 331, 335, 336, 338, 343, 344, 345, 346, 347, 350, 352, 356, 360, 373, 377, 378, 382
mechanical models, 390
mehta, 12, 49, 55, 56, 57, 59, 120, 132, 193, 348
melatonin, 121, 132, 385, 388, 402, 405, 407, 408, 409, 410, 411
melatonin deficiency, 388, 407
metal composition, 304
Milwaukee, 56, 59, 60, 158, 159, 160, 169, 170, 172
minimally invasive, 189, 206, 210, 215, 231, 232, 241
minimally invasive surgery, 231, 232, 241
mixed anomalies, 30
modifier, 28, 35, 39, 40, 41, 42, 218, 276, 287
monitoring devices, 380
morphine, 239, 381, 382
mortality, 11, 28, 47, 58, 194, 226, 240, 294, 332, 365, 390
mosaic, 1
motor-evoked potentials, 381
multidisciplinary, 91, 331, 336, 377
multidisciplinary approach, 331, 336, 377
muscle-splitting approach, 231

N

natural history, 30, 32, 34, 36, 37, 59, 87, 95, 101, 155, 156, 158, 162, 163, 169, 200, 214, 240, 270, 322, 328, 329, 331, 332, 333, 334, 335
nausea, 65
navigation, 206, 215, 234
neurocentral synchondrosis, 3, 12, 411
neuroendocrine models, 388
neurologic assessment, 378
neurologic complications, 65, 307, 308, 314, 342
neurological assessment, 339
neurological models, 388
neuromonitoring, vi, 72, 91, 96, 307, 310, 311, 314, 316, 317, 318, 339, 342, 343, 347, 381, 382
neuromuscular, vi, 11, 12, 27, 28, 29, 31, 34, 36, 48, 56, 58, 60, 65, 67, 69, 70, 75, 87, 92, 99, 115, 121, 131, 193, 239, 294, 295, 296, 300, 303, 305, 319, 323, 324, 325, 326, 327, 329, 331, 332, 333, 335, 337, 338, 341, 342, 343, 344, 345, 346, 347, 348, 349, 350, 351, 352, 355, 378, 379, 380, 381, 382, 383, 384, 386, 388, 389, 390
neuromuscular disease, 48, 295, 319, 323, 324, 325, 332, 338, 378, 380, 381, 382
neuromuscular scoliosis, vi, 11, 12, 31, 34, 58, 65, 67, 70, 92, 99, 115, 193, 239, 294, 295, 296, 303, 305, 319, 323, 324, 326, 327, 329, 331, 333, 335, 337, 338, 341, 342, 343, 344, 345, 347, 348, 349, 350, 351, 379
neutral vertebra (NV), 36, 83, 161, 268, 269, 270
night-time, 161, 338
nocturnal hypercapnic hypoventilation, 338
non-ambulatory, 4, 104, 340, 342
non-invasive, 51, 53, 163, 338, 366, 401, 410
non-operative treatment, 155, 156, 169, 319, 324, 329, 335
non-selective thoracic fusion, 252
nonstructural, 186, 204, 206, 286, 287
NSAIDs, 381
nutrition, 10, 137, 156, 163, 295, 379
nystagmus, 65

O

obesity, 25, 232
observation, 29, 60, 127, 128, 142, 143, 156, 169, 170, 191, 199, 270, 319, 324, 325, 335, 360, 366
occiput, 50, 247, 249
operating time, 240
operative treatment, 33, 67, 155, 204, 275, 319, 324, 335, 371
opioids, 380, 381

osteopathology, 395, 398, 401
outcome, vi, 13, 23, 24, 35, 57, 60, 62, 101, 108, 143, 156, 169, 170, 182, 199, 204, 205, 206, 211, 212, 213, 217, 220, 239, 253, 255, 259, 287, 317, 321, 328, 346, 347, 352, 377
outcome of treatment, 211
ovoid, 6

P

pain, vii, 53, 65, 128, 130, 139, 149, 152, 155, 163, 169, 170, 192, 197, 201, 205, 206, 212, 215, 220, 227, 232, 238, 239, 245, 247, 266, 293, 296, 297, 298, 299, 321, 334, 335, 343, 366, 377, 378, 381, 382
pain management, vii, 130, 239, 377, 381, 382
paracetamol, 381
parasol effect', 7
paravertebral muscles, 121, 123, 270, 393, 407
part-time, 60, 158, 171
patient-controlled analgesia, 381
peak height velocity (PHV), 14, 15, 18, 20, 21, 22, 23, 24, 104, 176, 177, 195, 201, 214
pediatric growth, 13
pedicle screws, 74, 89, 186, 187, 188, 189, 200, 233, 234, 235, 236, 249, 250, 251, 252, 254, 273, 276, 291, 292, 305, 310, 340, 341, 343
pelvic level, 335
pelvic morphology, 244, 246
pelvic obliquity, 31, 63, 92, 142, 321, 323, 331, 334, 335, 336, 338, 339, 340, 341
pelvis, 3, 12, 31, 50, 51, 63, 88, 92, 104, 130, 136, 147, 152, 157, 159, 176, 177, 243, 244, 246, 247, 255, 256, 258, 261, 262, 295, 323, 325, 331, 333, 334, 336, 337, 339, 340, 341, 348, 350, 355, 357, 363, 367, 380, 387, 391, 394
percussive pain, 297
perimeter, 6
perivertebral arthrodesis, 3, 4
phenomenon, vi, 7, 12, 18, 48, 49, 95, 107, 194, 211, 246, 261, 267, 269, 274, 276, 281, 287, 292, 343
phoenix, 75
physical examination, 36, 203, 323, 336, 369
physical therapy, 114, 137, 138, 139, 146, 161, 163, 167, 171, 238, 239, 324, 328
physiotherapeutic scoliosis specific exercises (PSSE), 113, 114, 116, 119, 125, 126, 127, 128
pilates, 135, 136, 137, 138, 139, 140, 141, 142, 143, 144, 145, 149, 150, 151, 152
pilates method, 135
pilates method exercise, 135
pin, 64, 65, 187

pinealectomy, 132, 388, 392, 401, 402, 403, 404, 408, 409, 411
plaster, 50, 51, 52, 59, 171
Ponseti-Friedmann classification, 37
poor prognosis, 53, 338
positioning, 50, 142, 179, 354, 355, 362, 368, 377, 380
posterior instrumented fusion, 74, 215, 262
posterior spinal fusion, 12, 134, 209, 211, 231, 232, 255, 257, 266, 291, 293, 294, 381, 382
posterior spinal instrumented fusion, 199, 200
postoperative, vi, 15, 65, 73, 75, 77, 82, 91, 97, 98, 115, 129, 130, 134, 143, 146, 147, 159, 181, 182, 184, 187, 190, 192, 203, 204, 207, 208, 209, 211, 212, 213, 215, 224, 232, 238, 239, 243, 245, 246, 247, 251, 252, 255, 256, 259, 261, 262, 263, 264, 265, 266, 267,268, 269, 270, 274, 275, 276, 277, 278, 283, 290, 291, 292, 293, 294, 296, 299, 300, 305, 316, 318, 336, 337, 338, 343, 344, 347, 378, 379, 380, 381
post-operative complications, 15, 343
postoperative protocol, 238
post-operative shoulder imbalance, 261, 262, 275
precocious arthrodesis, 2, 3, 177
preoperative assessment, 331, 336, 343, 351, 378
preoperative correction, 61, 63, 65
preoperative evaluation, 232, 336, 362, 377, 378
preoperative planning, vi, 199, 200, 203, 204, 217, 219, 233, 261, 273, 336
preoperative traction, 341
pressure points, 380
prevention, 17, 116, 132, 139, 153, 215, 266, 268, 294, 317, 334, 343
prognostic criteria, 55
progression, 5, 7, 10, 14, 15, 18, 19, 20, 22, 23, 24, 26, 28, 29, 30, 31, 33, 34, 37, 46, 53, 55, 80, 101, 102, 103, 106, 107, 108, 109, 110, 111, 114, 115, 116, 120, 123, 124, 126, 127, 131, 133, 138, 155, 156, 157, 161, 162, 163, 164, 169, 175, 176, 177, 178, 182,193, 194, 199, 200, 201, 218, 248, 267, 268, 276, 283, 290, 300, 302, 304, 319, 321, 322, 324, 325, 328, 331, 333, 334, 335, 336, 345, 349, 350, 351, 360, 364, 365, 366, 368, 370, 388, 405, 408
progressive, v, ix, 2, 4, 15, 16, 29, 33, 45, 46, 48, 49, 51, 53, 55, 56, 58, 59, 67, 70, 79, 81, 84, 87, 91, 98, 101, 114, 116, 120, 124, 126, 130, 131, 133, 151, 155, 158, 161, 169, 170, 186, 187, 188, 196, 199, 211, 270, 276, 283, 287, 290, 302, 321, 333, 336, 344, 349, 379, 385, 402, 403, 407, 410
prone position, 91, 380
Providence, 162, 172

proximal, 16, 19, 21, 39, 40, 50, 62, 71, 75, 76, 79, 80, 81, 85, 88, 89, 90, 91, 92, 93, 95, 96, 97, 100, 103, 201, 202, 204, 205, 207, 211, 213, 215, 236, 249, 250, 258, 262, 264, 265, 269, 270, 273, 274, 275, 277, 278, 283, 290, 291, 339, 343, 361
proximal junctional kyphosis, 75, 76, 79, 81, 85, 95, 211, 213, 215, 249, 258, 339
proximal kyphosis, 92, 343
proximal wedge angle, 265
proximal-fusion–level, 264
puberty, 2, 3, 4, 5, 6, 9, 13, 14, 15, 16, 20, 22, 23, 24, 26, 48, 101, 102, 103, 104, 105, 106, 107, 108, 109, 111, 155, 176, 177, 193, 199, 214, 385
pullout, 97, 339, 343
pulmonary assessment, 338
pulmonary function, 2, 7, 11, 12, 16, 46, 49, 55, 58, 64, 65, 66, 67, 70, 72, 85, 87, 89, 94, 99, 134, 170, 193, 217, 221, 226, 228, 229, 324, 334, 338, 378, 379

Q

quadrupeds, 385, 401

R

radiation exposure, 234, 365, 366, 371
radiation-free, 365, 366, 367, 370, 371, 375
radiologic assessment, 353
radiological evaluation, 262, 263
rasterstereography, vii, 365, 366, 367, 368, 369, 370, 371, 373, 374
reduction tubes, 233, 235, 236, 238
reliability, 22, 35, 38, 42, 43, 81, 132, 172, 215, 216, 309, 359, 362, 363, 365, 366, 368, 370, 371, 372, 373, 374, 375, 406, 412
respiratory failure, 6, 11, 28, 379
respiratory insufficiency, 2, 4, 7, 47, 48, 49, 177
restrictive pulmonary disease, 46, 70
retroverted, 246
retroverted pelvis, 246
rhesus monkeys, 395, 398, 401, 406
rib cage, 46, 54, 70, 71, 129, 159, 371
rib hump, 200, 218, 219, 220, 367, 369
rib-vertebral-sternal complex', 7
rigidity, 66, 121, 250, 254
risk factors, 80, 83, 97, 99, 100, 101, 106, 211, 215, 241, 255, 261, 264, 265, 268, 269, 270, 273, 274, 288, 295, 304, 305, 319, 321, 322, 328, 333, 398
Risser, 5, 13, 14, 18, 19, 20, 21, 23, 25, 45, 49, 58, 101, 104, 105, 106, 107, 108, 109, 110, 127, 156, 158, 160, 161, 162, 167, 177, 178, 182, 183, 186, 188, 190, 194, 201, 202, 264, 265, 269, 270, 289, 290, 355, 360, 361, 363
Risser sign, 5, 13, 14, 18, 19, 23, 25, 101, 104, 105, 106, 107, 108, 158, 160, 161, 162, 167, 177, 201, 264, 289, 355, 360, 361, 363
rod rotation, 200, 218, 222, 236, 237
rotation, 33, 50, 56, 60, 80, 117, 118, 123, 141, 142, 145, 146, 161, 166, 168, 178, 183, 191, 203, 204, 205, 214, 217, 218, 219, 236, 248, 257, 261, 262, 356, 359, 360, 362, 363, 366, 371, 372, 373, 375, 383, 384, 385, 390, 401, 403
rotational dimension, 35, 42

S

sagittal, vi, 35, 39, 40, 41, 42, 64, 71, 73, 74, 79, 80, 81, 83, 85, 91, 94, 118, 119, 121, 130, 131, 138, 145, 153, 157, 187, 188, 189, 201, 203, 204, 205, 206, 207, 211, 213, 217, 218, 219, 220, 226, 228, 236, 243, 244, 245, 246, 247, 248, 249, 250, 251, 252, 253, 254, 255, 256, 257, 258, 259, 261, 262, 269, 335, 347, 355, 357, 358, 359, 362, 363, 368, 369, 372, 374, 385
sagittal alignment, vi, 42, 201, 206, 243, 244, 245, 247, 248, 249, 250, 252, 253, 254, 256, 257, 258, 259, 363
sagittal plane, 35, 42, 64, 91, 118, 119, 121, 130, 145, 188, 189, 206, 213, 218, 220, 226, 236, 250, 252, 254, 256, 259, 385
sagittal profile, 81, 83, 85, 204, 205, 206, 217, 218, 219, 220, 226, 236, 245, 249, 250, 251, 252, 355
sagittal thoracic modifier, 39, 40, 41
satisfaction, 212, 220, 232, 243, 244, 253, 262, 278
Schulthess classification, 36, 37
scientific publications, 55, 56, 115
scoliometer, 142, 143, 152, 369
scoliosis and exercise, 135
scoliosis surgery, 115, 129, 183, 206, 214, 215, 218, 227, 228, 231, 232, 241, 257, 258, 262, 299, 302, 304, 311, 317, 338, 342, 372, 377, 379, 381, 382, 403
scoliotic phenotypes, 386
scoliotic risk, 53, 103
screening, 142, 143, 152, 156, 164, 171, 172, 320, 332, 373, 395
seating modification, 319, 323, 324, 327, 335
segmental derotation, 220
segmentation, 29, 34, 36, 405
selection, 13, 23, 42, 43, 155, 204, 205, 206, 208, 211, 264, 268, 270, 276, 281, 283, 287, 288, 290, 292, 346, 356, 403
selective dorsal rhizotomy, 321, 328, 333

selective thoracic fusion, 38, 42, 204, 214, 215, 252, 269, 283, 286, 363
serial, v, 45, 46, 47, 49, 51, 53, 54, 55, 56, 57, 58, 59, 60, 71, 76, 83, 94, 99, 177
Shilla procedure, 8, 74, 75
short lumbar brace, 319, 324, 325, 326
shoulder, vi, 98, 138, 142, 143, 149, 151, 160, 203, 204, 205, 206, 211, 212, 215, 219, 261, 262, 263, 264, 265, 266, 267, 269, 270, 273, 274, 275, 277, 278, 279, 280, 281, 282, 283, 284, 285, 286, 291, 292, 323, 367
shoulder balance, vi, 203, 204, 205, 206, 211, 215, 261, 262, 263, 264, 266, 270, 273, 274, 275, 277, 278, 282, 283, 284, 285, 286, 291
shoulder height, 203, 262, 277, 278, 279, 280, 281, 283
shoulder imbalance, vi, 204, 211, 261, 262, 264, 265, 266, 267, 269, 273, 274, 275, 277, 278, 283, 291
sitting height, 1, 3, 4, 5, 6, 9, 15, 16, 17, 23, 48, 103, 104, 176
skeletal age, 5, 22, 26, 104, 105, 201
skeletal maturity, 2, 3, 4, 5, 6, 8, 9, 11, 13, 15, 18, 19, 20, 23, 26, 36, 53, 55, 79, 102, 104, 105, 106, 107, 132, 158, 161, 163, 176, 177, 182, 186, 193, 200, 201, 328, 334, 360, 361, 364
snow ball effect, 9
soft brace, 163
somatosensory evoked potentials (SSEPs), 307, 308, 310, 311, 312, 316, 318, 342, 380, 397, 400, 401, 405, 406
spinal asymmetry, 135, 136, 138, 141, 144, 145
spinal balance, 65, 334
spinal cord injury, 31, 307, 308, 310, 312, 318
spinal deformity(ies), ix, 1, 2, 3, 4, 5, 6, 7, 8, 9, 10, 11, 12, 16, 22, 25, 28, 29, 31, 36, 45, 46, 47, 48, 49, 52, 54, 55, 56, 58, 61, 62, 64, 65, 66, 67, 70, 71, 82, 87, 88, 93, 95, 99, 100, 102, 103, 132, 155, 156, 163, 176, 193, 199, 215, 244, 247, 255, 256, 261, 262, 270, 293, 298, 300, 301, 306, 307, 308, 310, 312, 314, 317, 318, 319, 323, 324, 327, 328, 329, 333, 335, 336, 338, 339, 363, 366, 367, 368, 372, 374, 375, 377, 378, 382, 385, 386, 387, 388, 390, 391, 406, 407, 411
spinal disorders, 384, 409
spinal fusion level, 277, 286
spinal penetration index, 6, 11, 194
spinal segment, 3, 4, 16, 91, 179, 205
spine growth, 1, 5, 10, 11, 94, 193
spine surgery, 9, 10, 129, 214, 241, 304, 308, 310, 317, 318, 342, 382
SpineCor, 56, 59, 163, 172, 173, 192
spinopelvic alignment, 245, 246, 255, 259
spinopelvic parameters, 243, 255, 363

split cord, 50, 71
spontaneous electromyography, 308, 310
stable vertebra, 37, 38, 205, 208, 210, 268
Stagnara, 61, 116, 160, 171, 316
standing height, 4, 5, 15, 16, 23, 48, 102, 103, 104
staples, 80, 88, 178, 179, 181, 182, 183, 184, 186, 195, 394, 403
stapling, 54, 71, 80, 83, 85, 175, 176, 178, 181, 192, 195, 196
structural, 7, 33, 38, 40, 41, 42, 59, 114, 115, 125, 136, 146, 151, 162, 163, 164, 179, 203, 204, 205, 206, 218, 219, 264, 266, 267, 287, 323, 383, 398, 403, 405, 410
subcutaneous hematoma, 240
superficial wound infection, 240
surface topography, 143, 365, 366, 367, 369, 372, 374
surgical approach, ix, 219, 378, 385
surgical complications, 54, 56, 342, 348, 379
surgical scar, 239
surgical site infection, 54, 241, 293, 294, 295, 296, 297, 299, 300, 304, 305, 306, 338, 342, 343
surgical treatment, 29, 33, 37, 56, 61, 64, 65, 69, 85, 87, 93, 99, 115, 155, 156, 163, 171, 199, 200, 211, 228, 232, 240, 243, 244, 247, 254, 259, 261, 262, 267, 270, 273, 286, 293, 298, 305, 317, 324, 329, 331, 332, 385
suture granuloma, 240
swelling, 102, 139, 296, 297, 298
syndromic, 27, 28, 29, 31, 32, 55, 56, 69, 70, 71, 80, 81, 87, 92, 93, 294, 295

T

T1 tilt, 37, 203, 262, 263, 266, 278, 280, 281
T1-S1, 3, 4, 10, 48, 69, 71, 72, 73, 75, 81, 83, 94, 176
T1-T12, 2, 3, 7, 10, 53, 58, 75, 81, 176, 177, 358, 378
tachypnea, 46, 70, 378
Tanner, 5, 13, 14, 15, 19, 23, 24, 102, 103, 105, 111, 136, 149, 156, 177, 194, 201, 360, 361
Tanner and Whitehouse (TW), 19, 102, 192, 363
Tanner classification, 13, 14
temperature, 182, 297, 312, 318, 377, 399
tenderness, 157, 295, 297, 298, 299
tethers, 80, 88, 122, 403
thoracic cage, 1, 2, 3, 5, 6, 7, 8, 9, 10, 25, 28, 46, 47, 48, 49, 51, 53, 54, 58, 70, 82, 109, 176, 177, 193, 379
thoracic cage compliance, 49
thoracic cage excursion, 49
thoracic cage volume, 5, 48

thoracic depth/thoracic width, 6
thoracic growth, 1, 2, 3, 6, 10, 11, 49, 55, 97, 177, 194
thoracic insufficiency syndrome, 2, 6, 10, 12, 27, 28, 47, 48, 79, 81, 83, 176, 194
thoracic kyphosis, 41, 81, 91, 97, 99, 178, 203, 204, 207, 208, 217, 219, 221, 226, 244, 245, 247, 248, 249, 252, 253, 254, 256, 258, 322, 343, 357, 358, 361
thoracic perimeter, 4, 6
thoraco-abdominal window, 51
thoracoplasty, 10, 99, 194, 378
thoracostomy, 7, 83, 194
thoracotomy, 82, 219, 228, 406
three dimensional deformity, 42, 332
three-dimensional, 7, 9, 10, 11, 33, 45, 46, 47, 113, 114, 115, 125, 138, 144, 175, 194, 199, 200, 212, 217, 219, 220, 257, 261, 262, 363, 365, 366, 367, 371, 372, 373, 374, 385, 395, 403, 411, 412
three-dimensional classification, 33, 42
timing, 18, 22, 25, 26, 72, 102, 109, 176, 266, 299
TLSO, 159, 160, 161, 169, 172
tracheomalacia, 46, 70
traction, v, 50, 51, 61, 62, 63, 64, 65, 66, 67, 117, 189, 214, 219, 270, 271, 308, 323, 337, 339, 341, 346, 349, 350, 351, 355
traction films, 219, 339, 355
transcranial motor evoked potentials (TcMEPs), 307, 308, 309, 310, 311, 312
treatment modality, 54, 116
triggered EMG, 308, 310
trunk, 2, 4, 5, 9, 10, 16, 46, 48, 49, 53, 63, 65, 70, 78, 95, 103, 107, 119, 130, 132, 133, 142, 147, 152, 153, 162, 164, 166, 203, 211, 242, 261, 262, 274, 319, 321, 323, 324, 325, 327, 332, 333, 335, 338, 339, 340, 341, 356, 367, 371, 373, 374
tumor, 72, 378
TW3 maturity stages, 20

U

UIV, 204, 205, 206, 211, 249, 251, 266, 278, 281, 282
ultrasonic bone scalpel, 234
upper instrumented level, 277
upper instrumented vertebra, 204, 251, 266, 278
upright sitting ability, 334
urinary catheter, 178, 183, 380

V

VAC sponge, 300
validity, 215, 216, 368, 373, 374, 375
ventilation-perfusion maldistribution, 379
ventricular tachycardia, 46
vertebrae, 7, 8, 11, 29, 30, 88, 89, 92, 123, 124, 177, 178, 184, 189, 201, 220, 221, 233, 244, 246, 249, 267, 268, 269, 298, 356, 387, 390, 391, 394, 404, 410
vertical expandable prosthetic titanium rib (VEPTR), 10, 12, 58, 71, 73, 79, 81, 84, 85, 88, 94, 99, 295, 305
vital capacity, 2, 4, 7, 9, 47, 82, 94, 155, 159, 324, 338, 378

W

waistline asymmetry, 270, 367
Wake-Up test, 315, 316
weight, 4, 9, 10, 13, 14, 15, 24, 46, 62, 64, 65, 70, 94, 104, 111, 136, 139, 140, 143, 144, 146, 147, 168, 194, 201, 323, 324, 338, 379, 390, 398
wheezing, 378
white blood cell count, 297
wrench, 236, 237
wrist radiograph, 21, 178

Orthopaedic Biomechanics: A Trainee's Guide

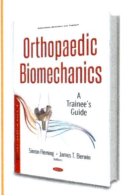

Editors: Simon Fleming and James T. Berwin (Barts Health, Trauma and Orthopaedics, Spr, UK)

Series: Orthopedic Research and Therapy

Book Description: This book focusses specifically on Orthopaedic Biomechanics. It's been written for orthopaedic trainee's, by orthopaedic trainees and is designed to give you a little more than the broad brushstrokes many other books deliver, whilst also holding back from being an in-depth engineering text.

Hardcover ISBN: 978-1-53612-877-2
Retail Price: $230

The Medial Collateral Ligament and the Posteromedial Corner: A Comprehensive Analysis

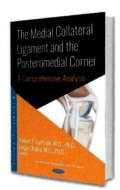

Editor: Robert F. LaPrade, M.D., Ph.D., and Jorge Chahla, M.D., Ph.D. (Complex Knee Surgeon, The Steadman Clinic and Chief Medical Officer, Steadman Philippon Research Institute, Vail, CO, US, and others)

Series: Orthopedic Research and Therapy

Book Description: From anatomical and biomechanical foundations to clinical treatment, surgical pearls, or rehabilitation principles, the authors believe that this textbook represents a significant advancement on the topic of MCL injuries with highly detailed and easy-to-read chapters, presented with vividly illustrated guidance on how best to manage medial sided knee pathology.

Hardcover ISBN: 978-1-53614-178-8
Retail Price: $195

3D Applications in Hip Surgery

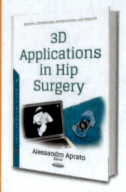

Author: Alessandro Aprato (Trauma and Orthopaedic Hospital of Turin, University of Turin, Torino, Italy)

Series: Surgery - Procedures, Complications, and Results

Book Description: Recent studies demonstrated the utility of advanced imaging techniques including 3D CT collision modeling, MRI 3D reconstruction and 3D fluoroscopy in hip surgery. Collision modeling including software based on a CT scan and 3D fluoroscopy are able to predict the specific zone of femoral-acetabular impingement and are useful tools to plan the bone resection in preserving hip surgery.

Hardcover ISBN: 978-1-53612-292-3
Retail Price: $160